THAT'S
GOTTA
HURT

Dr. David Geier

THAT'S GOTTA HURT

THE INJURIES THAT CHANGED SPORTS FOREVER

ForeEdge

ForeEdge

An imprint of University Press of New England

www.upne.com
Manufactured in the United States of America

Designed by Mindy Basinger Hill

Typeset in Minion Pro

For permission to reproduce any of the material in this book,
contact Permissions, University Press of New England,
One Court Street, Suite 250, Lebanon NH 03766;
or visit www.upne.com

Library of Congress Cataloging-in-Publication Data

Names: Geier, David, Dr., author.

Title: That's Gotta Hurt : The Injuries That Changed Sports Forever /
Dr. David Geier.

Description: Lebanon, NH : ForeEdge, 2017. |
Includes bibliographical references and index.

Identifiers: LCCN 2016042501 (print) | LCCN 2017007926 (ebook) |
ISBN 9781611689068 (pbk.) | ISBN 9781512600698 (epub, mobi & pdf)

Subjects: LCSH: Sports injuries—History. | Sports medicine—History. |
Athletes—Health and hygiene. | Athletes—United States—Biography. |
Sports—United States—History.

Classification: LCC RD97 .G44 2017 (print) | LCC RD97 (ebook)
DDC 617.1/027—dc23

LC record available at https://lccn.loc.gov/2016042501

5   4   3   2   1

For Marshall and Madeline

CONTENTS

INTRODUCTION

March 7, 1970

"I realized that something was wrong," Bogataj would recall years later to *Philadelphia Daily News* columnist Rich Hoffman. "I tried not to go, tried to stop myself. But the speed was too big, about 105 kilometers an hour [roughly 65 miles per hour]. So I did everything I was able to do."[1]

You might not know the name Vinko Bogataj, but you know who he is—or at least you know his crash.

Earlier that day, Bogataj had left the chain factory in Yugoslavia where he worked, along with his three friends, to drive to Oberstdorf, West Germany. Growing up on a farm in a family with eight children, the 22-year-old set out on that snowy day to compete in a passion of his: ski flying.

Despite working full time, Bogataj was fairly accomplished in the sport that would later become known as ski jumping. He competed more for fun than prize winnings, as his greatest career "paydays" included $200, a stove, and a color television.[2]

Little did he know as he set out for Oberstdorf that he would soon become famous—or infamous—depending on one's perspective.

Having already fallen once, Bogataj faced worsening weather conditions heading into his second jump. Now he faced swirling winds and new snow on the ramp. Race officials shortened the jump out of safety concerns. "These days, they wouldn't even compete in those conditions," Bogataj told Dave Seminara of *Real Clear Sports* 40 years later.[3]

Bogataj sped down the ramp, but he lost his balance before he reached the end of the platform. He placed his right hand down, but his legs gave way. He flipped off the side of the jump in a spectacular fashion. He somersaulted through the air, ripping through a sign that read OBERSTDORF at the bottom of the ramp, and nearly crashing into nearby broadcasters, spectators, and race officials.[4]

"I could've gotten up, I didn't feel hurt, but they wouldn't let me," Bogataj told Seminara. "They insisted on carrying me off on a stretcher, which I wasn't happy about because my family was watching on TV."[5]

His family would soon learn that Vinko would be fine, despite crashing at over 60 mph. Bogataj told Hoffman that the violent appearance of what happened had scared the medical staff and onlookers.

"I didn't feel any pain at first. I was just angry it happened. People kept telling me that it had to hurt. It looked so dangerous."[6]

The video footage of that dangerous crash would immortalize Vinko Bogataj. As he would ask in a ceremony to honor the 25th anniversary of the show on which Bogataj's crash was broadcast, legendary sports host Jim McKay asked the audience, "Do you know this man? Probably not. He doesn't even own a credit card."[7]

Each Saturday for 37 years, *Wide World of Sports* opened the same way. It featured video clips of a variety of athletic competitions to an instrumental musical fanfare. Host Jim McKay read a narration that became timeless:

> Spanning the globe to bring you the constant variety of sport.
> The thrill of victory
> and the agony of defeat.
> The human drama of athletic competition.
> This is ABC's "Wide World of Sports."

Vinko Bogataj and his spectacular crash were "the agony of defeat."

When *Wide World of Sports* first aired in 1961, producers ran footage of Irish hurlers colliding during "the agony of defeat." In 1970 Dennis Lewin, the coordinating producer for *Wild World of Sports* between 1966 and 1996, and executive producer Roone Arledge decided to pair Bogataj's crash footage with the words "agony of defeat."[8]

Despite frequently changing the clips throughout the remainder of the opening montage, the show kept the footage of Vinko Bogataj to represent "the agony of defeat" for the next 28 years. It is difficult to imagine anyone thinking of *Wild World of Sports* without recalling Bogataj spinning wildly off the ski ramp in Oberstdorf, West Germany. Not everyone appreciated that fact, though.

Doug Wilson produced the show in Oberstdorf for ABC. He recalled that leaders in the sport of ski jumping were never particularly happy about Bogataj's crash being prominently featured in the *Wide World of Sports* opening montage. They believed it created a ripple effect week after week, causing hesitation among athletes considering the sport.[9]

Ken Anderson, founder of the website SkiJumpingUSA.com and a former ski jumper himself, argued that ski jumping has never recovered from the damage inflicted by the *Wide World of Sports* opening montage. "Well, absolutely," Anderson said about the damage done by that footage. "It's a well-known sport everywhere else in the sports world, but in North America, the U.S. and Canada, it's not a sport that is very well known. Because people see something like that, that becomes their whole perception. They don't see much of the sport. It's poorly covered here, so that's all they know about it. It definitely affected recruiting."[10]

According to Anderson, ski jumping has struggled in the United States for reasons other than the *Wide World of Sports* footage. Only a few sites maintained their jumping facilities, and most eventually closed them. Only a handful of ski-jumping clubs currently exist in the country. They are spread out across the United States, so young athletes rarely compete against each other. Travel costs for competitive jumpers, a lack of recreational participants, and the growth of winter sports like snowboarding and freestyle skiing have all contributed to the sport's decline.[11]

Despite the widespread perception that ski jumping is dangerous, Anderson argued that it is a safe sport. He noted that a study by the International Ski Federation (Fédération Internationale de Ski, FIS) tracked six snow sport disciplines, including Alpine, freestyle, snowboard, ski jumping, Nordic combine, and cross country, and according to the FIS Injury Surveillance System, only cross-country skiing is safer than ski jumping.[12]

"ABC never did a good job of saying, 'Yeah, but he wasn't really seriously hurt, and he went back to jumping.' They just left it there, left it hanging and let people's perceptions be whatever they might be," Anderson complained.[13]

Wilson recognized the value of the crash footage. "Instantaneously, as it happened, I thought it would be a great 'Agony of Defeat.'" He pointed out that Bogataj "could have been very, very badly hurt. If that had happened, it would have been inappropriate to show week after week as the 'Agony of Defeat.'"[14]

That's Gotta Hurt examines the intersection of sports and medicine over the last 50 years. While millions of people have seen the footage of Vinko Bogataj's ski-jumping crash, few viewers saw its outcome. Aides carried the Yugoslav jumper away on a sled and transported him to a local hospital, where he was admitted overnight. Amazingly, Bogataj suffered only a mild concussion.[15] The video of that high-speed trauma, though, might have changed a sport forever.

In the ensuing chapters, I explore a series of injuries that changed their sports—or sports in general—forever. I examine how emerging surgeries, treatments, and prevention strategies affected athletes in many sports.

I discuss how sports medicine has had a tremendous influence on athletes and sports—perhaps more than any change in coaching or training has had. I also examine how sports medicine will continue to influence sports and the athletes who play them for years to come.

It would be fair to say that sports and medicine have always been closely associated. In a 1984 article in the *American Journal of Sports Medicine*, George A. Snook, MD, presented a thorough review of the history of sports medicine from ancient Greece to the mid-1900s. He asserted that the first recorded sporting competition, the first incident of rule breaking, and the first sports injury were described in the book of Genesis:

> And Jacob was left alone; and there wrestled a man with him until the breaking of the day. And when (the man) saw that he prevailed not against (Jacob), he touched the hollow of his thigh; and the hollow of Jacob's thigh was out of joint as he wrestled with him.[16]

In the second century AD, Galen of Pergamon, a prominent surgeon and philosopher of the Roman Empire, was appointed as the first "team physician." Pontifex Maximus appointed Galen to serve as physician to the gladiators. He was reappointed to that position five times. He later served as physician to Emperor Marcus Aurelius. During his career, Galen performed extensive anatomical dissections and physiology research, publishing numerous works.[17]

Sports medicine likely owes its American origins to Amherst College. In 1854 Edward Hitchcock, MD, became Amherst's first instructor of physical education and hygiene. Dr. Hitchcock created a physical education system that included running, basketball, and baseball, earning him the label "father of physical education." He collected data on sports, diseases, and injuries at the college, publishing a textbook and well over 100 articles. As such, it's fair to say he was America's first sports medicine physician and team doctor.[18]

In the early 20th century the sport of football faced intense scrutiny for its high injury rate. The government considered banning the sport altogether. Dr. Edward Nichols published two papers on injuries in football, one in 1905 and a second in 1909 after the National Collegiate Athletic Association (NCAA) adopted changes to its rules to make the sport safer. Nichols's work largely helped to save football.[19]

Dr. Mal Stevens played football at Yale University and later became the team's head coach. Stevens coached football during medical school and while working as an intern, resident, and fellow. He later became president of the American College Football Coaches Association and coauthored a textbook on football injuries. In that work, he advocated pneumatic padding in football helmets. Stevens later became the team physician for the New York Yankees.[20]

Dr. Augustus Thorndike of Harvard University published what is considered to be the first American sports medicine textbook in 1938, *Athletic Injuries: Prevention, Diagnosis, and Treatment*. Harvard developed a model for athletic care that largely represents the modern sports medicine team. Harvard's sports teams had team physicians, athletic trainers, and therapists to treat and rehabilitate injuries and educate the athletes about proper fitness and equipment.[21]

Another key member of the Harvard faculty, Dr. Thomas B. Quigley, served on the American Medical Association's Committee on the Medical Aspects of Sports. As the committee's chair, he helped to publish "The Bill of Rights for the College Athlete," which pushed for preseason physicals, doctors at sporting events, and physicians being closely involved in the care of the athletes. Dr. Quigley emphasized the need for quality equipment, facilities, officiating, and coaching. He stressed that the medical needs of the athlete should take precedence over any other concerns.

From gladiators in ancient times to gladiators on the gridiron, we know that injuries occur. As Dr. Quigley explained whenever asked about his interest in sports medicine, "Whenever young men gather regularly on green autumn fields, or winter ice, or polished wooden floors to dispute the physical possession and position of various leather and rubber objects according to certain rules, sooner or later somebody is going to get hurt."[22]

Wide World of Sports aired from 1961 to 1998. The program usually featured sports other than mainstream American sports like football and baseball. Instead, it featured Olympic sports such as skiing and figure skating as well as less traditional sports such as Mexican cliff diving, powerlifting, and firefighters' competitions.

The show first broadcast sports competitions that went on to become noteworthy in their own right. Wimbledon, the British Open, the Daytona 500, the Indianapolis 500, and the Little League World Series are just a few of the events first broadcast on *Wide World of Sports*.

As television coverage of sports exploded in the second half of the 20th century, broadcast and cable networks siphoned off much of the programming that had made *Wide World of Sports* habitual Saturday viewing for decades.[23] *Wide World of Sports* alone did not cause the increasing prominence that sports acquired in American society, but it certainly accompanied that growth.

A few statistics from different sports reveal how sports—and society—have changed since 1970, the year Vinko Bogataj crashed in West Germany.

In 1970 the average player salary in Major League Baseball (MLB) was $29,303.[24] The game's highest paid player, Willie Mays, earned $135,000 that season.[25] Contrast those numbers with 2013, when the average salary reached $3.39 million,[26] and Alex Rodriguez collected $29 million.[27]

The Buffalo Braves National Basketball Association (NBA) franchise was founded in 1970. The team moved to San Diego in 1978. Three years later, Donald Sterling bought the San Diego Clippers for $12.5 million. Steve Ballmer bought the Los Angeles Clippers in the summer of 2014 for $2 billion.[28]

On January 11, 1970, approximately 44.3 million viewers in the United States watched the Kansas City Chiefs defeat the Minnesota Vikings in Super Bowl IV. Approximately 111.5 million people tuned in to see the Seattle Seahawks crush the Denver Broncos in Super Bowl XLVIII on February 2, 2014.[29]

Many more kids play sports today than played decades ago. In fact, more than 1 million young athletes currently play high school football, and 2.58 million children between the ages of 6 and 14 played tackle football in the United States in 2013.[30]

As any National Football League (NFL) fan can tell you, injuries are a normal part of sports. It should be no surprise that along with the growing popularity of the athletes comes a heightened prominence for the doctors who treat their injuries.

Doctors travel with their teams as they play all over the country. They obtain magnetic resonance images (MRIS) minutes after injuries occur. Websites feature medical analysis of injuries and try to predict when athletes will return to play. And fans can rarely watch an hour of ESPN's *SportsCenter* without hearing that a player will travel to undergo surgery by Dr. James Andrews.

In fact, I will be doing an interview on SiriusXM Fantasy Sports Radio later today (on the day I am writing this introduction). We will discuss all of the injuries in the NFL this weekend: Robert Griffin III, Jamaal Charles, DeSean Jackson, A. J. Green, and others.

The fact that fantasy sports exist at all and are so popular—and that people want to hear from an orthopaedic surgeon to explain the injuries—shows how much sports and sports medicine have changed.

That's Gotta Hurt discusses the injuries that brought sports—and sports medicine—to where we are today.

I examine key injuries that changed the athletes and subsequently the treatment of athletes and active individuals: Joan Benoit's arthroscopic knee surgery 17 days before she competed in the US Olympic marathon trials; Bernard King's anterior cruciate ligament (ACL) injury and unprecedented rehabilitation and return to sports; and Hines Ward's use of a novel treatment—platelet-rich plasma—for a medial collateral ligament (MCL) injury of the knee days before playing in the Super Bowl.

I also discuss injuries that changed their sports, leading to rules changes, adoption of protective equipment, or even calls for the elimination of the sport: the death of cricket star Phillip Hughes and severe injuries from the ball striking players in cricket and baseball; Marc Buoniconti's quadriplegia after a tackling injury and changes to decrease catastrophic cervical spine injuries; the death of freestyle skier Sarah Burke and snowmobiler Caleb Moore and the dangers of "extreme" sports; and Dave Duerson's suicide and the role of concussions and repetitive subconcussive blows to the head, leading to chronic traumatic encephalopathy (CTE).

The discussion then turns to injuries that have impacted athletes and sports generally and will affect treatment of future athletes in all sports: Sam Bowie and the complex evaluation of athletes to try to predict whether they will stay healthy; Michael Jordan's navicular fracture and the difficult issues that arise when trying to determine appropriate return to play for professional athletes; the sudden cardiac death of college basketball star Hank Gathers and the intense debate over mandatory cardiac screening of athletes; Minnesota Vikings tackle Korey Stringer's death from exertional heat stroke; ACL injuries among Brandi Chastain, other members of the US Women's National Soccer Team, and young female athletes generally, and the development of injury prevention programs to decrease them; and Tommy John's landmark elbow surgery and the epidemic of youth pitching injuries decades later.

I wrap up this journey by exploring what could lie ahead for sports and the field of sports medicine, looking ahead not only to new treatments and prevention strategies, but also to where we could be headed in terms of ethics, legal dilemmas, and conflicts of interest.

And within this entire discussion of the influence of sports medicine on sports—and vice versa—at the elite level, I show how these changes have influenced and will continue to influence the far more numerous youth athletes and adult weekend warriors.

Wide World of Sports remained a staple of American sports for 37 years. The umbrella title ABC's *Wide World of Sports* was used for a number of years after that, so the footage of that crash in Oberstdorf remained in the opening montage decades after the event happened.

"Maybe it was 10 years later, about 1980, there was a suggestion that maybe it was time to replace Vinko's fall," Wilson recounted. "Roone Arledge, in his brilliance, sort of tugged at his sweater, as was his habit when he didn't want something to happen or wanted to make a point. Basically he said, 'Why are we doing that?' What that meant was we shouldn't do it, and we didn't. It stayed in the rest of the history of Wide World. There was a moment where people were talking about replacing it, and Roone put a stop to that. He knew what he had. He had a signature thing. I mean, everybody remembers it. Everybody who ever watched the show. You mention the 'Agony of Defeat,' and people think of the ski jumper."[31]

Bogataj became somewhat of a celebrity, although it was years before he realized it. "He found out that he was famous, or his fall was famous, in Oscar's, the coffee shop in the Waldorf," Wilson recalled. "We brought him over with an interpreter and his wife, and put them up in the Waldorf. He was a forklift driver in an iron foundry in Yugoslavia. He was speaking Serbo-Croatian in the coffee shop, and some of the waiters coincidentally in Oscar's were Serbo-Croatian. They don't normally hear their language, so when they stopped and they heard that language, they inquired. When they found out who he was, they went nuts. They went over to the restaurant saying, 'See the guy in the booth there? He's the 'Agony of Defeat.'"[32]

We might not remember Vinko Bogataj by name, but we will always remember "the agony of defeat" guy. In fact, at the 20th anniversary celebration for *Wide World of Sports* in 1981, Bogataj received a standing ovation and the loudest applause, more than Nadia Comaneci and the 1980 US Olympic hockey team. Muhammad Ali asked Bogataj for his autograph.[33]

Vinko Bogataj has settled back into his life as a forklift operator and a painter in Lesce, Slovenia. Despite his relative "fame," he hopes that athletes take home one message from watching his crash: "Every time you fall, you have to get back up."[34]

1 / JOAN BENOIT
The Advent of Arthroscopic Surgery

May 12, 1984

Olympia, Washington, was the site of what would be a historic race. In all, 238 runners left the starting line in the US qualifier for the 1984 Olympic marathon. That marathon would soon become a milestone as well, marking the first ever women's marathon in the Olympics.[1]

One of those 238 competitors made the race historic for an entirely different reason. Joan Benoit left the starting line only 17 days after undergoing knee surgery.

Benoit started the race quickly, staying in the front of the pack. Due to her recent injuries, she ran cautiously for the first 12 miles.

After running 5:40 miles for almost half of the race, Benoit increased the pace and quickly built a large lead. She knew, though, that the race wasn't over. Three days before the trials, Benoit had told Kenny Moore of *Sports Illustrated*, "Those last six miles are scary. Anything can happen."[2]

Benoit had a 400-yard lead at the 17-mile mark. There, standing on the side of the road, stood her Athletics West coach, Bob Sevene. Sevene, who had helped guide her through her race preparation and recovery from surgery, tried to gauge her status.

"Sev, I'm all right," Benoit told him.

Her coach jumped for joy right there on the side of the road. "When she says that," Sevene told Moore, "you can go wait in the bar. The race is over."[3]

Benoit might have been all right, but the race was far from over. With those last six scary miles left, Benoit's legs became weak, including her surgically repaired right knee. She slowed her pace to six-minute miles, but she hung on to win the race in 2:31:04.[4]

Many years later, in an interview with Amby Burfoot of *Runner's World*, she called the 1984 Olympic trials "the race of her life."[5]

Sevene professed that Benoit's mental strength, especially in races, was unlike anything he has ever seen. "The sport is 90% ability and attitude, 5% coaching, and 5% luck. In her case, her ability is mental as well as physical."[6] Benoit's ability to fight through 26.2 miles and beat the entire field of healthy runners serves as a testament to that mental strength.

With her win, she went on to compete in Los Angeles against many of the best marathoners in the world. In 1984 the Soviet Union and its satellite states in Eastern Europe boycotted the Olympic Games in response to the US pullout from the 1980 Games over the Soviet invasion of Afghanistan. Even without the athletes from the boycotting Communist nations, Benoit would soon face some of the top female athletes in the world, including Norway's Grete Waitz and Ingrid Kristiansen and Portugal's Rosa Mota. She knew she still had work to do.

"I feel I've really been tested," said a relieved Benoit to Moore after the trials. "The knee, the operation, the hamstring, the emotional ups and downs. Somehow, with all the people who helped, all the people who love me, I made it. I can't believe it. Now I'm looking forward to two months of solid training."[7]

Sevene became emotional as he described the end of the Olympic trials and Benoit's TV interview after she won. He still has a picture of her in his arms after that race. He held her because she didn't want to be seen on television crying.[8]

Bob Sevene knew Benoit could train and win the Olympic marathon, since she had just overcome a bigger obstacle than any competitor. As she crossed the finish line, Sevene held Benoit and exclaimed, "The greatest damn athlete in the world."[9]

Often considered the greatest marathoner of all time, Joan Benoit was widely known to be a religious trainer early in her career. She ran about 200 miles each week. Perhaps it was that volume of training that led to the knee injury that almost kept her out of the Olympics.

As the 1984 Olympic trials approached, Benoit quit her job and moved to her home state of Maine to train full time. Rumors spread throughout the running world that she was training 130 miles per week with sub-five-minute interval miles.[10]

Sevene claimed that Benoit was doing some "scary" workouts to prepare for the trials. Since it was winter in Maine, she trained on the flat 200-meter indoor track at Bates College. "I would tell her to run 4:55 in practice, and she was running 4:40s for the mile," he remembered.[11]

On March 16, just under two months before the race in Olympia, a normal training run threatened to derail her quest.

When she was 14 miles into a 20-mile run, Benoit felt a catching sensation in her right knee. Within a mile she developed pain that completely shut her down. It was the first time she had ever quit a training run.

"Joanie was training in Maine, and I was out in Eugene, Oregon, with Athletics West," Sevene recalled. "I got a call at 7:00 in the morning of all things. Joanie had just gone out on her run. She told me that her knee locked up, and of course I just said, 'Don't worry about it. It's probably an IT band problem,' because it was on the lateral knee. Of course Joanie knew her body."[12]

As many runners do with new onset pain, Benoit took a few days off. The pain improved, but it returned quickly once she resumed training. She decided to try a cortisone shot, which gave her 10 days of relief. But soon she had to stop another training session and walk.

After a second cortisone injection into her ailing knee and five more days of rest, she still had pain.[13] She flew to Eugene, Oregon, the hometown of her coach. Sevene arranged a consultation with an orthopaedic surgeon in Eugene, Dr. Stan James.

Dr. James prescribed five more days of rest and Butazolidin, an anti-inflammatory medication. Benoit, who had finished 10 marathons and risked missing the 11th, was not pleased.

"Joanie immediately came outside and for the first time I ever heard her swear in her life," Sevene remembered. "She was so pissed off because she said, 'Sev, there's something in my knee.'"[14]

After five days of rest, Benoit's fears proved to be true. During the 10-mile test run Dr. James had suggested she do on April 24, she only completed 3 miles before she had to walk. When she told him of her setback, he gave her a final option.

"He said I only had one option—surgery," she told Moore. "Actually I was hoping he'd say that because I thought there was something there. But to do it with so little time . . ."[15]

They chose to proceed with arthroscopic surgery the next day, April 25, just 17 days before the Olympic trials.

As the surgery approached, Dr. James remained pessimistic that the 26-year-old world record holder could recover quickly enough to qualify for the Olympics. He told Frank Litsky of the *New York Times*, "It is possible, not probable, she can run in 12 to 14 days. We'll have to play that by ear. It would be nice if the trials were six weeks away and not three weeks, so we're pressing the issue."

Benoit's record time of 2:22:43 in the Boston Marathon a year earlier would have won every Olympic marathon contest before 1960—for men. And it was fast enough to earn her a spot on the 1980 Olympic team, only four years earlier, based on the times finished by the men's qualifiers.

Now knee surgery threatened to keep her off the team that would compete in the first-ever Olympic marathon for women. But she entered the operating room that day with a backup plan.

"If I don't qualify for the marathon," Benoit told Litsky prior to going under the knife, "I think I'll try the 3,000. I have a possibility of making the team. But it's not the same. My chances in the Olympic marathon are pretty good, but in the 3,000 I'm not world class."[16]

At the time, she held the American record for 25 kilometers, 10 kilometers, 10 miles, and the half marathon in addition to the world record for the marathon. She had her heart set on the marathon, though. Now this knee injury threatened her chance of winning a gold medal for her country.

"This injury is bad," Sevene warned Litsky ahead of the procedure, "not so much for her as for the country. She had the best chance of any American woman, even Mary Decker, to win a gold medal in track."[17]

Arthroscopic knee surgery was practically unheard of in the world of athletes and orthopaedic surgery until the mid-1970s. Its use grew quickly in the years leading up to Benoit's surgery.

Traditionally when an athlete suffered a musculoskeletal injury, such as a torn ligament or meniscus in the knee, the orthopaedic surgeon sliced open the knee, making an incision six to eight inches long to look inside the knee, determine what structures were damaged, and treat them.

Many of these open surgeries served their underlying purpose, but they were invasive. Recovery took months—not just time spent overcoming the ligament or meniscal work, but also to recover from the skin and muscle damage the surgery inflicted.

Arthroscopy promised to deliver equal ability for surgeons to fix whatever damage had led to the surgery with less trauma to the knee. Instead of one or more long incisions, the surgeon made two or three small incisions barely big enough to insert instruments the size of ink pens. Theoretically, with less soft tissue trauma, the patient would regain range of motion and strength much more quickly than after an open surgery.

The role of arthroscopy in the repertoire of orthopaedic surgeons was just developing around the time Dr. James used an arthroscope to look into Benoit's knee.

One of the challenges facing an orthopaedic surgeon treating an athlete's injury in those days was figuring out exactly what the injury was. X-rays only show bones. They are very helpful, to be sure, but often a young competitor has a more complex injury than simply a broken bone around the knee or arthritis.

What X-rays do not show are the soft tissue structures of the knee. These structures include the meniscus, or the C-shaped piece of cartilage between the femur and tibia that serves a shock-absorbing function. Articular cartilage, or the cartilage lining of the bones, also plays a role in absorbing impact and helps the bones glide over each other smoothly as the knee goes through a range of motion. The ligaments that stabilize the knee are likewise not visualized on X-rays.

Orthopaedic surgeons often used arthrograms to improve their diagnostic capabilities. An arthrogram is a radiology test in which contrast material injected into the knee is used to enlarge the joint and provide better images of small structures within it. Arthrography gave physicians a better ability to confirm or refute their impressions of injuries based on an athlete's history and physical examination, but it still did not diagnose many joint injuries.

Magnetic resonance imaging was first available for use in health care in the early 1980s, but it was not a commonly used diagnostic tool by orthopaedic surgeons in Benoit's day.

Now a minimally invasive surgery provided surgeons an opportunity to look inside a patient's knee and figure out exactly what the cause of his or her symptoms was. If the surgeon found the cause of the pain, popping, or buckling, it could be treated on the spot.

This diagnostic and therapeutic option would change the care of athletes—and the field of sports medicine—forever.

If a marathon runner developed a sharp knee pain and catching sensation in her knee today, as Joan Benoit did on that training run, how might the diagnosis and treatment differ?

First of all, nagging knee pain with running can be a very common malady for avid runners. She might notice a localized pain in one part of her knee only with activity—pain with jogging but also physical activities like going up and down stairs or with squats or leg presses in the gym. She likely wouldn't have pain at rest. There also could be symptoms other than pain, like a catching or snapping sensation in a specific location in her knee. Swelling could accompany these symptoms.

Thinking her pain is not serious, she probably would take a few days off from running or switch to biking or swimming to see if her troubles resolved. To be fair, many runners are extremely determined—some might even say stubborn—so she might try to run through the pain. She might use over-the-counter anti-inflammatory medications, ice, or a knee sleeve. Only when she cannot run at all or at least can't run as well as she would like does she decide to see her doctor or an orthopaedic surgeon.

In that first orthopaedic surgery visit, the surgeon performs a history and physical examination. The surgeon asks a number of questions and performs a host of exam tests to determine the cause of the pain. He will usually obtain X-rays of the knee as well. Often the X-rays are negative, but they can show bony changes like osteoarthritis or stress fractures in runners.

Depending on the location of her pain and other knee symptoms, the orthopaedic surgeon might suspect an overuse condition such as patellofemoral pain, iliotibial band syndrome, or a painful plica. Often the surgeon does not order an MRI at the first visit unless he suspects an injury that requires surgery, like a meniscus tear. Occasionally though, the surgeon might obtain an MRI for a high-level athlete to ensure that he or she is not doing any further harm to the knee.

The surgeon might send the runner to work with a physical therapist if he does not suspect structural damage. In the case of a runner with a plica, physical therapy can often be effective, but it can take some time before the runner can completely recover.

In the initial visit, a physical therapist often works to decrease soft tissue inflammation and pain. The therapist might use soft tissue mobilization, myofascial release techniques, or even dry needling. He might use modalities like ultrasound or electrical stimulation. He will also emphasize stretching to any tight muscle groups, like the hamstrings or hip flexors. And the therapist will give the patient some basic exercises to perform each day on her own.

As the runner's symptoms improve, the physical therapist will likely add strengthening exercises for the lower extremity, focusing on closed-chain exercises. These are exercises in which the foot remains fixed to the floor or foot plate of a machine. They use multiple joints and work multiple muscle groups at the same time. The exercises could include wall slides, step ups, step downs, and double leg presses. The therapist might also emphasize hip and gluteal strengthening to restore lower extremity function and take some of the stress off the quadriceps and hamstrings. The therapist will focus on proper technique and control through the exercises.

As the runner progresses, she likely can move to more advanced rehab techniques like plyometrics. She can also begin running, and the therapist can help correct poor running mechanics if they are present. Some physical therapists might even try kinesiology tape to relieve pressure on aggravated areas in the knee and to better balance the muscle forces pulling on the knee.

If the runner modifies her activities and completes her course of physical therapy and home exercise, yet she still cannot run without the pain, then the orthopaedic surgeon will likely pursue a more aggressive path. He might consider a cortisone injection into the knee, although concerns about the effects of cortisone on the articular cartilage have decreased their use somewhat in younger patients. Cortisone, though, can help decrease inflammation within the knee and lower pain.

The surgeon might order an MRI at this point, since traditional measures aren't helping. Magnetic resonance imaging has a high sensitivity for detecting injury to tendons, ligaments, articular cartilage, menisci, and other structures within the knee. Orthopaedic surgeons perform diagnostic arthroscopy, or surgery to look inside the knee to make a diagnosis and treat the problem, far less often now than they did in the 1980s and 1990s. An MRI can detect the injuries seen on these arthroscopic procedures without the risks of surgery.

April 25, 1984

Bob Sevene entered the operating room with his star athlete and Dr. James. "He was in there with the scope looking around. Sure enough, all of the sudden it looked like a piece of steel cable was right there. It was all locked up. He actually just snipped it and that was the extent of it."[18]

During what the *New York Times* would describe as "microsurgery" in its report of the procedure the next day, Dr. Stan James hoped he had found the cause of Joan Benoit's pain.

"There was no obvious cause," James told *Sports Illustrated*'s Moore. "I got in there and saw this little vertical suspension, just a slender little band of collagen fibers in front of the fibular collateral ligament. It didn't look like it could be causing all her problems. And it wasn't inflamed. But it was where the pain was, so I snipped it. It was guilt by association."[19]

By looking in Benoit's knee with an arthroscope, Dr. James determined the cause of her pain to be an inflamed plica. This tight, inflamed band of tissue was only 3 or 4 mm in diameter, but it was located exactly where the runner felt her pain.

Just a year before Dr. James operated on Benoit, Wesley M. Nottage and others had published a study in the *American Journal of Sports Medicine* describing plicae and their symptoms and treatments:

> Prior to the advent of arthroscopy, little attention was paid to the (synovial) plicae within the knee joint. Tight bands were noted at arthrotomy and dismissed as "adhesions" and were not felt to be capable of producing an internal derangement of the knee. Increased arthroscopic experience has led to the identification of several characteristic plicae which have been implicated as causing acute and chronic knee pain.[20]

This band of tissue was the cause of Benoit's training setbacks, and arthroscopy had given Dr. James the ability to find and treat it.

A plica is a remnant of a septum that separates the knee into compartments in embryos. In utero, the plicae are gradually resorbed, and the knee becomes one undivided cavity. If resorption of the plica is incomplete, then a synovial plica remains in the knee of children and adults.

It is thought that 20% to 60% of adults have plicae within their knees. In most people, these plicae are asymptomatic. In a small percentage of people, repetitive stress on the knee with athletic activities like running can cause a normal plica to become inflamed and painful.

A runner with a pathologic plica often complains of knee pain located along the course of the tissue. Often she notices a popping sensation as she straightens her knee.

Currently, to make the diagnosis of plica syndrome by MRI, the plica would have to be one that exists where the patient experiences consistent pain. A large percentage of the population has plicae within their knees that aren't symptomatic, so the surgeon would look for the plica to appear thickened and inflamed on the study in order to suggest that it could be the cause of the patient's symptoms.

Even with a painful plica, the orthopaedic surgeon might still try to treat the patient without surgery. He might try physical therapy if the patient didn't do it previously, and the therapist could focus more attention specifically on the part of the knee where the plica is aggravated. The surgeon might inject cortisone directly into the plica to decrease the inflammation within it, possibly decreasing discomfort from the plica rubbing on nearby bones.

Occasionally nonsurgical treatments fail to work. The orthopaedic surgeon can arthroscopically treat the plica. He would look throughout the knee for any other pathology that could be present and then use a shaver to remove the inflamed band of tissue.

In a runner with a painful plica in the knee who has symptoms that limit her activities and who isn't improving with more conservative measures, arthroscopic surgery can effectively help her get back on the road.

In 1991 John D. Dorchak and his team of researchers published their long-term results of treating patients with symptomatic plicae arthroscopically. Thirty-eight of their fifty-one patients reported good or excellent results.

When they studied their patients who had poor results after the arthroscopic surgery, they learned that most of the failures resulted from an inaccurate diagnosis.[21] That is a key challenge with knee pain thought to be caused by an inflamed plica.

Many people have a plica in their knees, and they don't even know it. Just because it's there doesn't mean it is responsible for a patient's pain. The surgeon must rule out any other possible causes of knee pain before considering a plica as the culprit.

On that April day, Dr. James hoped a plica was the cause of Joan Benoit's pain. Even if it was, it seemed ridiculous to most running experts that she would be ready to compete 17 days after surgery.

Joan Benoit was anxious to use all of those 17 days to train. In the hours after her surgery, while still under the influence of anesthesia and pain medications, she asked her coach if she could start training the next morning.

"She was looking up at me in the fetal position, 'Sev, can I start tomorrow?'" Sevene recalled.[22]

While Sevene wouldn't let her run, he redesigned an exercise bike, turning it upside down so that she could pedal with her arms. She used it for the first few days after her operation. He also limited her to walking on a treadmill.[23]

Benoit could have taken an easy route—one that avoided training so soon after knee surgery—to make the Olympic team. "The TAC had called her and said, 'Joanie we may put you directly on the team,' because she was the world record holder at the time," Sevene mentioned. "She said, 'No way in hell. I'm not telling some kid that finishes third in the race that she's not going to be on the team because I was selected for the team.' She was the real deal."[24]

On Monday, April 30, just five days out from arthroscopic knee surgery,

Benoit ran for the first time. Her first 55-minute run through Eugene, Oregon, gave her an enormous lift. She ran without pain.

Sevene still recalled that first run. "I remember I went on her first run with her, which was supposed to be 4–5 miles, just easy to see how it was. I remember getting to 6 miles going, 'Joanie, we've got to turn around. Stan James is going to kill us.' To this day, I remember the look in her eyes. She said, 'We don't have time to screw around.' She ended up running 9 miles on her first run."[25]

She ran again later that day with her coach, and Sevene told *Sports Illustrated* that she sped up to six-minute miles to test herself. "She was on an emotional high. In retrospect, that was the biggest mistake, letting her loose too early," Sevene told Moore.

Only three days later, she suffered another injury setback. During a run approaching two hours, she felt a pull in her other leg. She had overcompensated and strained her left hamstring.[26]

On Tuesday, May 8, now just four days before the trials in Olympia, Benoit needed to find out if her limited training was enough to compete. She ran 17 miles.

She decided she was ready, although she understood the challenge in front of her. At a press conference before the trials, Benoit told reporters, "I'll be running strictly to make the team. I'm aware of my problem, but I wouldn't be here if I didn't think I could handle it."[27]

It has been over 30 years since Dr. James looked into Joan Benoit's knee to release a plica from the lateral side of her knee. The surgery itself hasn't changed much since then. Have the rehabilitation and recovery changed?

After undergoing arthroscopic knee surgery, the patient usually rests the day of surgery and often the day after it. She usually can put all of her weight on that leg, although surgical pain might lead her to use crutches for a day or two. She would ice her knee and elevate her leg to get the knee swelling down. She might take narcotic pain medications if needed.

Soon after surgery, she could start home exercises to increase her knee motion and lower extremity strength. Often the surgeon might encourage an active person to work with a physical therapist, especially if she aims to return to sports quickly.

As far as exercise after surgery, she could likely start using a stationary bike to get some cardiovascular exercise. Soon she might try an elliptical trainer, which resembles running but causes less impact on the knee. These activities might also improve her knee range of motion. As her surgical incisions heal, she could start swimming. Within two to six weeks, she could start jogging. While jogging earlier wouldn't cause structural injury to the knee, the repetitive impact might cause her knee to swell and ache. Many joggers who try to return very early after knee surgery often feel that it sets them back, making recovery take longer than it otherwise might have required.

At the first clinic visit, the orthopaedic surgeon removes sutures from the skin. He checks the patient's knee range of motion and leg strength. He evaluates for any signs of a problem, such as a blood clot in the leg, and he will advance the physical activity she can do.

Generally, when a patient has full range of motion and lower extremity strength, no knee swelling, and can walk without a limp, she can try to jog. At first she just tries to get used to it, figuring out if she has any pain. She likely can't run at her preinjury speed or distance right away. She can gradually increase her distance, speed, and duration within training as she tolerates them. This gradual progression can help her avoid setbacks.

Often full jogging takes four to six weeks, but it can take several months for the patient's knee to feel normal and for her to return to normal training and competition.

Bob Sevene explained Benoit's determination to accelerate the challenging rehab process after surgery. "A lot of it was her—I don't want to say not listening—but being able to read her knee and know what she could do and couldn't do. In other words, she rehab-wise pushed ahead of the curve just because of knowing her own body."[28]

Arthroscopic surgery is one of the three greatest advancements in the history of orthopaedic surgery, along with fracture fixation and joint replacement. Instead of far more invasive surgeries that required months of recovery and risked an athlete never being able to return to sports, these surgeries allowed a much quicker return to activity. At the time of Joan Benoit's surgery, however, orthopaedic surgeons were just beginning to realize its potential.

The origins of arthroscopy, or looking inside of a joint, came from the ancient Romans.[29] Their curiosity to examine and learn about the human body led to the use of a speculum and other instruments to look in various body cavities like the mouth, ears, and vagina.

In 1806 a German doctor named Phillipp Bozzini developed the first cysto-scope to look at the interior of the bladder. Decades later, Desormeaux refined this cystoscope to improve the visualization of the bladder. His cystoscope is regarded as the first endoscopic instrument.

Thomas Edison's invention of the lightbulb in 1879 significantly aided these efforts to see inside human cavities, replacing the candles and turpentine and gasoline mixtures of earlier cystoscopies. Using this equipment, Max Nitze took the first photograph of the interior of the bladder in 1890. With better light and the use of mirrors, physicians could see into the human body as never before.

Endoscopy did not make its way to the joints of the body until 1912. Danish physician Dr. Severin Nordentoft used a laparoscope to look inside the knee. He presented his studies at the 41st Congress of the German Surgical Society in Berlin. He called this new procedure "arthroscopy." It is not known if Dr. Nordentoft ever used his arthroscope in the care of patients.

Kenji Takigi, a Japanese professor, adapted the cystoscope specifically to look inside the knee. He used that cystoscope to look inside a cadaver's knee in 1918. Over the next 13 years he developed 12 arthroscopes of different sizes and with different viewing angles. He also created small instruments that would allow him to perform some procedures within the knee.

In 1921, three years after Takigi looked inside a cadaver knee, a Swiss physi-cian named Eugen Bircher performed an arthroscopy. He used an abdominal laparoscope like that used by Nordentoft to perform about 60 of what he called arthroendoscopic procedures. Historians often refer to Takigi and Bircher as the "fathers of arthroscopy."

In 1931 Michael Burman, a resident at the Hospital for Joint Diseases in New York City, attempted to use an arthroscope in the anatomy laboratory at New York University. He left New York to study with George Schmorl in Germany. When he returned later in 1931, he published his results in a paper called "Ar-throscopy or the Direct Visualization of Joints."

Throughout the remainder of his career as an orthopaedic surgeon at the Hospital for Joint Diseases, Burman studied his procedure to produce an "Atlas of Arthroscopy." This work was reportedly never published, as Burman could not find an editor willing to share it.

Arthroscopy stagnated through World War II, until Masaki Watanabe used the optics and electronics developed in Japan after the war to develop much more sophisticated endoscopic equipment. Watanabe's No. 21 arthroscope became the model that surgeons in the United States would use in the coming years.

Not only did Watanabe develop the improved arthroscope, but he showed that it could be used to treat patients as well. He removed a tumor from a patient's knee on March 9, 1955. On May 4, 1962, he performed the first-ever arthroscopic partial meniscectomy. Now this surgery, which involves trimming out a portion of meniscus that is torn, is one of the most common operations in all of orthopaedic surgery. Watanabe rightly deserves the title "father of modern arthroscopy."

In 1964 Canadian doctor Robert W. Jackson traveled to Japan to study with Watanabe. Upon his return, Jackson convinced the University of Toronto to purchase a No. 21 arthroscope for $675. He used the device in several cases and subsequently gave the first instructional course lecture on arthroscopic surgery at the American Academy of Orthopaedic Surgeons meeting in 1968.[30]

In 1969 Richard O'Connor, MD, studied under Watanabe. He later created instruments and arthroscopes that allowed him to perform the first partial meniscectomies in North America, in 1974.

Arthroscopy blossomed in the 1970s as fiber optics and television equipment developed. Instead of having to look through the arthroscope directly, surgeons could now move the scope with their hands and project the images onto television monitors. With their hands free, they could perform a wider array of procedures.

By the mid-1980s, around the time Dr. James arthroscopically excised a plica within Joan Benoit's knee, orthopaedic surgeons started to collect data showing that arthroscopic surgery might have better results than open procedures. Surgeons began to demonstrate that complex surgeries might be possible with smaller incisions, shorter recovery times, and lower costs.

Today, arthroscopic surgery is the standard, not the exception. Over 4 million knee arthroscopies are performed worldwide each year, according to the American Orthopaedic Society for Sports Medicine.[31] Approximately 1.4 million arthroscopic shoulder procedures are performed.[32] Hip, elbow, and ankle arthroscopy have exploded, and just about every joint in the body can be visualized arthroscopically. And very few surgeries of the joints require the open incisions of prior generations.

In Joan Benoit's Olympic days, the public at large still didn't understand the breakthrough that arthroscopy had provided. We were still seeing retired professional athletes with eight-inch incisions on their knees walking with terrible limps. We had never seen athletes undergo knee surgery and return—and excel—17 days later.

While Joan Benoit gave us an example of an athlete's tremendous determination and resilience to compete despite seemingly insurmountable obstacles, she also offered a glimpse into the future of the treatment of all athletes.

August 5, 1984

A team from Nike gathered in a room in Los Angeles to watch one of its star athletes compete for the gold medal in the first ever women's marathon in the Olympic Games. Joan Benoit was one of the first athletes Nike had sponsored.

After all, she worked with Nike coaches. She wore Nike shoes. She even underwent surgery by a Nike consultant, Dr. Stan James.

Now her sponsors were watching her pull away from the top female runners in the world. Only blocks from the Los Angeles Coliseum, the Nike staff heard the crowd erupt as Benoit entered the stadium. She had won the gold medal.

Nike founder Phil Knight has been at the center of the explosion of sports as a fundamental aspect of our society. Despite all of the superstars with whom he and Nike have worked, Knight has a special fondness for Benoit.

When he was asked recently if he had a favorite moment in sports, he responded simply, "Yes, when Joan Benoit emerged from the tunnel in Los Angeles."[33]

Later, Benoit would call that Olympic race—still only months removed from her knee surgery—the biggest win of her life.[34]

Even with the advances in arthroscopic surgery, could a runner today expect that she could complete a marathon—or even win it—17 days after undergoing surgery?

It wouldn't be impossible, but it wouldn't be likely, either.

Even though arthroscopic surgery only requires the surgeon to make two or three very small incisions, it can take one or two weeks for a patient's swelling to subside. The orthopaedic surgeon runs liters of fluid through the knee to help with visualization. The soft tissues of the knee absorb some of this fluid, increasing postoperative swelling. Swelling within the knee can cause quadriceps weakness. The patient can ice, elevate the leg frequently, and use anti-inflammatory medications to decrease swelling, but eliminating it still takes time.

Likewise, regaining full strength of the quadriceps, hamstrings, and hip muscles often takes weeks, or sometimes a few months. Working with a physical therapist can speed up this process, but patients are often surprised how long it can take for the knee to feel normal after a seemingly minor surgery.

Also, there is a huge difference between being allowed to run and being able to do it well. Depending on the duration of symptoms, it might take a long time to reach the same level of performance that a runner had prior to being injured. A marathoner might successfully start jogging three or four weeks after surgery, but she might need two or three months before she could run 15 miles at her previous pace.

Orthopaedic surgeons see this recovery time frequently with professional athletes in sports like football or basketball. A team doctor might perform an arthroscopic partial meniscectomy on one of the team's players, scoping the knee to trim out a meniscus tear. For the reasons mentioned, the athlete might be able to return to the field or court four or six weeks after surgery, but it might take three months before he performs at 100% of his abilities.

A high-level runner today could theoretically enter and complete a marathon within six weeks of arthroscopic knee surgery. Maybe one of the best athletes in the world, with a very short amount of time between the onset of symptoms and surgery, could do it 17 days after the procedure. Completing a marathon and running well enough to beat the best female runners in the country, however, would be just as amazing today as it was in 1984.

Joan Benoit's career has been marked by accomplishments and overcoming challenges. Benoit entered the Boston Marathon as a college senior and won it. In that race, she broke the world record by 10 minutes.[35]

In 1983 she again set the world record in the Boston Marathon. In that race, she started at a pace no one believed any runner could maintain.

"People were saying things like, 'Wow, that's really fast,'" she told Amby Burfoot. "And, 'You'd better slow down. You're not going to be able to hold this pace to the finish.'"[36] Benoit's 10K split of 31:45 would equal a 2:13:00 pace. At 10 miles, she clocked in at 51:38 (a 2:15:12 pace). She won the race in a time of 2:22:43.

What made that Boston Marathon more remarkable was the fact that Benoit had only recently undergone surgery on both Achilles tendons.

Sevene first met Benoit in 1981. She was fighting terrible Achilles tendonitis in both legs, so much in fact that she thought her career was over. She contacted Sevene, who was coaching at Boston University. She told him that she wanted to start coaching. When she arrived, they started training together.

Sevene had previously undergone surgery to resect the sheath around his Achilles tendon and claimed it had helped him keep running. At age 72, he still runs 70 miles per week.

He convinced Benoit to see Dr. Robert Leach. Leach, the team physician for Boston University, agreed to operate on Benoit on December 10. On the morning of surgery, she failed to show up.

Sevene convinced Leach to reschedule the surgery, and he drove Benoit to the hospital on December 27. Leach resected the sheath around both Achilles tendons. Fearing that she would try to run too early, Leach put her in casts.

Benoit started training the following March. Just before running a marathon, she took off her watch and handed it to Sevene. He asked why she didn't want to track her splits.

She said, "Sev, I'm going as hard as I can, as long as I can. If I don't break 2:30:00, I'm retiring."

"She was dead serious," Sevene recalled. "She went out and ran 2:26:11. The world's record at the time was 2:25:30. Literally, the next time out of the blocks in Boston the following spring is when she broke the world record and ran 2:22:43."[37]

In 2008 Boston hosted the US Women's Olympic marathon trials. Joan Benoit, now Joan Samuelson, entered her fourth and final marathon trials. She publicly declared her goal of finishing faster than 2:50 at the age of 50, and she accomplished it, finishing in a time of 2:49:08.[38]

Sevene said that Benoit still sets goals for her running to this day. She has never failed to finish a marathon. In fact, the only time she failed to break three hours was in a marathon she ran with her daughter.[39]

In 2013 she competed again in the Boston Marathon, 30 years after her landmark race there. Given the anniversary, she aimed to finish within 30 minutes of her 1983 time of 2:22:43. She finished in 2:50:37.[40]

One week before that race, she had developed inflammation in her knee.

No matter how many goals she sets and obstacles she overcomes, none will surpass what Joan Benoit achieved in Olympia, Washington, in 1984. Not only did she return from knee surgery to win a marathon barely two weeks later, but she also showed millions of people that they might be able to do it too.

Instead of operations in which surgeons make large incisions to cut open the knee that require months of recuperation, she was proof that a surgeon can perform arthroscopy of the knee to find a cause for knee pain and treat it. She could return to training and competition more quickly than ever before. And now this technology could help millions of runners and other athletes just like Joan Benoit.

2 / BERNARD KING

Return to Elite Sports after ACL Injury

March 23, 1985

One minute and twenty-four seconds remained in a late season game between the New York Knicks and the Kansas City Kings.

Bernard King was by far the best player on the floor. He was leading the NBA in scoring that season, averaging 32.9 points per game so far. He had set a record for his hometown Knicks on Christmas Day, scoring 60 points.

Boston Celtics legend Larry Bird called King "the best scorer I've ever seen or played against," that season.[1]

"He was so far above everyone else that it looked like he was playing on an 8-foot basket," teammate Ernie Grunfeld later recalled.[2]

A proficient scorer, King is often remembered for back-to-back 50-point games in 1984 against the San Antonio Spurs and Dallas Mavericks. He was the first player to achieve that feat in 20 years.

Later that season, King steered his Knicks to a win in game 5 of a playoff series against the Isiah Thomas–led Detroit Pistons. King averaged 42.6 points in the series and played through the flu and dislocated fingers in both hands in that decisive game.

Fittingly, he was named NBA most valuable player (MVP) in that 1983–1984 season.

King had already scored 37 points in the March 1985 game against Kansas City. As he ran back on defense, he jumped to block a shot by Kings guard Reggie Theus. When King landed from that jump, he immediately grabbed his right leg. He would later describe that he felt as though his knee had exploded.

On that seemingly routine play, Bernard King tore the ACL in his knee. His season—and possibly his career—ended.

King's journey to the NBA began in Brooklyn, New York. He learned to play basketball on playgrounds only a short distance from Madison Square Garden, the home of the New York Knicks.

Basketball later led him to the University of Tennessee, where the six-foot-seven small forward earned Southeastern Conference (SEC) Player of the Year honors three times.

Success on the court came with trouble off it. King battled an opponent greater than an injury in his early years. Alcohol-related mood swings reportedly led to disorderly conduct arrests during his time at Tennessee and in his first few years in the NBA.[3]

Despite being drafted seventh overall in the 1977 NBA draft by the New Jersey Nets and winning the NBA Rookie of the Year award in 1978, King was traded to Utah after two seasons. The following year, Utah traded him to Golden State. The Warriors then traded him to the Knicks in 1982.

King overcame his struggles with alcohol and shone under the bright lights of Madison Square Garden.

Perhaps it was this difficult journey from the asphalt playground courts to playing in one of the most legendary venues in all of sports, or maybe his off-the-court battles, that strengthened his resolve even further.

King would need all of that courage and determination in the spring of 1985.

"At that time, I was told my career was over," King told *Newsday*'s Andrew MacDougall about his ACL tear. "Obviously, I didn't believe anyone."[4]

"My attitude and thought was always, No. 1, I am from Brooklyn," King told Sean Deveney of *Sporting News* years later. "I grew up on the toughest basketball courts in the world in one of the toughest communities in the nation. And my thought was, if I can make it all the way from there to the top in the NBA, and rise to the top of my profession, I can handle this with regard to coming back from my ACL. This is nothing."[5]

If anyone told Bernard King that his career was over—and it's likely that everyone told him it was—it was for the simple reason that elite athletes did not return from ACL injuries.

For example, a decade earlier Philadelphia 76ers forward Billy Cunningham had entered the 1975–1976 season as a four-time NBA All-Star, three-time first-team all-NBA selection, and a member of the 76ers' championship team.

On December 5, 1975, Cunningham drove down the left side of the lane guarded by New York Knicks point guard Butch Beard. When Cunningham stopped quickly, his knee locked. The small forward out of the University of North Carolina crumpled to the Spectrum floor.

"I've never felt pain like that before," Cunningham told reporters after the injury. "I thought my knee had left me."[6]

Cunningham felt like his knee had left him because essentially it had.

The ACL is a thick ligament that runs in the center of the knee between the femur (thigh bone) and tibia (shin bone). It stabilizes the knee, preventing the tibia from shifting out from under the femur. The ligament provides both front-to-back stability of the knee as well as rotational stability of the knee.

After an ACL injury, an athlete of any age and skill level can take steps to improve his pain, swelling, and basic function. As an example, let's use a 17-year-old high school basketball player who tears his ACL playing in a preseason practice. He can ice his knee and use compression wraps to decrease the knee swelling. He can work on knee range of motion on his own, pushing to get the knee fully extended and flexed, or he can work with a physical therapist on motion. The therapist can also help him regain full lower extremity strength, which can help him return to daily activities and often some basic physical activities such as jogging.

The challenge with an ACL-deficient knee, though, is the instability that many athletes experience. Despite even normal strength of the quadriceps, hamstrings, hip flexors, and other lower extremity muscles, the tibia can shift out from under the femur during athletic activities.

Two common athletic scenarios present a risk for knee instability. The recreational basketball player might jump to take a shot or grab a rebound. When he lands from that jump, the lack of an ACL might allow the tibia to displace in front of the femur. His knee buckles, and he crumples to the ground.

Or he could run down the court dribbling the ball. To evade a defender, he plants his foot on that injured knee in order to change direction. His foot stays planted while his knee rotates awkwardly. Again, his knee gives way.

The instability is obviously a major barrier to the athlete's ability to function the way he wants in sports. Worse, each time his knee gives way, he can do more harm to the knee. When his tibia slides out of position, he could potentially injure the meniscus—the C-shaped shock-absorbing cartilage between the femur and tibia—or the articular cartilage—the cartilage lining on the ends of the bones that provides cushion and helps the ends of the bones glide through a range of motion.

On October 18, 1976, less than one year after his devastating injury, Billy Cunningham retired from basketball at the age of 33.[7]

Bernard King was just 28 years old when he left the court in Kansas City. If King's career had ended after his knee buckled, as Cunningham's had done, Knicks fans would probably still revere him today for his on-court accomplishments up to that point. His return from that injury, though, is largely what makes him a legend today.

March 25, 1985

After suffering his knee injury in Kansas City, Bernard King returned to New York City, where he was hospitalized.

Dania Sweitzer, a physical therapist who had worked with King when he was recovering from an ankle sprain a year earlier, remembered exactly when she learned of King's injury. "I had been at a tennis match in the city, and someone said to me, 'Oh my God! Bernard King went down with an ACL!'" She knew her life had changed right then.[8]

King interviewed several orthopaedic surgeons at his bedside and asked each of them questions. "How are you going to do this? What are your guarantees? What do you think I'll look like?" He ultimately chose Dr. Norman Scott, the New York Knicks team physician.

Then he informed Dr. Scott, "and I want Dania."[9]

Dr. Scott took the star forward to the operating room for a diagnostic arthroscopic surgery.

"Our concern is about a torn ligament," Dr. Scott informed the media prior to that surgery. "The arthroscopy will provide a definite diagnosis and we'll go from there."[10]

The diagnostic surgery soon revealed the full extent of the injury that jeopardized King's career. Dr. Scott determined that King had torn his ACL and cartilage in the knee and broken a bone.

"Bernard will make the decision on whether he will have surgery," Dr. Scott informed the media after that arthroscopic surgery. "There are options. The ligament won't heal by itself, but muscle around it can compensate for the loss of the ligament. The cartilage is no problem, the ligament is."[11]

Dr. Scott wanted King to understand these options and even discuss them with other players and orthopaedic surgeons. He offered King some time to rest in the hospital before making the decision about a possible second—a much more invasive—surgery.

"We're going to talk about the surgery tomorrow," Dr. Scott said. "I will present all the options to him. Bernard was a little uncomfortable after the anesthesia, and in all fairness to him there is no emergency. We want him to think it over. If surgery is performed, there will be an extensive rehabilitation period over the summer. But either way, we expect that he will be back healthy for next season."[12]

Many years later, King described his determination to not only recover from his injury, but also return to play in the NBA.

"At the time, I was told my career was over," King told *Newsday*'s Andrew MacDougall years later. "Obviously, I did not believe anyone. I knew I was going to come back. It wasn't a question of whether I was going to come back. I was going to come back and be an All-Star again. That's the goal I set for myself. There was no deviation, ever. I had a goal in mind and I had tunnel vision, and I was not going to stop until I reached that goal."[13]

Just before the surgery on April 1, 1985, Dr. Scott spoke to reporters. "Bernard is going to have a reconstruction of the anterior cruciate ligament. Essentially we are making him a new ligament by moving a structure to serve as a new ligament," Dr. Scott told them. He estimated that King's surgery would last two hours.[14]

Ninety years before Bernard King underwent ACL reconstruction by Dr. Scott, A. W. Mayo Robson performed what is believed to be the first ACL repair. Robson described his treatment of a 41-year-old miner who had been injured three years earlier. The miner continued to experience knee weakness and instability after his injury. Robson repaired both "crucial" ligaments—now known as cruciate ligaments. He sewed them to their attachment sites on the femur. According to Robson's case description, the patient walked without a limp and never missed another day of work due to his knee.[15]

Eight years after Robson first tried to repair the torn ligament, a German surgeon attempted to replace it. F. Lange used silk suture attached to one of the hamstring tendons—the semitendinosis—in an attempt to substitute for the ACL. Lange's technique did not prove to be successful.

In 1917 Ernest W. Hey Groves performed the world's first ACL reconstruction. He used a strip of the iliotibial band on the lateral side of the knee to make a new ligament. He made a large horseshoe incision on the front of the knee and cut the bony attachment of the patellar tendon to expose the inside of the joint. After harvesting a strip of the IT band, Hey Groves passed it through tunnels drilled in the femur and tibia before sewing it to the bone and soft tissue. He then reattached the tibial tubercle with nails.[16]

Over the next 50 years, surgeons all over the world attempted to improve ACL reconstruction techniques. In 1935 Willis C. Campbell used a graft constructed from portions of the patella tendon, prepatellar retinaculum (soft tissue over the kneecap), and quadriceps tendon. Harry B. Macey used the semitendinosis tendon in 1939. In 1963 Kenneth G. Jones first harvested the central portion of the patella tendon with a portion of bone from the patella still attached to the graft. And in 1969 Kurt Franke first used a graft harvested from the patella tendon with a bone block from the patella and the tibia left attached.[17]

One of Franke's patients participated in the Olympics as a wrestler five months after ACL surgery.

In the 1970s the procedure became more complex, as orthopaedic surgeons attempted to surgically correct the rotational instability of an ACL-deficient knee and not just the front-to-back instability. D. L. MacIntosh used a fascia lata graft from the outside of the thigh and routed it through the knee. He and J. L. Marshall used a similar extra-articular technique but used the central third of the patella tendon and quadriceps tendon. These extra-articular reconstructions had mixed success.[18]

All of these reconstructions required harvesting tissue from the patient's knee—autografts—to create a graft that would become a new ligament. As such, these procedures inflicted a fair amount of trauma on the soft tissues around the knee. Even though Lange's attempt to use a silk suture with the semitendinosis tendon had failed, surgeons wondered if a synthetic ligament substitute would stabilize the knee with little morbidity.

In 1981 D. J. Candy used a graft reinforced with carbon fiber. Unfortunately, this graft led to carbon deposits in the tissue lining the knee as well as the liver, so this procedure was abandoned. Soon surgeons were experimenting with grafts made of Dacron or Gore-Tex. These grafts also failed, due to both high rates of re-rupture as well as frequent cases of inflammation of the lining of the knee joint.[19]

Heading into the mid-1980s, surgeons returned to using autografts for ACL reconstruction, usually bone-patella tendon-bone grafts or hamstring grafts. While surgeons have modified these techniques somewhat since the 1980s, ACL reconstruction today closely resembles the operations performed by surgeons three decades earlier.

April 1, 1985

The ACL reconstruction Scott performed on Bernard King required an arthrotomy. He essentially made a large incision on the knee to look inside. Scott used the iliotibial band, a tendon on the outside of the knee, and rerouted it through the knee to create a new ligament.[20]

The extensive procedure required a very lengthy recovery period. "Just by opening the joint and all the surgery, it took a long time for that healing process to occur. . . . While it was successful, it took a long period of time for all that and the subsequent rehabilitation to take place," Dr. Scott explained years later to *Hoop Magazine*.[21]

In the 1980s elite athletes who tore their ACLs largely did not expect that they would return to play sports. Often surgeons allowed the knee to become stiff, which actually improved knee stability. Unfortunately, only nonmobile centers could play with stiff knees with any effectiveness.

In the early 1980s surgeons often placed athletes in long-leg casts with the knee bent in about 30 degrees of flexion for up to six weeks. And it would take 6 to 12 weeks to regain somewhat normal knee motion. Then months of strengthening work followed.[22]

Scott did not put King in a cast. In fact, Sweitzer used a continuous passive motion (CPM) machine to help restore his knee motion. Patients place their injured legs in a CPM machine for many hours a day, allowing the machine to slowly bend and straighten out the knee to gradually improve knee range of motion.[23]

Still, King faced a lengthy rehab process. "We'd all love to say it was only a year," Dr. Scott remembered. "It was probably, for elite athletes, closer to two years than it was to one."[24]

While current ACL reconstructions are largely similar to the techniques of the 1980s, two significant modifications occurred shortly after Dr. Scott performed surgery on Bernard King.

Unlike Scott's arthrotomy, in which he made a large incision to completely open the knee joint, surgeons began performing these procedures arthroscopically. Instead of making a six- to eight-inch incision across the knee and causing significant injury to the muscles and tendons to get inside the knee, the surgeon could look at the injured ACL through an arthroscope placed through two or three small incisions barely large enough to fit a pen. An arthroscopic-assisted reconstruction using a patella tendon or hamstring autograft still required a small incision, usually between one and two inches long, to harvest the graft. With less soft tissue damage, though, the patient had less postoperative pain and usually regained motion and strength faster and easier.

Dr. Scott also noted another important evolution in his *Hoop Magazine* interview: "[F]ixation in that era was not as good as we'd like. Now that we have great fixation, we could put a substitute [tendon] in there that was more of a free substitute."[25]

In the late 1980s M. Kurosaka showed that a graft's weakest point was its fixation inside the knee. Surgeons then began using metal and bioabsorbable screws to fix the bone plugs on either side of the patellar tendon graft within the tunnels in the femur and tibia.

Toward the end of the 1980s a variety of fixation techniques, including bioabsorbable screws, screws and washers, cross-pins, and buttons, were developed for hamstring grafts.

Today, between 100,000 and 150,000 ACL reconstructions are performed annually in the United States alone. Surgeons continue to look for better techniques, grafts, and fixation.

However, for athletes trying to return to high-level sports, most orthopaedic surgeons perform arthroscopic-assisted ACL reconstruction using patellar tendon or hamstring autografts, similar to the surgeries performed on athletes soon after Bernard King's procedure.

Dr. Scott opened King's knee, reconstructed the ACL, fixed torn cartilage, and fixed a broken bone, but it seemed unlikely that Bernard King would return to the basketball court. At his first physical therapy visit, Sweitzer asked King to perform a straight leg raise, lifting his leg off the bed. King lacked the quadriceps strength to do it.

"To go from playing the game every day at the speed that I played it at, running on the fast break, to be reduced to someone helping you raise your leg a few inches off the bed was disconcerting," King explained to Sean Deveney of *Sporting News*, "to say the least."[26]

King wanted to come back to basketball at his previous level of play. Fortunately, the New York Knicks allowed him to take as long as necessary, rehabbing the knee on his schedule. The team installed a Cybex machine, a treadmill, and other equipment in his home for King to use in his rehab. Sweitzer even taught Bernard how to swim so that he could walk and run in place in a pool. King and Sweitzer worked six days each week, often for up to five hours a day, to progress through the steps of his rehab:

> I was working full time in New York City, and so I worked from 7:30 to 2:30. I
> wouldn't have lunch. I would work straight through. I was on the way to my car.

The deli knew to have my lunch ready. I would bring my lunch, and I would eat it as I was crossing the G.W. Bridge, just trying to eat to make sure that I was perfectly on time to work with Bernard for the next couple of hours.

It was a big commitment on both of our parts. He had to commit to what he was doing, and he was great, and I had to commit also. He was expecting me to be as committed as he was to his rehab.[27]

Sweitzer fondly remembered how motivated King was. "Bernard wanted to come back the way he was before. He didn't want to come back as some of the other NBA players who tried to come back but didn't look quite the same."[28]

Rehabilitation from ACL reconstruction is a long, painful process for any athlete. The patient works to decrease his knee swelling and pain. He pushes to regain his knee motion over many weeks. He works to build his quad strength and the strength of other muscles around the knee. He walks, and later, he jogs. If each step goes well, he progresses to sport-specific activities. At some point, he might—yes, might—return to sports.

Just as the surgical techniques involved in ACL reconstruction evolved over more than a century, the rehabilitation process after surgery did as well.

In the late 1970s and early 1980s orthopaedic surgeons used a long process to slowly restore knee range of motion and strength in order to protect the ACL graft. They usually immobilized the patient's knee in some amount of flexion. They also limited weight bearing for up to six weeks. The patient often wore a brace for about four months. Strengthening of the leg advanced slowly over the ensuing months. If a patient had regained full motion and most of his strength when compared to the uninjured leg, then he could start progressing to sport-specific activities, usually after nine months.

In the late 1980s Dr. Donald Shelbourne, an orthopaedic surgeon in Indianapolis, Indiana, observed that patients were often dissatisfied with their knee function and could not return to preinjury activities. Many athletes struggled to regain the ability to fully straighten the knee. They also often complained of pain in the front of the knee and the long delay in return of strength.

Instead of electing not to reconstruct the ACL and casting the knee to make it stiff, these ACL reconstructions did improve the stability of the knee. That stability, however, came at the expense of increased pain and inability to fully extend the knee.

Dr. Shelbourne wanted to find a way to correct an athlete's ACL deficiency without causing motion problems after surgery. He stopped using casts. Patients started working with a physical therapist before surgery to decrease swelling and improve knee range of motion. They used a CPM machine after surgery and worked on regaining full knee extension immediately after the procedure.

Perhaps ironically, Dr. Shelbourne noticed that patients who were not compliant with this rehabilitation protocol actually seemed to do better than those patients who followed the physical therapy plan. One of his medical students interviewed the first 200 patients. He learned that few of the patients were using their crutches or wearing their removable splints to bed, despite being instructed to wear them 24 hours a day except when working on knee motion.

Shelbourne then switched his post-ACL reconstruction rehabilitation protocol to allow immediate weight bearing after surgery. He did not immobilize the patient's knee at all. He progressed the patient's strength and functional activities to allow return to sports as soon as four to six months after surgery.

When he compared results from patients who used the two different protocols, Shelbourne observed that patients who had the "accelerated" rehabilitation had better outcomes by all measures, with no decrease in graft stability.

"I could not tell people to ignore me, but I could follow the ones who were ignoring me and see if they were having detrimental outcomes because of the ignorance of my advice. I realized that the less they listened to me, the better off they were. I didn't experiment on my patients. They experimented on themselves, and I was just smart enough to be around and get them to fess up," Dr. Shelbourne explained.[29]

Dr. Stephen Lombardo, an orthopaedic surgeon and team physician for the Los Angeles Lakers, called King's recovery and return to the NBA a "landmark." Much of the credit for the surgery's later success among numerous high-level athletes should be given to the advances in the rehabilitation of the athletes after surgery. Dr. Shelbourne's shift to early knee motion was an important part of that process.

"They are dramatic improvements that we've made to allow players to go back to compete at a high level in a very functionally demanding sport. It's sort of equivalent to Tommy John surgery for the elbow," Dr. Lombardo argued.[30]

Let's return to the example of a 17-year-old basketball player who tears his ACL in preseason training for his high school team. He and his parents see an orthopaedic surgeon, who discusses the treatment options. They proceed with ACL reconstruction in order to stabilize his knee and allow him to return to playing basketball.

Depending on the tissue he and the surgeon choose to use as a graft, the timeline for return to play differs. Using autografts, in which the surgeon uses tissue from the patient's knee, generally leads to quicker return to play times than allografts, or tissue from a donor. The graft incorporates more quickly, and failure rates are generally lower. Patellar tendon grafts and hamstring grafts are the autografts most commonly utilized for younger athletes.

Within the first week after surgery, the young athlete starts physical therapy. In addition to efforts to decrease his pain and swelling, the therapist works to restore knee range of motion over the first four weeks, aiming for full range of motion, symmetrical with the opposite knee. He also works to get the patient's quadriceps muscles firing appropriately. He stresses normal gait and lower extremity motor control so the athlete can perform activities of daily living normally.

In the next phase, usually between 4 and 12 weeks, assuming the athlete has regained full knee range of motion, he enters a strengthening phase. He can perform functional exercises like double-leg squats, single-leg stance, and gluteal and hamstring strength exercises. The therapist may have him run in a pool to increase movement without body weight. The athlete can work on his stride without actually running. And the therapist works to restore balance and neuromuscular control.

Around 12 weeks after surgery, or longer if the patient is slower to regain motion and strength, the therapist may start straight-ahead jogging. He also adds plyometric exercises, including working on landing symmetrically. The patient may gradually progress through double-leg plyometric exercises, to single-leg work, to bounding and hopping. He may even start jumping, changing directions, and decelerating. Since the athlete is a basketball player, the therapist may work on basketball activities like jumping for layups and rebounds and changing directions to defend opponents.

At approximately six months, the patient may advance through a return-to-sports phase, often working with other athletes or patients in a small group environment. Generally, if all aspects are improving appropriately, the basketball player may progress from noncontact activities with the team, to controlled contact drills, to training with the team, to full competition.

In the past, many orthopaedic surgeons gave patients an estimate that return to sports required six months after surgery. Julie Eibensteiner, a physical therapist in Minneapolis, Minnesota, who rehabs athletes after ACL reconstruction almost exclusively in her practice, explained that the six-month deadline is an absolute minimum with her patients. Every aspect of the patient's recovery, such as his motion, strength, and movement, has to return to normal in order to play that quickly.[31]

Dania Sweitzer performed King's physical therapy after ACL surgery, and she still rehabs athletes after these surgeries today. "The recovery is like night and day. It really is. I mean we still look for the same aspects at the end, that the patient goes back to full function and looks the way he did before. But it's easier to accomplish that now as compared to back then."[32]

Bernard King's entire journey from operating room to Madison Square Garden took two years. Sweitzer gave much of the credit for King's returning to the court to him. King was engaged in every aspect of his therapy, questioning every aspect of his rehab. He was as motivated as any patient she has ever had.

"My physical therapist, we worked six days a week, five hours a day," King told *Newsday*'s Andrew MacDougall. "To me, that's the epitome of determination, hard work, self-motivation and discipline. And I did that every single day. I knew I was going to come back. It was not a question whether I was going to come back.

I'm proud of that, and to me, that's what defines my career."[33]

It was less the ACL surgery Bernard King underwent that defined his career than the return to play in an NBA game almost exactly two years later.

On April 10, 1987, in front of his hometown crowd, King played 23 minutes in his team's loss to the Milwaukee Bucks. He scored seven points.

King, who was now 30 years old, played in six games at the end of his return season. Despite scoring 30, 29, and 31 points in his last three games, the Knicks elected not to re-sign him. Reportedly the Knicks did not believe that his knee could hold up. Midway through the exhibition schedule for the 1987–1988 season, the Washington Bullets offered him a two-year contract worth $2.5 million.

Despite his return to play, the ACL injury sapped some of his prior explosiveness. Instead, King developed his inside game to score points. In his first full season back, King played in 69 games and averaged 20.7 points per game for the Bullets.

During the 1990–1991 season, King averaged 28.4 points, 5.0 rebounds, and 4.6 assists per game. Despite games of 52 points against Denver, 47 points against New Jersey, and 44 points against Chicago, his 49-point performance against his former team personified his comeback. Shortly after his dazzling display at

Madison Square Garden, King was named to the All-Star Game for a fourth time, at the age of 34.

Bernard King was the first NBA player to return to an All-Star team after having an ACL reconstruction.

"To most guys, playing in the All-Star Game is an honor. But for me, it's totally different. It's so much more than that," King told the media before the game. "It's the culmination of a dream that only three people thought possible. This will be the happiest day of my life."[34]

Bernard King is widely touted as the first athlete to return to an elite level of competition after an ACL injury. Fittingly, Dr. Norman Scott and Dania Sweitzer attended the All-Star Game that completed his unprecedented return.

Sweitzer still fondly remembered the invitation to the All-Star Game and King's appreciation of the work she and her husband, also a physical therapist, did to get him back on the court. "In my office, I have a signed ball that says, 'To Dania and Ron—we made history together.' It's a special ball. It reminds me of motivation, about how hard we worked. It's special."[35]

Bernard King's was the first famous athlete "success" story, but by no means the last. Now it is widely expected that professional athletes return to play at the same level.

Soon after King returned to basketball, athletes became more enthusiastic about the procedure. Players witnessed the improved rehab. At the same time, orthopaedic surgeons learned to use the arthroscope to look inside the knee and reconstruct the ACL without having to make a long incision to open the knee. Gradually players developed higher expectations for their abilities after this injury and surgery.

Multiple studies have shown encouraging results for top athletes after ACL reconstruction. A 2013 study by Joshua D. Harris, MD and others looked at return to sports among NBA players. They analyzed data from 58 NBA players who underwent ACL reconstruction between 1975 and 2012. They wanted to determine not only the rate of return to play for NBA players, but also their performance if and when they did return.

Fifty of the fifty-eight (86%) NBA players returned to play in the NBA after ACL reconstruction. And 12% returned to the International Basketball Federation (FIBA) or the NBA D-league.

Of the players who returned to play in the NBA, 98% did so the season following surgery, with return to play at an average of 11.6 months from injury. These athletes played for an average of 4.3 years after surgery.

Performance after ACL reconstruction declined among these NBA players. Games played per season dropped compared to games played before the injury. Likewise, points, rebounds, field-goal percentage, and minutes per game dropped significantly. Not surprisingly, many fewer players were selected for All-Star teams after surgery than before surgery.

However, when the authors of the study compared these reconstructed NBA players to uninjured, age-matched control players, the non-ACL tear control players demonstrated similar declines in on-court performance.[36]

Given these results, it is not surprising that sports medicine physicians and orthopaedic surgeons now expect elite athletes to return to sports after ACL reconstruction. In 2002 NFL team orthopaedic surgeons completed surveys about ACL surgery for football players. As part of that survey, the team doctors were asked, "What percentage of players actually return to play in the NFL following ACL reconstruction?" In response, 90% of the surgeons selected 90% to 100%, while 10% chose 75%.[37]

Simply because an athlete can return that quickly to an elite level of play doesn't mean it is the norm. Professional athletes do have certain advantages over high school kids and adult weekend warriors in recovering from these surgeries, such as time and money for top-quality therapists and equipment. On the other hand, they must compete with other athletes in elite physical condition to reclaim their spots on the rosters.

When a sports fan watches the star of his favorite team go down with an ACL injury, he usually assumes the athlete will return as good as new the following season. Despite some studies showing high rates of return to sports, like Harris's NBA study, others are more cautious.

A 2010 study of 49 NFL players who underwent ACL reconstruction found that only 63% returned to play in an NFL game.[38]

A 2006 study of 31 NFL running backs and wide receivers who underwent ACL reconstructions observed that 21% never returned to play in an NFL game. Interestingly, much as performance appears to decline for NBA players after ACL surgery, player performance dropped by about one-third among the wide receivers and running backs who did make it back to play.[39]

Kirk A. McCullough, MD, and others followed 147 high school and college football players who underwent ACL reconstruction, finding that 69% of college football players successfully returned to play, and 63% of high school players returned to the field. Only 43% of the athletes felt that they were able to play at their preinjury level of performance.

Interestingly, about half of the high school and college football players who did not return to sports acknowledged a fear of reinjury or fear of further injury to their knees.[40]

In 2013 Vehniah K. Tjong, MD, and other researchers at the University of Toronto interviewed patients between the ages of 18 and 40 who had participated in sports at varying levels before ACL surgery. They found that fear was a predominant theme among the athletes who did not return to their preinjury level of performance.

The majority of the patients who didn't return to sports after ACL surgery battled a fear of reinjury, not being able to compete at the same level, and even constant thoughts about the original injury. These fears often kept those patients from rehabbing effectively. They struggled to return to play their sports and to push through to achieve their preinjury level of play.[41]

Physical readiness to play after surgery does not always come with psychological readiness to do so.

Dr. Erin Shannon, a doctor of clinical psychology and energy medicine practitioner who has worked with the St. Louis Rams and other top athletes, believes that fear of reinjury is a real issue for many athletes after surgery. Memories of the original injury often create a barrier.

"Anybody that's had a significant injury and then has to reenter the field of battle where they had the injury occur, for example if you're a football player and you got the injury on the football field and then you are thrust back into the game, you're going to have some mild post-traumatic stress-type memories of the injury that are going to haunt you as you reenter the sport," Dr. Shannon explained.[42]

Open communication between the medical staff and the injured athlete is crucial for all athletes—pros, high school athletes, and adult weekend warriors. Often the athletic trainers and physical therapists recognize a problem before the surgeons. Many patients feel more comfortable talking about their fears to the therapist and athletic trainers, since they spend so much more time with them than with the doctors.

It's important that these members of the care team be involved in the discussions with the athlete, surgeon, and sports team. They can help set the athlete's expectations before surgery and even direct that player to other athletes who have successfully returned from these surgeries.

Sports medicine physicians and orthopaedic surgeons must learn to recognize fear of reinjury and other psychological barriers athletes face if we want to improve the rates of return to sports. In the coming years, we will likely see orthopaedic surgeons using personality and mood assessments during the injury evaluation process. Athletes working with counselors or sports psychologists as part of the ACL rehab process could become standard as well.

Bernard King returned to All-Star form after suffering a devastating ACL injury. Athletes of all sports, ages, and skill levels must remember that it took him two years, working hours in the gym almost every day. He likely encountered the same fear of reinjury along the way that so many athletes experience. All athletes could use a sign like the one that hung in Bernard King's gym—"I shall not be denied"[43]—to help them push through the grueling rehab process.

Bernard King was inducted into the Naismith Memorial Basketball Hall of Fame on September 8, 2013. It's hard to know how great King could have become as a player had he never suffered his brutal knee injury back in 1985. But we know how and why he will always be remembered.

Reggie Theus, whose shot King tried to block on that fateful play in Kansas City, summarized King's return to an All-Star caliber of play: "Before he got hurt, Bernard was well on his way to becoming known as one of the best of all time. For him to come back and pick up where he left off is a humongous, unbelievable accomplishment."[44]

Bernard King understands his legacy and what he represents to all of the injured athletes who have come after him.

"You can go back and look at my career—whether it's back to back 50 [point games], whether it's first-team all-pro, whether it's as averaging 32 points a game, whether it's 60 points in a game, my peers in the NBA in 1983-84 voted me MVP of the league," King explained to the *Washington Post*'s Michael Lee after his Hall of Fame induction. "You can look at all of those things, but as a player, strictly as a player, my personal legacy is what I did for five hours a day, six days a week, to come back from an injury that players were not coming back from. That was a death knell for players' career. That's my basketball legacy."[45]

3 / HINES WARD

Use of Platelet-Rich Plasma and Stem Cells for Active People

January 18, 2009

Normally finishing a game with only three catches for 55 yards would be a disappointment for a top player like Pittsburgh Steelers wide receiver Hines Ward. Ward's first catch in that playoff win against rival Baltimore gained the Steelers 45 yards and set up a field goal. With that catch, Ward had caught at least one pass in 13 straight postseason games.

It would be his second reception that had a lasting impact on sports medicine, although no one could have known that at the time.

With 6 minutes, 54 seconds left in the first quarter, Ward caught an 11-yard pass on third down, keeping the Steelers' drive alive. Cornerback Frank Walker tackled the receiver, who got up slowly and limped off the field. Ward went to the locker room with a right knee injury. The team announced his return as questionable, but the former University of Georgia receiver lived up to his tough reputation. The 32-year-old reentered the game at the beginning of the second quarter.

His third catch would prove to be his last. Ward was listed as "doubtful" to return. He missed the rest of the game with what would later be diagnosed as a grade 2 MCL injury.

Medial collateral ligament injuries are some of the most common in sports. This is a ligament on the inside of the knee (the side of the knee closest to the midline) that stabilizes the knee against stress from the side. Athletes often suffer these injuries when they are hit on the outside of the knee. Fortunately, almost all of them heal without surgery. Recovery takes anywhere from one to six weeks, depending on the severity of the injury.

Unfortunately for Hines Ward, his knee injury occurred during the AFC Championship game. Super Bowl XLIII would take place only two weeks later.

February 1, 2009

Andrea Kremer, an NBC sideline reporter, nervously prepared to go on the air just before kickoff of Super Bowl XLIII. The fact that 98 million viewers[1]—the largest television audience for a sporting event ever at that time—were watching accounted for only part of her jitters.

"Truthfully there is rarely any news that comes out right before the Super Bowl because you've had the most intense media scrutiny for two weeks," Kremer explained.[2]

At 5:29 p.m. Kremer stood on the sidelines and explained a novel treatment used on Hines Ward to help him play in the Super Bowl. She described a procedure in which a doctor drew blood from Ward, removed cells, and concentrated them before injecting them into his injured knee.

Kremer had received a tip from someone in the medical profession whom she trusted implicitly. He (or she) described the procedure, how it works, and why it could potentially be effective.

The day before the Super Bowl, the Steelers held a walk-through practice. Head coach Mike Tomlin allowed friends and family members to watch and take pictures. This practice would be Kremer's only opportunity to get Hines Ward to confirm what she had learned about his platelet-rich plasma (PRP) procedure.

Unfortunately, the team's public relations official told Kremer that while she could go anywhere that day, she had to leave the players alone and not talk to them. She felt obligated to abide by those restrictions because she needed access on game day.

After practice, she stood on the side of the field as the players walked by. When Ward asked Kremer how she was doing, she took the opportunity to ask him if he had undergone a PRP procedure. He told her, "Yeah, I did." In 90 seconds or so, Andrea Kremer had confirmed her breaking news.

"Seriously I have been in this business a very long time, but I am a news junky. If I could have danced in honor of Mr. Rooney, the owner of the Steelers, the Irish jig on the field at that moment I would have. Because I confirmed it with the one person, whose name I could use, who had the most credibility."[3]

Kremer's report certainly got the attention of football fans, although the unusual nature of Kremer's story might have caught many by surprise. *Pro Football Talk*'s Mike Florio quipped, "It's unknown whether Ward also spent the week wearing a necklace of garlic cloves."[4]

After fellow sideline reporter Alex Flanagan next compared Arizona Cardinals quarterback Kurt Warner to an F. Scott Fitzgerald quote, Reid Kerr of examiner. com remarked, "It's like NBC is trying to sneak a semester of community college into their broadcast."[5]

Hines Ward finished that game with two catches for 43 yards in the Steelers' Super Bowl victory. His performance in the Super Bowl wasn't the subject of Internet chatter nearly as much as the fact that he played at all.

Kremer has covered over 20 Super Bowls. She also teaches journalism at Boston University, so she understands how interviews can make an impact. "I was aware of how big it was because of the place in which it was delivered. Usually those pre-kick reports are filled with platitudes. 'Here's what the coach told everybody last night.' That sort of thing. So that's, of all the reports I've ever done, probably the biggest, most impactful one."[6]

Immediately questions about the legal and ethical ramifications of Ward's procedure surfaced. Was the treatment Andrea Kremer described to millions of viewers equivalent to blood doping?

Essentially, no. When we think of blood doping, we think of a performance-enhancing procedure used by elite cyclists. In blood doping, an athlete has a large amount of blood removed and stored while his body naturally replaces the red blood cells. When that blood is later put back into his body—usually before a competition—the added blood increases his red blood cell count to much higher levels than normal. Since red blood cells carry oxygen throughout the body, the higher levels should improve his endurance.

Platelet-rich plasma, on the other hand, has a very different purpose than blood doping. Unlike adding additional red blood cells to improve performance, PRP improves the body's healing from an injury through the platelets and their growth factors.

National Football League spokesman Greg Aiello acknowledged that Ward did not violate the NFL's drug policy by using PRP.[7]

Dr. James Bradley, the team physician for the Pittsburgh Steelers, described the circumstances that had led him to use PRP on Hines Ward before the Super Bowl. Five days before the Steelers played the Baltimore Ravens in the AFC Championship game, he had had conversations with Arthrex, a medical device company. Arthrex had developed a new biologic, a form of platelet-rich plasma called "autologous conditioned plasma," or ACP.

I believe that to be an orthopedic physician there is a burden of craft to the patient that requires you to stay up to date on new medical advances. Thus, I had been reading about platelet-rich plasma and possible uses. I read the studies, and I agreed with the findings. I had just received one of the first kits in the United States used to prepare PRP, because I wanted to begin incorporating this treatment into my practice. I thought platelet-rich plasma was a reasonable treatment given the amount of data available at the time.

Shortly after reading on this subject, I was on the sidelines in AFC Championships game against Baltimore, and Hines Ward, our star receiver, went down. After examining him, I diagnosed him with a grade 2 MCL injury. Serendipitously we still won the game and were now going to the Super Bowl. However, winning really put the heat on the medical staff to help get Hines back onto the field.

Hines was pretty adamant that I was going to give him a steroid injection to help him get back in the game. I refused the idea because he was too young, and so I didn't. Having recently reviewed the literature on platelet-rich plasma, I said to him, "There's this new biologic that I think has a lot of potential. So if you have any chance of getting back, I think that is the thing you should at least look at because I know it's not going to hurt you. It's your own platelets, and it's your own plasma."

After learning about the biologic treatment, Hines agreed to proceed with the biologic option. We injected him, and then rested him one week. Then I injected him again a week later. After the first two injections, I released him to practice in 10 days, and then injected him a third time. Using that basic science and our knowledge of biology at the time, we thought this treatment and the sequence of injections were reasonable. Sure enough, he got right back in the game and played very well. He caught the first pass of the game. We kept the treatment silent, because we didn't want anyone else to know, quite frankly. However, the silence was broken when he mentioned the treatment to Andrea Kremer. Andrea Kremer then said it on TV in front of ninety-two million people. That's when my cell phone exploded.[8]

Dr. Neal ElAttrache, an orthopaedic surgeon at the Kerlan-Jobe Orthopaedic Clinic in Los Angeles, explained the treatment to Colin Dunlap of the *Pittsburgh Post Gazette* in the days after the Super Bowl. "When you injure yourself, it promotes a cascade of events that eventually leads to healing. But, with ACP, you take some of your own blood out, centrifuge the blood into the injured area. You might take out 20 or 30 ccs, treat it, and then inject back a very nutrient-rich 3 or 4 ccs."[9]

Dr. ElAttrache had used PRP on Dodgers pitcher Takashi Saito for a partial ulnar collateral ligament injury of the elbow months earlier. ElAttrache argued that Dr. Bradley had made a smart decision in trying this procedure on Ward's MCL injury.

"I think it was genius for Bradley to think about doing this," ElAttrache told the *Pittsburgh Post-Gazette*. "This was the perfect use for ACP. There was no potential downside to using it on Hines Ward and it probably helped him a great deal. Now, there is no way to prove that Hines Ward wouldn't have gotten better without Bradley having this done to him, but I think we can all come to the conclusion, without a doubt, that it helped Hines Ward be able to participate in the Super Bowl."[10]

Dr. Bradley insisted that he would not inject steroids (cortisone) into Ward's knee due to the effects of cortisone on tissue. Instead he hoped that biologics—in this case PRP—would potentially help the MCL heal faster, with no chance for rejection or adverse effects on the ligament.

Years later, and after extensive studies on PRP, Bradley observed that the benefits of the procedure to Ward likely had nothing to do with making the ligament heal faster. He pointed out that PRP has been shown to act as a natural anti-inflammatory and antibiotic. It works on substance P and interleukins 1, 8, and 15, which are chemical mediators in the body involved with pain. Bradley asserted that his use of PRP served to modify Ward's pain response, helping him rehab.[11]

Platelet-rich plasma had been used in other fields of medicine—dentistry, plastic surgery, maxillofacial surgery, and even veterinary medicine—before catching on in orthopaedic surgery.

A surgeon or physician creates PRP by taking the athlete's blood and placing it in a centrifuge. In the first phase of spinning, the plasma and platelets are separated from the red blood cells and white blood cells. The second, faster phase of spinning further concentrates the platelets in the plasma. The physician then injects this PRP into the injured area.

This process concentrates the platelets in PRP to levels between 2.5 and 8.0 times their levels in normal blood. Platelets are the first cells to arrive at the site of injury and are critical in the inflammation that starts the healing process.

Platelets contain growth factors, such as platelet-derived growth factor and transforming growth factor-$\beta 1$. They also contain proteins and other substances that play a role in the tissue-repair process.

One theory behind PRP use, then, centers on tissue healing. Delivering large concentrations of platelets into an area of ligament or tendon injury early in the healing process will potentially help the athlete heal more quickly and reliably and return to play faster.

Hines Ward credited the unproven treatment with helping him return more quickly from injury.

"I was next in line, the next guinea pig," Ward told Alan Schwarz of the *New York Times*. "I think it really helped me. The injury that I had was a severe injury, maybe a four- or six-week injury. In order for me to go out there and play in two weeks, I don't think anyone with a grade-2 M.C.L. sprain gets back that fast."[12]

"I have diagnosed, conservatively treated and operated on several patients who suffered grade 2 MCLS," Dr. Bradley explained. "In my experience, they do not get better in two weeks, much less go onto to perform at an elite level. I'm telling you, it just doesn't happen. Luckily, with adding PRP as part of our treatment regimen for Hines, we got him back to his professional level of play. Looking back, I feel we were forced into trying this option because he was our starting number one receiver. If we lost him, we would have had to change our entire passing scheme for the game and been at a significant disadvantage. It was a big deal that he not only entered back into the game, but played well."[13]

The headline read "A Promising Treatment for Athletes, in Blood." The article, written by Alan Schwarz, appeared on the paper's first page—not of the sports section, but the front page of the *New York Times*.

If Kremer's mention of PRP piqued the curiosity of sports fans, the February 17, 2009, *New York Times* article put it front and center in the minds of orthopaedic surgeons and athletes. In fact, when Kremer saw the article, she knew that her Super Bowl report was big.[14]

Schwarz described the treatment in detail, including its possible uses. He noted the hope of orthopaedic surgeons that PRP could help patients with nagging injuries like tennis elbow and tendinitis of other joints.

"It's a better option for problems that don't have a great solution—it's non-surgical and uses the body's own cells to help it heal," Dr. Allan Mishra, of Stanford University Medical Center, pointed out to Schwarz. "I think it's fair to say that platelet-rich plasma has the potential to revolutionize not just sports medicine but all of orthopedics. It needs a lot more study, but we are obligated to pursue this."[15]

Despite a lack of scientific evidence showing good results for PRP, many surgeons quoted in the article still touted its use as a treatment option before resorting to surgery.

Among the benefits promoted by the experts was the lack of an allergic reaction, since PRP was created using the patient's blood. There was little chance of infection. By avoiding surgery, no surgical incision was made, and no scar developed. Theoretically, the patient recovered much more quickly than he would from surgery.

In his article, Schwarz did point out that PRP was an expensive treatment that largely was not covered by insurance. Treatments at the time were approximately $2,000.

From a cost perspective, PRP might appeal to a patient facing surgery for a musculoskeletal injury. Let's use the example of a 46-year-old golfer who has battled tennis elbow pain for several months. Nonsurgical treatments, including a brace, anti-inflammatory medications, and physical therapy, have not reduced his pain. Now he struggles to play, and it bothers him when he tries to do yard work at home.

Now he wants to proceed with surgery, but first he discusses PRP with his orthopaedic surgeon.

Let's say that the total cost of surgery for lateral epicondylitis (tennis elbow)— surgeon's fee, anesthesia, hospital or surgery center fee, and so forth—comes to roughly $15,000. The golfer might not consider $2,000 dollars for PRP, even if it comes out of his own pocket, unreasonable if it provided a good chance of making surgery unnecessary.

For a professional sports team, this cost-benefit analysis could be even more attractive. In his article, Schwarz pointed out that in the 2008 season, 519 players on the 30 MLB teams spent a collective 28,602 days on the disabled list. When factoring in their lost salaries, teams had $455 million in players' salaries sitting on the bench.

If PRP helped a pro athlete return even a week or two sooner, his team would win big. "Let's say a soccer player is out six weeks—if you can cut a week or two off, that equates to two, three, four games," explained Dr. Michael Gerhardt, the team physician for the Los Angeles Galaxy Major League Soccer team, in the article.[16]

Let's do the math with recent NFL numbers. In 2012 the average NFL player's salary was $1.9 million.[17] If a wide receiver making that salary suffered an injury like Hines Ward's—a grade 2 MCL injury—the team doctor would likely treat him with rest, a brace, and physical therapy. We would expect that injury to heal in roughly four weeks. That's $475,000—$118,750 per week multiplied by four weeks—standing in street clothes on the sidelines.

Now let's assume that the team doctor used PRP as part of the treatment. The team would pay the cost of the treatment—currently $250 to $1,000. If the treatment worked and actually helped his body heal the injury faster, the athlete might return one or two weeks faster. The team would "save" $118,750 or $237,500.

The *New York Times* article's real impact, though, might have been to raise awareness among athletic people outside of professional sports.

"It's not just the professional athlete who needs to get back to their game," Dr. Mishra argued in that article. "Everyone wants to get back to what they do for play or for work."[18]

Alan Schwarz admitted that he hadn't gotten any feedback from readers and was surprised when he learned the impact his article had had. "I honestly received no reaction from readers that I can possibly recall, but they weren't going to contact me about this. They were going to go to their doctors. The doctors were the ones who could actually help."[19]

Kremer recalled the story of a nonathlete asking about PRP soon after the Super Bowl. "This is how it sort of sinks in the American consciousness. My producer, my Sunday Night Football producer, is playing golf. He lives in Connecticut, and he's playing golf on one of these tony golf courses they have up there. And he's on the course, and one of the guys that he's playing with says, 'Hey, I heard about that PRP procedure. Do you think it's any good? Do you think I should get it?'"[20]

For many weekend warriors, Alan Schwarz alerted them to a possible miracle cure. Marathoners, triathletes, and others who love to play sports or exercise religiously deal with nagging aches and pains all the time.

Most of the time these injuries heal with a short period of rest or activity modification. Maybe a few weeks of physical therapy are needed. In most cases, athletes recover from these overuse injuries and return to their regular activities.

Unfortunately, some of these injuries are tough to overcome. Small areas of degeneration within a tendon, like the patellar tendon of the knee or Achilles tendon of the ankle, can cause pain with jumping or running that limits activity.

What do you do if you're in the 5% to 15% of patients who don't get better despite rest or physical therapy? Cortisone injections often don't help, and they can make some injuries worse. For instance, cortisone injected directly into the patellar tendon or Achilles tendon for chronic tendon disorders could actually increase the chance of that tendon rupturing. Surgery doesn't guarantee successful return to sports or exercise either, and it could take months to recover from it.

For athletes with difficult chronic maladies, PRP offered hope.

In her September 4, 2011, *New York Times* article, "As Sports Medicine Surges, Hope and Hype Outpace Proven Treatments," Gina Kolata told the story of Tina Basle. Tina ran marathons until she suffered a hamstring injury. She tried everything: physical therapy, ultrasound, laser therapy, cortisone injections, and even PRP.

Nothing helped, and eventually Tina gave up.

Interviewing many sports medicine orthopaedic surgeons, Kolata described how PRP—like many treatments—is used with little proof that it works. Also, the fact that surgeons use PRP on pro athletes entices other athletic people who have been struggling with injuries to try it as well.

In fact, in the article Dr. John Bergfeld, an orthopaedic surgeon at the Cleveland Clinic, labeled PRP the "Orthopedic triad." Famous athlete. Famous doctor. Untested treatment.[21]

Even before Kolata pointed out that the hype of PRP might have been unjustified, leaders within sports medicine were arguing for a cautious approach to its use.

Bruce Reider, MD, editor of the *American Journal of Sports Medicine*, wrote an editorial in 2009 titled "Proceed with Caution." Reider pointed out that PRP could become an orthopaedic panacea. Surgeons were using the treatment for all kinds of acute and chronic musculoskeletal injuries. Nonhealing fractures, articular cartilage injuries, ligament and tendon tears, chronic tendon degeneration, and osteoarthritis have different characteristics and might not respond to PRP in the same way.

Reider argued that clinicians should base treatment decisions on published data. Surgeons should consider limiting use of PRP to patients in whom the accepted treatments have not worked or might not be expected to work. He urged more surgeons to collect data and perform comparative studies on PRP.[22]

In an editorial, "Sport Science vs. 'Boutique Medicine,'" Edward M. Wojtys,

MD, editor of *Sports Health: A Multidisciplinary Approach*, pointed out the potential ethical dilemmas that PRP and stem cell treatments could present:

> These dilemmas force clinicians to decide on their type of practice and reputation. Are they knowledgeable clinicians who are up-to-date on the science and applicability of emerging technologies and therapies? Will they rely on solid research to make evidence-based decisions and recommendations for their patients? Or, are they willing to use unproven, untested forms of treatment to claim being "on the cutting edge" or for financial gain?[23]

Kolata argued that the examples set by pro athletes like Hines Ward receiving PRP essentially served as testimonials. Patients across the country were requesting the treatments from their orthopaedic surgeons. And many sports medicine surgeons were obliging.

Dr. Edward McDevitt, an orthopaedic surgeon in Arnold, Maryland, shared his experience in the *New York Times* piece: "Patients come in and say, 'I want the same thing that Tiger Woods had.' "I say, 'It really hasn't been proven.' And they say, 'Well, I don't care.'"

In his experience, if patients insisted on receiving PRP and he refused, "They usually say: 'No offense, Doctor. You seem like a nice guy, but I will go to see one of the many, many other doctors who will do it.'"[24]

S. Terry Canale, MD, an orthopaedic surgeon at the Campbell Clinic and former president of the American Academy of Orthopaedic Surgeons, explained to Kolata, "The bottom line is that most think it works. The operative word is 'think.' They don't know if it works. They have a feeling it does."[25]

Many years have passed since Dr. Bradley drew blood from Hines Ward, spun it in a centrifuge, and reinjected it into the receiver's knee. Orthopaedic surgeons now have studies on the use of PRP for a number of orthopaedic conditions.

What have we learned?

Unfortunately, there are no clear answers. The benefits of PRP appear to vary widely depending on what injury or condition is being treated.

Let's start with MCL injuries, like the one Hines Ward suffered in the 2009 AFC Championship game. Bert R. Mandelbaum, MD, and Michael B. Gerhardt, MD, treated 22 professional soccer players with single PRP injections for grade 2 MCL injuries within 72 hours of injury. Compared to a control group of players with similar injuries who were treated with only rest and rehabilitation, players who received PRP returned to play 27% faster.[26]

That study is encouraging for acute knee ligament injuries common in sports, but it is a retrospective study and not a randomized controlled trial in which the researchers assign patients into treatment or control groups, which are thought to provide less biased results. As of this writing, this study has not been published.

As I discuss in the Tommy John chapter, ulnar collateral ligament (UCL) injuries of the elbow are devastating to throwing athletes. Pitchers with complete UCL tears almost always require Tommy John surgery to return to the mound.

Luga Podesta, MD, and others at the Kerlan-Jobe Orthopaedic Clinic used PRP to treat 34 overhead athletes (27 baseball players, 3 softball players, 2 tennis players, and 2 volleyball players) with partial UCL injuries in their elbows. Thirty of the thirty-four athletes (88%) returned to play in an average of 12 weeks.[27]

Mohamad Shariff A. Hamid, MBBS, PhD, and others used PRP to treat hamstring injuries. They took 24 athletes who were determined to have suffered partial tears of the hamstring muscle fibers. Half of the athletes received a PRP injection in addition to progressive agility and trunk stabilization exercises, while the remaining athletes only used the rehabilitation exercises.

The mean time for return to play in the control group was 42.5 days, compared to a mean return to play time of 26.7 days for the athletes who received PRP. This was a short-term study that did not assess the risk of reinjury, which is a common problem with hamstring injuries. Still, the study might indicate that PRP could play a role in treating hamstring injuries in professional athletes.[28]

Two other randomized controlled studies that looked at the use of PRP for acute hamstring injuries had less encouraging results.

Bruce Hamilton and others found no significant benefit for professional athletes who received a single PRP injection over intensive rehabilitation for acute hamstring injuries.[29] Likewise, Reurink and others found no benefit of PRP injected into a hamstring muscle injury compared to placebo injections of saline. The results were not statistically different at two months or one year after injury in terms of return to play or reinjury rate.[30]

Dr. Bradley presented a study at an NFL Physicians Society meeting on his use of PRP in NFL players with hamstring injuries. He found that using the biologic within 24 to 48 hours significantly decreased the number of retears.

"The PRP does not hurt the player. It has only been shown to help," Dr. Bradley argued. "I think orthobiologic treatments are the wave of the future."[31]

As promising as these studies on acute ligament and muscle injuries might be, some critics point out that these are injuries that usually heal with standard treatment options.

Unlike acute injuries, chronic injuries with areas of degeneration within the tendon often afflict weekend warriors and competitive athletes alike. Problems like lateral epicondylitis (tennis elbow), Achilles tendinopathy, patellar tendinopathy, and rotator cuff tendinopathy often resolve for a majority of patients with rest, activity modification, and physical therapy. A small percentage of these patients fail to improve, so PRP has been tried as a treatment in these refractory cases.

For tennis elbow, some studies have shown a benefit with PRP. Allan K. Mishra, MD and others at 12 orthopaedic centers treated 230 patients and randomized them into either PRP or control groups. At 24-week follow-up, patients treated with a single PRP injection had less elbow pain.

Likewise, two studies published by Dr. Mishra compared results of PRP treatment to cortisone injections at one-year and two-year follow-up for patients with lateral epicondylitis. The PRP offered better improvements of pain than the cortisone. In addition, the benefits of PRP appeared to be maintained over time, while the outcomes in patients treated with cortisone slowly declined over time.[32]

On the other hand, in a randomized controlled trial Krogh and other Danish researchers found no benefit of PRP compared to saline injections for lateral epicondylitis after three months.[33]

Other chronic tendon disorders have been proven to be less amenable to PRP treatment.

Comparing PRP to saline for chronic Achilles tendinopathy, de Jonge and others found no difference in clinical outcomes at 24 weeks. That same group found no significant difference between PRP and saline administered in addition to a rehab program for 54 patients followed for one year.[34]

For tendinopathy of the patellar tendon of the knee, PRP has had mixed results. Jason L. Dragoo, MD, and others at Stanford compared patients with patellar tendinopathy randomized to PRP to patients treated with dry needling. The PRP group had improved significantly more than the dry needling group by 12 weeks, but the benefit of PRP slowly dissipated by 26 weeks.[35]

And a Turkish study compared patients with chronic rotator cuff tendinopathy treated with PRP injection into the shoulder to patients treated with saline. The authors of the randomized controlled trial found no improvement in quality of life, disability, pain, and shoulder range of motion in the patients treated with a PRP injection compared to those treated with saline.[36]

So where do these data leave us?

Clearly PRP is not a definitive cure for all of the difficult musculoskeletal problems facing athletes and active individuals. But we need much more research to know exactly where it should fit into our treatment plans.

There is much more we need to learn. When should it be administered after an acute injury, like an MCL injury or hamstring injury? Should it be administered within two to three days for all athletes? Should the physician or orthopaedic surgeon perform a single injection or a series of three or more? Most of these injuries would heal without PRP, so should we wait and use it weeks later on those people who seem to be struggling to heal and return to sports and exercise?

We also need to figure out the exact nature of the PRP treatments being used. Different PRP products (and the bodies of different people) create different numbers of platelets. What is the ideal concentration of platelets that should be administered? Should the white blood cells be removed from the blood or left in the treatment and reinjected into the injury site? Most studies differ in the nature of the PRP preparation, and these differences complicate the results of research studies.

Dr. Bradley and other proponents of PRP and orthobiologics often point out that these studies are misleading. For starters, it is problematic to compare one PRP product or system to another. Each one delivers different concentrations of platelets. For instance, Bradley has observed that in several studies that showed no benefits to PRP, the researchers used such a high number of platelets that they would inherently create a negative feedback.[37]

In addition, patients create different amounts of platelets and growth factors in their bodies. Controlling for all of the different patient variables in a research study would be extremely difficult.

It will be a long time until we have conclusive evidence about the effectiveness of PRP for these different musculoskeletal injuries.

"The problem is, people (patients, doctors, athletes, etc.) keep asking questions and expecting concrete answers about PRP," Dr. Bradley claimed. "Right now, we just don't know all the answers. In order to get the answers, a lot of trials need to be performed, and good investigative research needs to be performed. I think we all have to be patient. I tell that to my players. When will we get all the answers? I don't know, but we are getting there, and we already know a lot more than we did. Relatively speaking, this is still a new and emerging treatment. This reminds me of ACL reconstructions in the knee. We have been doing them for a long time. Yet, there are hundreds of studies that continue to be performed and papers that continue to be written."[38]

Finally, how should orthopaedic surgeons use PRP? Should they use it as a marketing tool to show that they are willing to try the latest, cutting-edge medical treatments? Or should they refuse to use it until conclusive evidence from well-designed, randomized controlled trials exists for the injuries that their patients have?

Surgeons charging large amounts of money to perform the procedure could create problems with both public perception and getting insurance companies to pay for it. If a surgeon's practice buys the kit for $150 from a company like Arthrex and then adds a small amount for nursing costs and supplies like the needles and bandages, then he could charge the patient $200 or so. Instead, many practices charge patients close to $1,000 for the procedure. Not only does that cost discourage many people who must pay for it out of their own pockets, but it likely also dissuades insurance companies from paying for it.

"We should be making this treatment affordable for patients, as well as getting insurance companies to recognize and cover this treatment as potentially saving them on surgical costs, as it has helped several of my patients avoid surgery. I feel insurance companies would see this as revolutionary if they knew its potential," Dr. Bradley argued.[39]

Is a middle ground acceptable, in which orthopaedic surgeons try PRP for patients with chronic injuries, like tennis elbow, who don't seem to be responding to conventional treatments?

Going back to the example of the hypothetical 46-year-old recreational golfer, would it be acceptable to try a largely unproven treatment when nothing else has worked for him? The PRP might not work either, and an orthopaedic surgeon should inform him of that possibility. But it has little risk in terms of side effects. The biggest risk is the cost, as the golfer might spend hundreds of dollars out of his own pocket for a treatment that might not make him better. If it helps him avoid surgery, though, he, like many other people, would likely take that chance.

This experience with PRP—from Hines Ward to the weekend warrior—provides a glimpse of the dilemma orthopaedic surgeons will face as we begin to use another controversial sports medicine treatment.

Stem cells are largely believed to represent the next frontier of musculoskeletal injury healing. How aggressive should orthopaedic surgeons in the United States be in trying stem cells, when little research has been published on using them for various injuries in human patients?

Let's consider these treatments with one of the most common musculoskeletal problems adult athletes and active people face.

Arthritis is one of the most common joint maladies—and one of the most crippling. According to statistics from the Centers for Disease Control and Prevention (CDC), arthritis in all forms currently afflicts about 52.5 million American adults. Arthritis limits the activities of 22.7 million people, or almost 10% of all adults in the United States. It comprises the country's most common cause of disability.

As the population ages and stays active, arthritis will become an even bigger factor in our health. The CDC predicts that 78 million adults will be diagnosed with arthritis by the year 2040. That is over one in every four adults. The CDC also estimates that 44% of adults with arthritis will have limited activity due to arthritis.[40]

The most common form of arthritis is osteoarthritis, currently affecting more than 27 million adults. At some point in their lives, half of all adults will experience symptoms from osteoarthritis of the knee. Of adults with knee OA, 11% require assistance with personal care, and 14% need help with daily activities. Each year, 11.1 million patients make outpatient physician visits for osteoarthritis. The CDC estimated the total societal costs due to arthritis from all causes, including the direct costs of medical care as well as indirect costs such as lost wages, to be approximately $128 billion in 2003. That amount equals 1.2% of the 2003 US gross domestic product.[41]

In simple terms, osteoarthritis results from the breakdown of the articular cartilage of the joint. For example, the femur (thigh bone), tibia (shin bone), and patella (kneecap) are the major bones of the knee. Articular cartilage is the cartilage lining on the ends of these bones that helps them glide over each other for smooth knee motion. When this cartilage breaks down, more stress transfers to the underlying bone. Secondary changes, such as bone spurs and joint space narrowing, slowly develop.

The end result is often bone-on-bone arthritis. Pain often gradually increases as the arthritis progresses until both are so severe that the patient and the surgeon agree to proceed with a knee replacement.

Joint replacement surgeries are increasing rapidly in the United States. Between 1999 and 2008, the US population increased by 11%. The number of total knee arthroplasties performed during that same period skyrocketed 134%.[42] Projections estimate that by 2030, close to 3.5 million total knee replacements will be performed each year in the United States.[43]

According to the American Academy of Orthopaedic Surgeons, orthopaedic surgeons performed more than 645,000 knee replacements in 2011, up from about 321,000 in 2000.[44] They performed more than 306,000 primary hip replacements in 2011, compared to just over 176,000 in 2000.[45] According to data from the National Hospital Discharge Survey, around seven million Americans were living with a hip or knee replacement in place in 2010.[46]

These surgeries aim to replace worn-out bone and cartilage with metal and plastic. Knee replacements are extremely effective for relief of osteoarthritis pain. According to the American Academy of Orthopaedic Surgeons, over 90% of patients who undergo total knee arthroplasty obtain significant pain relief and improvement in the ability to perform activities of daily living. Likewise, greater than 90% of the knee replacements are functioning well 15 years after surgery.[47]

Unfortunately for athletes and athletic individuals, knee replacement is not a reasonable surgical option to allow return to sports. Repetitive impact, such as the running and jumping a professional athlete does, would likely cause the prosthesis to wear out much quicker than in more sedentary patients. It is also very unlikely an athlete would even be able to run as fast or jump as high to compete at an elite level.

If knee and other joint replacements are not feasible options to relieve an athlete's pain and improve function, then what can he or she try?

Imagine a 53-year-old marathon runner who wants to continue to train and compete despite pain from osteoarthritis in her knee.

Current nonoperative treatment options for osteoarthritis would be similar for her as for a high-level athlete. Anti-inflammatory medications could decrease her pain and knee swelling after her runs. Physical therapy could improve the strength around her knee. She might try over-the-counter supplements like glucosamine and chondroitin. Activity modification, such as switching to a lower impact activity like swimming, can be an option but would not satisfy someone trying to compete in endurance races.

Injecting corticosteroids—commonly referred to as cortisone injections—has been a popular treatment for decades. These medications aim to decrease pain for months by decreasing inflammation in the joint. While they can offer pain relief, they do not reverse the cartilage damage. In addition, concerns have existed for many years that injections of these steroids into a joint, especially if done on a repeated basis, could further damage the joint's articular cartilage.

The runner could also try a series of injections called viscosupplementation. There are many of these products, such as Synvisc, Supartz, Hyalgan, and Euflexxa. These injections consist of substances made in the lab to chemically replicate hyaluronic acid, a main component of joint fluid. Research into the efficacy of these injections has failed to show a significant long-term benefit, but many patients claim to get pain relief from them.

Platelet-rich plasma has recently been tried for osteoarthritis of the knee as well. There are not many studies on the use of PRP for knee osteoarthritis. While a few studies have shown a benefit of PRP compared to viscosupplementation or placebo, others have failed to show a significant improvement.[48]

Dr. Bradley uses PRP for early arthritis. "Even if the PRP doesn't work for the patient with early arthritis, you haven't caused further damage or aggressively treated them with steroids which causes further articular cartilage damage. Steroids are a horrible first line of defense against arthritis. That doesn't happen in my office. I start with platelet-rich plasma. That's the first thing we give them before we give them any viscosupplementation or anything else."[49]

Here lies one of the essential problems with osteoarthritis. These nonoperative treatments might provide some degree of pain relief. Unfortunately, none of them actually rebuilds damaged articular cartilage.

What about surgical options? For years orthopaedic surgeons performed arthroscopic debridements of the knee—"cleanup" procedures—as patients often recall their surgeons explaining the operation. Essentially the surgeon uses a shaver to try to smooth out areas where the articular cartilage is frayed or fragmented.

Over the last decade, researchers have shown that these arthroscopic debridements might not work.

In 2002, a landmark study was published in the *New England Journal of Medicine*. J. Bruce Moseley, MD, and others randomly assigned 180 patients with osteoarthritis of the knee into three different treatment groups. One group underwent arthroscopic debridement, in which a surgeon arthroscopically smoothed out damaged cartilage, while another underwent arthroscopic lavage, or surgery to just run fluid through the knee arthroscopically. The third group had placebo surgery, in which the surgeon made skin incisions but did not insert the arthroscope. Both the researchers and the patients were blinded as to which treatment was performed. The patients were studied at multiple points over 24 months using three self-reported pain scores, two reporting function, and one objective test for walking and stair climbing.

At no point in those 24 months did either the arthroscopic debridement group or arthroscopic lavage group report less pain or better function than the placebo surgery group. The authors concluded that arthroscopic surgeries—either debridement or lavage—provided no better outcomes than placebo surgery.[50]

An equally important study, led by Alexandra Kirkley, MD, was published in 2008, also in the *New England Journal of Medicine*. The researchers randomly assigned patients with moderate-to-severe osteoarthritis of the knee into two groups. One group of patients underwent arthroscopic lavage and debridement in conjunction with physical and medical therapy, while the other group received only physical and medical therapy. They assessed each patient's WOMAC score, a self-administered scale assessing pain, stiffness, and physical function from osteoarthritis, administered at regular periods throughout a two-year follow-up period.

Other than a transient improvement at three months after surgery, patients who underwent arthroscopic surgery had no additional improvement compared to the group that received only medical and physical therapy throughout the two-year study period. The authors concluded that for osteoarthritis of the knee, arthroscopic surgery confers no additional benefit to physical and medical therapy.[51]

Going back to the hypothetical 53-year-old marathon runner, imagine her articular cartilage as pavement on a road. Now imagine a pothole in that pavement. If you somehow tried to smooth out the pothole, it might make the edges of the hole smoother, but the hole would still be present. You have not filled in the hole with new pavement.

Despite a lack of long-term success, surgeons still perform these arthroscopic cartilage debridements occasionally, including on elite athletes. In theory, the scope might provide a short period of time—a few months or maybe a year or two—that the athlete can play. After his career is over, he could undergo a more definitive procedure, such as a knee replacement.

Orthopaedic surgeons rarely accept the fact that they cannot fix a problem, even one as seemingly inevitable and invincible as osteoarthritis. They have devised a number of surgeries to attempt to replace or rebuild damaged articular cartilage.

Dr. Richard Steadman first described microfracture surgeries in the late 1980s. These arthroscopic procedures involve the surgeon taking what looks like an ice pick and poking holes in the bone under the damaged articular cartilage. These holes allow the inflow of blood. Theoretically, the blood starts an inflammatory process that ultimately leads to the formation of fibrocartilage.

Even if fibrocartilage does fill the defect, that tissue is not as durable as the hyaline cartilage that makes up the normal articular cartilage surface of the joint. Fibrocartilage is more brittle than hyaline cartilage and breaks down faster. It is better than having no cartilage with exposed bone in an athlete, but it won't last forever.

Despite initial studies showing good results, even in high-level athletes, concerns about microfracture surgeries have increased in recent years. A 2009 study in the *American Journal of Sports Medicine*, performed by Surena Namdari, MD, MMSC, et al., evaluated 24 NBA players who had undergone microfracture surgeries between 1997 and 2006. Eight of twenty-four, or 33.3%, never returned to play in an NBA game. Players who did return played limited minutes in the first season after microfracture surgery. They tended to be less productive in terms of points, rebounds, and assists per game.

The authors concluded that microfracture surgery presents a significant risk for ending an NBA player's career, although it is difficult to conclude whether it is the surgery or the underlying cartilage injury itself that is the critical factor.[52]

Other surgical options are even more invasive. For cartilage damage limited to a small area within the knee, surgeons often try to transfer one or more cylinders of healthy bone and cartilage from a non-weight-bearing location in the knee into the defect. For larger defects, the surgeon possibly could transfer a larger cylinder of bone and cartilage from a donor.

Largely limited to patients with a single focal area of cartilage damage and not diffuse arthritic changes, these procedures have not been used frequently in athletes. In addition, concern about the ability of the transferred bone and cartilage to withstand the repetitive stress of sports is significant.

Attempts to grow new cartilage continue to evolve. Harvesting small samples of healthy articular cartilage and generating chondrocytes—cartilage cell precursors—in the lab offers promise. These chondrocytes can be implanted back into the defect to try to develop more normal hyaline cartilage.

Despite modifications to these surgeries, definitive evidence that surgeons can surgically create new, healthy cartilage just doesn't exist. Articular cartilage does not have a blood supply. The lack of a blood supply is thought by most orthopaedic surgeons to provide the largest obstacle to creating new articular cartilage.

Despite the advances in orthopaedic surgery and sports medicine, we just have not found a cure for arthritis. With athletes placing so much stress on their bones and joints during their careers, it is no wonder that arthritis and debilitating pain and deformity often follow the athletes after they stop playing.

If an orthopaedic surgeon can develop a procedure—a surgery, an oral or injectable medicine, or a substance or cartilage cells injected into a joint—that doesn't just provide pain relief but actually reverses the degenerative process, he or she would have found the Holy Grail of sports medicine.

For all of the benefits sports medicine physicians and surgeons have provided to athletes—longer careers in particular—wear and tear on the cartilage is most often the injury that ends those careers. A procedure or treatment that reverses this damage, or prevents it in the first place, would unquestionably be the greatest accomplishment in the history of sports medicine.

Expect orthopaedic surgeons to increasingly turn to orthobiologics—substances used to treat musculoskeletal injuries and improve healing of bones, muscles, tendons, and ligaments—to treat osteoarthritis and other debilitating musculoskeletal conditions. They are made from substances found within your body. Platelet-rich plasma, stem cells, and even Regenokine—treatments performed by Dr. Peter Wehling for which many famous athletes have traveled to his clinic in Germany—are prominent examples of orthobiologics.

For example, Dr. Bert Mandelbaum, an orthopaedic surgeon in the Santa Monica Orthopedic and Sports Medicine Group, believes that we will soon use these substances on a regular basis to manage arthritis and other injuries.

"Why do we think that you can do an operation one time and correct all the biology when biology is happening every day, all the time? We're going to begin to think of ourselves as temporal interventionists.

"These are going to have a tremendous effect on all our practices. How we think about it and how we further facilitate our operative procedures are going to change."[53]

Dr. Bradley believes that physicians in many other countries are ahead of orthopaedic surgeons in the United States because they have been studying orthobiologics for a longer period of time.

"I know people who get on their planes and have sought their orthobiologic treatments in Russia, Korea, and even the Cayman Islands. Medical tourism is a big thing. However, I don't think that is fair. I think that these treatments need to be available to the general public, right here in the United States. It's not that difficult."[54]

Whether or not the United States and our orthopaedic surgeons are far behind the rest of the world is not the issue as much as how we choose to move forward. Platelet-rich plasma is just the beginning. Orthopaedic surgeons and sports medicine doctors will have to decide what role experimental treatments such as PRP and stem cells play in the care of athletes—not just professional athletes, but people who just want to run, lift weights, and play recreational sports.

The use of orthobiologics could be viewed through the lens of the popular social science diffusion of innovation theory. Developed by E. M. Rogers, this theory aims to explain how an idea or product—in this case PRP—spreads through a specific population, in this case sports medicine physicians and orthopaedic surgeons. It categorizes people based on how and when a person adopts an innovation.

There are innovators who want to be the first to try the new product. Next, the early adopters embrace change and new opportunities. Then the early majority adopt the new idea but usually after they see evidence that the product works. The late majority only adopt the innovation after a majority of the population has made the change. And finally, the laggards are extremely resistant to change. Most of a population falls into the early or late majority.[55]

Dr. Bert Mandelbaum feels that the use of PRP and other orthobiologics fits this continuum, and we are somewhere between the early adopters and early majority when it comes to orthopaedic surgeons in the United States using it. "We need to continue to shift that pendulum. Continue to educate, motivate, inspire our population with different platforms to do that," Mandelbaum advised. "I personally believe that with our orthobiologic approach, we're just getting to the tip of the iceberg."[56]

Dr. Bradley pointed to resistance to the use of the arthroscope, discussed in the chapter on Joan Benoit, as an obstacle. "Remember when [legendary shoulder surgeon] Charlie Rockwood said that the arthroscope was the work of the devil? That was his direct quote. Today, I would say that the arthroscope is invaluable. Many physicians feel the same way as Rockwood about biologics. To that I say, wait and see."[57]

In the coming years, orthopaedic surgeons and sports medicine physicians might use different orthobiologic products for different injuries. For example, if a patient has a chronic tendon disorder like patellar tendinosis or lateral epicondylitis, we might use a system that augments and delivers certain cells like monocytes in order to intentionally increase the inflammatory response to help the tendon heal.

"With steroids I feel like we are napalming the knee and destroying viable cartilage prematurely. I feel that with PRP we are in a sense nourishing the knee and creating a better environment. In three or four years from now, or five years, we're going to be able to pinpoint, with laser-like accuracy, the exact platelet number and how many white cells would provide the most effective treatments. We will also be able to develop more specific protocols and evidence-based guidance on how to use orthobiologics," Bradley predicted.

"Orthobiologics has got to run its course. The right respected professionals, hopefully, will get involved. They will realize that they don't need to charge exorbitant prices for the science. We'll find out what's good and what's not good. Obviously, with all the research, we will learn there are going to be some things about biologics you shouldn't do. But we will also learn that there are going to be some things that are really, really good."[58]

4 / PHILLIP HUGHES
Use of Protective Equipment in Sports

November 27, 2014

Professional cricketer Phillip Hughes was batting for South Australia in the Sheffield Shield match against New South Wales in Sydney. He was 63 not out when bowler Sean Abbott delivered a bouncer. Hughes swiveled his body to try to hook the ball but missed it. The ball slammed into the back of his head.

Hughes, wearing a helmet, collapsed on the field.

Hughes was resuscitated on the field, taken to St. Vincent's Hospital, and placed in a medically induced coma. Despite two operations in which surgeons removed parts of his skull to relieve pressure on his brain, Hughes never regained consciousness.

Australian team doctor Peter Brukner told the media that the impact of the bouncer, a quick, rising ball, caused a vertebral artery dissection when it hit the left side of Hughes's neck. The arterial injury then caused massive bleeding in his brain.[1]

Immediately after Hughes hit the ground, officials stopped the match. The scoreboard read, "PJ Hughes retired hurt 63."[2] He died two days later.

James Sutherland, chief of Cricket Australia, told BBC Sport, "It's a freak incident, but one freak incident is too many."[3]

Cricket is an inherently dangerous game.

A bowler hurls a ball weighing less than six ounces at a batsman only 20 meters away at speeds that often exceed 145 km/h (90 mph). Add to that speed the fact that the ball is covered in hard leather. A bowler can also throw at the batsman's head and body in an effort to intimidate him. Not surprisingly, serious injuries can occur.

Like many cricket supporters do, Dr. Brukner argued that danger is part of the sport of cricket and possibly one reason fans love it. "I think the fans love to see a great fast ball or a bowler against a great batsman. There are real battles, and I think that is certainly a component of what crowds enjoy, there's no doubt about that. The intimidating fast ball, it's a great part of the game."[4]

Likewise, *Game Theory*, a sports blog of *The Economist*, observed that while the danger is real, the sport must carefully balance the risk. "Yet part of the visceral attraction of the game comes from the knowledge that a batsman is facing down real danger. Watching a battle between a snarling fast-bowler and a fearless batsman at close quarters is one of the finest spectacles in sport precisely because of this tension. It is what makes them heroes to many. Cricket needs to be dangerous; it just should never be deadly. That is a fine line to walk."[5]

Shortly after Hughes passed away, questions about cricket safety focused on the mechanism of injury: bouncers. A bouncer is a fast ball delivered in such a way that it lands on the ground short of the batsman and rises up to the level of the batsman's waist or head. It is often used to drive a batsman back. A bouncer might confuse him as to whether to come forward or step back. A bowler might use bouncers to intimidate a batsman, many critics believe.

Bouncers have been a key tactic in cricket since the 1930s. In 1933 English bowlers repeatedly hurled short, fast balls directly at the bodies of Australian batsmen, inciting anger between the teams and diplomatic tension between the countries.

The current law with respect to bouncers does not forbid them but restricts the frequency with which bowlers can use them. "The bowling of fast short pitched balls is dangerous and unfair if the bowler's end umpire considers that by their repetition and taking into account their length, height and direction they are likely to inflict physical injury on the striker irrespective of the protective equipment he may be wearing."[6]

Currently the International Cricket Council limits bowlers to using bouncers for one of every six balls.

The law also allows umpires to take the skill of the batsman into account. In an interview with *Time* magazine, the head coach of Australia's Darren Lehmann Cricket Academy, Shaun Seigert, argued that the short ball should not be restricted at the youth levels. Essentially he believes that if young cricketers have no experience with short bowling, they might have difficulty facing it at the professional level.[7]

In professional cricket, bouncers are still commonly used as an intimidation strategy, especially against proficient batsmen like Hughes.

Proponents of bouncers argue that eliminating them from cricket entirely would not eliminate the risk of physical injury. A ball can fly off the top edge of the bat if the batsman mistimes his attempt to hook the ball, much like a foul tip in baseball. Many point out that these events can cause almost as many injuries as direct impacts to the batsmen.

Jason Gillespie, a former Australia fast bowler, told BBC Sport that Hughes's death should have little effect on the use of bouncers. "The bouncer will continue—it is part of cricket. I can't see a rule change about bowling short balls."[8]

"It's such an integral part of the sport," Dr. Brukner observed. "It'd be like saying you can't throw a knuckleball or curveball. It's a very basic part of bowling."[9]

Even if a bowler doesn't intend to hurt a batsman with a bouncer, a direct blow can cause a serious, albeit rare, injury. So if cricket officials want to leave bouncers as a key part of the game, then attention should be focused on the best way to protect the batsmen against the risk of injury.

That form of protection is seemingly straightforward: the helmet.

Manufacturers of sports helmets aim to design them to attenuate the energy from impact and distribute those forces. Given that 44.4% of children's injuries resulting from cricket and 16.6% of those in adults that presented to Australian emergency departments between 1989 and 1993 were head injuries,[10] helmet use is worth reviewing.

Considering the long history of the sport, however, the use of helmets is a relatively new practice. Many historians point to English batsman Dennis Amiss as the first cricketer to wear a helmet, in the 1978 World Series Cricket Tournament. In their early use, the helmets largely resembled motorcycle helmets.[11]

Modern helmets consist of a shell and a detached face guard, usually in the form of a grill. Usually only players at three positions wear helmets in cricket. The batsmen wear them. The wicketkeepers, who are roughly equivalent to the catchers in baseball, usually wear them as well. Balls can pop up and strike them in the face or head. Finally, "short legs," or fieldsmen near the batsmen, often wear them because they can be struck by balls hit hard directly at them.

In 2013 Craig Ranson and others published an analysis of batting head injuries in professional cricket. They analyzed video clips of 35 national- or international-level batters who were injured after being struck with the ball on the helmet, face, head, or neck while wearing a helmet.

They observed that 97% of the injuries resulted from direct impacts, as the ball struck the helmet or head without first hitting the batsman or bat. Interestingly, 10 of the 35 injuries (28%) resulted from the ball penetrating the gap between the peak of the helmet and the grill, or faceguard. Newer helmet designs have aimed to correct that problem.

Two of the thirty-five head injuries (6%) resulted from the impact of the ball at the occiput, or back of the head, and neck of the batsman with no helmet contact, as had happened to Philip Hughes.

The authors concluded that these incidents prove that cricket helmets, as designed currently, do not completely protect against head and neck injuries.[12]

It is possible that batsmen started taking more impacts to the head after the adoption of helmets than they did when they weren't wearing helmets. Part of that increase could be related to a change in how cricket is played.

In shorter formats, a batsman might try to score runs on every ball. In test cricket, on the other hand, a batsman would probably just duck out of the way the majority of the times a ball was bowled toward his head.

The combination of the different formats and the perceived protection that batsmen might feel from wearing helmets could account for the increase in batsmen being hit in the head today.

Perhaps ironically, some cricket experts feel that helmets might increase the chance of injury. Basically, wearing a helmet leads to more risk-taking behavior by the batsmen.

The helmet could eliminate the fear a batsman would feel when facing one of these fast bouncers. Instead of ducking or turning out of the way, the batsman might stay in harm's way and try to hook or pull the short ball.

Angus Porter, the Professional Cricketers Association chief, seemed to share that belief in comments he made to the *New York Times*: "We wouldn't want anyone wearing a helmet designed to the new standards to think that they were invulnerable. A cricket ball is a hard and potentially dangerous object, whatever protection you are wearing."[13]

Philip Hughes, whether he felt invincible or not, did try to play the bouncer rather than get out of its way.

If batsmen are susceptible to head, face, and neck injuries despite wearing cricket helmets, are athletes in a similar sport who wear helmets significantly thicker than cricket helmets better protected?

Let's look at batters in baseball.

September 11, 2014

In the fifth inning of a late season game at Miller Park, Miami Marlins slugger Giancarlo Stanton took a first-pitch fastball at his knees from Milwaukee Brewers pitcher Mike Fiers.

Stanton entered the game leading the major leagues with 105 RBIS. His 37 home runs led the National League. Clearly he was one of the most feared hitters in baseball.

Brewers catcher Jonathan Lucroy set up on the inside of the plate, and Fiers threw another fastball, one that traveled at 88 mph. Perhaps the overhand delivery Fiers uses, which hides the ball as he releases it, kept Stanton from realizing the pitch's continued upward and inward movement. Stanton began his swing before the ball struck him in the side of the face.

The umpire ruled Stanton swung at the pitch, making the count 0–2.

Stanton lay motionless on the ground as blood began to pool in the infield dirt. Athletic trainers for both teams rushed to his aid, placing him on a backboard. Fiers stood on the mound and watched with his hands on his head as fans watched the scene in silence. Stanton was transferred onto a stretcher and placed in an ambulance.[14]

Giancarlo Stanton's father witnessed his son taking the fastball to the face and traveled with him to the hospital.[15]

The Marlins ended up losing the game 4–2. They lost their MVP candidate for the rest of the season. X-rays and a computed tomography (CT) scan revealed that Stanton suffered multiple facial fractures and dental damage.

In an observation about Stanton's injury that is eerily similar to those about Hughes's injury, Lucroy admitted the incident was frightening, but Fiers was not trying to hurt the slugger. "[Fiers] gets a lot of [strikeouts] on fastballs up, and the ball just got away from him. You saw what happened. It was definitely a scary moment. You never wish that on anybody. It's just a freak accident."[16]

Dr. Gary Green, the medical director of MLB, acknowledged that these are low-frequency events. With roughly 750,000 pitches thrown each year in the major leagues, batters suffer only one or two serious head or face injuries each year.

He pointed out that MLB has upgraded the batters' helmets in recent years. The Rawlings S100 is now rated up to 100 mph. Few pitches exceed that speed.

"We wanted to make sure that they had full protection in terms of the head," Dr. Green asserted. "Now that doesn't mean that if you get hit in the head with a ball, you won't get a concussion. It just means you won't fracture your skull, get an epidural hematoma and die."[17]

He noted that batters can wear facial protection that extends from the helmet down to and around the jaw. The facial guard offers good protection, though some batters might complain that it impedes their ability to see the ball.

In the days after Stanton hit the ground in Milwaukee, critics began calling for equipment changes to prevent these types of injuries. Baseball writer Buster Olney of ESPN argued it was time to adopt helmets with facial protection:

> In the name of player safety, can more be done to protect hitters?
>
> The answer, without question, is yes.
>
> We know this because already we see players in Little League and softball and in cricket wear helmets that also include facial protection. . . .
>
> Face flaps for helmets are like safety belts in cars in the '70s—they are available, they could prevent serious injury, and as [Jason] Heyward and others have demonstrated, there is really no downside to wearing one, just as there was no strong counterargument to wearing a helmet, beyond personal comfort.[18]

The personal comfort argument has been used in baseball for decades. Basically players have played for years wearing only the traditional batting helmet, and they have become accustomed to playing that way. Not only would switching to helmets with added facial protection impair batters' comfort, but it could theoretically affect their performance.

If many batters would resist these modified helmets, though, the players throwing the pitches might resist them even more.

September 5, 2012

Almost exactly two years before Stanton's scary injury, a pitcher suffered one that was life threatening.

In the fourth inning of an afternoon game against the Los Angeles Angels, Oakland A's pitcher Brandon McCarthy hit the ground after taking a line drive off the bat of shortstop Erick Aybar. He sat on the mound, feeling his head, before he walked off the field. Medical personnel transported him to Alta Bates Summit Medical Center.

There, a CT scan proved how serious the 29-year-old pitcher's injuries were. McCarthy had suffered a skull fracture, an epidural hemorrhage, and a brain contusion. He was transferred that night to another Bay Area hospital, where he underwent a two-hour surgery to evacuate the blood and stabilize the fracture.[19]

A follow-up CT scan the next day reportedly showed the hematoma had resolved. Although he remained in the hospital critical care unit, the right-handed pitcher was in stable condition.[20]

Just over two months after fighting for his life, McCarthy completed an intensive rehab program before he was cleared to return to baseball. Dr. Michael Collins administered tests to the pitcher and determined he had returned to his baseline levels.[21] McCarthy signed a two-year contract with the Arizona Diamondbacks worth $15.5 million.

In June the following year, McCarthy suffered a seizure that doctors felt was related to his head injury.

McCarthy's head injury brought out calls for equipment changes, much like Stanton's injury would two years later. In 2007 a death in baseball did, in fact, lead to helmet use. It wasn't a player who died, though.

July 22, 2007

Mike Coolbaugh was still in his first month as a coach with the Tulsa Drillers, the Double A affiliate of the Colorado Rockies. His wife Amanda said that Mike took the job because his two sons—five-year-old Joseph and three-year-old Jacob—loved seeing their dad on the field.

Coolbaugh stood in the first base coach's box for the Drillers as they took on the Arkansas Travelers. In the ninth inning, with no outs and a Drillers player on first base, Tino Sanchez hit a foul ball that struck Coolbaugh in the head.

The Drillers coach was knocked unconscious. Medical personnel administered CPR on the field. An ambulance took him to Baptist Medical Center–North Little Rock Hospital, but Coolbaugh stopped breathing as he arrived.

Doctors pronounced Coolbaugh dead at 9:47 p.m. He was 35 years old. His wife Amanda was 32. She was pregnant with their third child.

Like cricket officials did after Philip Hughes's injury, Texas League officials suspended the game after Coolbaugh went down. Arkansas was awarded a 7–3 victory the following day.[22]

Amanda gave birth to the child—a daughter she named Anne Michael—in November. Only a day before her birth, MLB general managers voted to adopt head protection for first- and third-base coaches for the following season.[23]

The only MLB player killed during a game by a ball was Cleveland Indians shortstop Ray Chapman, who was hit and killed by a pitch in 1920. Many batters started wearing helmets after his death, although the conventional batting helmets were not mandated until 1971. Major League Baseball acted much faster for coaches after Coolbaugh's death.

Dr. Green insisted that implementing batting helmets for base coaches is important, despite coaches occasionally complaining about them on hot days. Base coaches are often focused on the batter, the pitcher, or the base runners, so they aren't always looking at the plate. They are often extremely vulnerable to a line drive off the hitter's bat.[24]

Despite the change for coaches, no change has resulted for pitchers, even after McCarthy's skull fracture and the injuries of several other pitchers, including Toronto Blue Jays pitcher J. A. Happ.

The logic was curious. Coolbaugh stood in the first base coach's box, roughly 90 feet from home plate, farther from home plate than the 55 feet the pitcher's mound is. Why then would baseball mandate helmets for base coaches and not pitchers?

Serious injuries to the head and face of the pitcher are rare—Dr. Green indicated that they occur roughly once or twice per season[25]—but they do occur, as Brandon McCarthy experienced.

McCarthy wanted some sort of protective headgear before he returned to pitch the following season. Major League Baseball determined that the average line drive comes back to the pitcher at roughly 85 mph, Dr. Green noted. The league worked with companies to develop products that could withstand impacts from balls traveling up to 85 mph.[26]

Major League Baseball would allow a pitcher to wear a helmet or padded cap if he chose to do so even though the league had not officially approved one.

In January 2014 MLB approved a protective cap for pitchers. IsoBLOX, a subsidiary of 4 Licensing Corporation, created the cap, which weighs seven ounces more than traditional baseball caps and is much thicker on the front and over half an inch thicker on the sides than normal caps. The isoBLOX caps have protective plates beneath the fabric made of plastic polymers arranged in hexagons, designed to absorb and disperse energy from the impact of a high-speed baseball.

McCarthy felt that the cap was an improvement but still not appropriate for major league pitchers. For one thing, the size and weight of the cap were such that a pitcher would overly notice it, possibly affecting his performance. In addition, the caps were hot.[27]

Even before the isoBLOX caps were approved, McCarthy had experimented with cricket helmets and found them encouraging compared to caps or helmets with hard shells, like those worn by base coaches after Coolbaugh's death.

"I purchased a couple of cricket helmets on my own to see if I could make something out of it, if it was something that worked," McCarthy told William Weinbaum of *Outside the Lines*. "I actually feel like even with the face mask and all, I could get used to that quicker than I could with a half-shell [hard] helmet [like first- and third-base coaches and some catchers wear]."[28]

Dr. Green noted that MLB has been working with companies to develop materials for caps that are lightweight and yet resist significant impact. The goal is to find a material that pitchers would find appealing to wear.[29]

There is one way in which a helmet similar to those used in cricket would prove superior to a padded cap. Many of the impacts pitchers have suffered in recent years—including McCarthy's—occurred below the level of a cap. Even if a padded cap minimized impact to a pitcher's skull, it would do little to protect the facial and orbital bones or the temple region, where a fracture could tear the middle meningeal blood vessels, possibly leading to an epidural hematoma.

A protective cap would not have aided Brandon McCarthy, because the ball struck him below the cap line.

The National Operating Committee on Standards for Athletic Equipment (NOCSAE) researches protective equipment in sports and develops performance standards for football helmets and face masks, baseball and softball batting helmets, lacrosse helmets and face masks, and baseballs and softballs.

Mike Oliver, the executive director of NOCSAE, argued that a player in the field has just as high a risk of injury as a batter. The ball usually comes off the bat faster than the pitcher delivers it. Therefore, the head protection should be equally robust as the batter's helmet.

With facial protection for pitchers and fielders, though, the face mask would have to be attached to something rigid, like a helmet, and not simply a soft cap. The NOCSAE does have a standard for a face guard, although no baseball organization requires equipment that meets that standard.

That facial protection would be different than a face mask on a football helmet, for instance. The equipment that would meet the NOCSAE standard would be what Oliver called "one-hit equipment." Basically, in order to keep it light, the face guard would deform on impact. If a pitcher gets hit in the face, the mask breaks or permanently bends, and he must then get a new one.[30]

Dr. Green shared the concern that it could be difficult to secure a face mask. If a company created a face mask that required a chinstrap, like a football helmet uses, it could interfere with a pitcher's head motion and vision.[31]

Major League Baseball allows pitchers to wear a padded cap. Alex Torres, formally with the Tampa Bay Rays, San Diego Padres, and New York Mets and now pitching in triple-A, decided to wear the isoBLOX cap after witnessing teammate Alex Cobb get struck in the head. Many teammates and members of the media poked fun at the pitcher for the cap's unusual appearance, Dr. Green recalled, but Torres still wore it.[32]

Brandon McCarthy might still have suffered a skull fracture and an epidural hemorrhage even if he had been wearing a padded cap. The ball would have struck him on an exposed part of his head.

The same scenario played out with Phillip Hughes.

Hughes swiveled his body to play the hook on a short ball. He missed it, and when the ball reached him, his head spun far enough that the ball hit an area on the back of his head and neck. Despite wearing a cricket helmet, the ball struck him in a vulnerable location, tearing the vertebral artery and causing the fatal bleeding.

Theoretically it would be possible to cover this area, either by extending the shell or adding a thick rubber pad. Protecting the back of the head and neck, though, would likely restrict a batsman's ability to rotate the head and neck. An additional foam piece that secures to the helmet is available commercially, and some cricket players wear them.

Just as baseball pitchers might resist the idea of wearing a helmet or padding that alters their vision, balance, or comfort even slightly, cricket batsmen would probably reject more protective—but also more restrictive—helmets, even if they prevent the rarest of the catastrophic injuries.

It could be possible that companies will continue to develop helmets and facial protection that are as strong as possible. In any sport with hard objects flying through the air, we might not be able to prevent every event. A freak accident might occur no matter how protective the equipment.

Such "freak accidents" are tragic in baseball, but they do occur.

Barry P. Boden, MD, and others reviewed the data recorded by the National

Center for Catastrophic Sports Injury Research on catastrophic injuries in high school and college baseball that occurred between 1989 and 2012. These included both fatal and nonfatal injuries as well as serious injuries, such as fractures of the cervical vertebrae, that didn't result in permanent disability.

Over the 21-year period, 41 catastrophic injuries occurred in high school and college baseball, or 1.95 catastrophic injuries per year. Given that roughly 8.975 million high school athletes and 467,000 college athletes played baseball during that period, the incidence of these direct catastrophic injuries proved to be 0.43 per 100,000 participants. There were 0.11 fatalities per 100,000 baseball players.[33]

These might be "freak accidents," but again, they do occur.

While collisions between two players proved to be the most common mechanism of injury for these catastrophic injuries, injuries caused by impact from the baseball were common as well. Some 34% of the catastrophic injuries resulted from a pitcher being struck by a batted ball. All of these injuries were head injuries and/or facial fractures.

Just under 10% of the injuries involved athletes, either base runners or infielders, struck by a thrown ball, and 7.3% of the injuries resulted from nonpitching players—fielders and baserunners—being hit by a batted ball. Two of the forty-one catastrophic high school and college baseball injuries, or 4.8%, occurred when a pitch struck a batter.

One injury might truly be considered a "freak accident." A pitcher was hit in the neck with a part of the wooden bat that broke after the batter's contact with the ball. The broken bat caused a tracheal injury, but a physician at the game provided airway support until the player was taken to the hospital. He underwent a tracheostomy that saved his life.[34]

In 2008 Christy L. Collins, MA, and R. Dawn Comstock, PhD, published data on injuries in high school baseball over a three-year period from 2005 to 2007. They observed that 11.6% of all high school baseball injuries, regardless of severity, resulted from a player being hit by a batted ball. Of these impact injuries, 48% affected the head and face, and 16% affected the mouth and teeth.

Interestingly, almost one-quarter (23.2%) of pitching injuries and over one-quarter (26.6%) of fielding injuries at the high school level were caused by players being hit with a batted ball.

Fortunately, over half of these injuries were minor and led to the affected athletes missing less than one week of baseball. But 12% of these injuries did cause a player to miss the remainder of the season.

On the basis of these findings, Collins and Comstock recommended that all baseball players at risk of head and face injuries, including pitchers, infielders, and batters, resulting from impacts from a batted ball wear helmets with face shields. At a minimum, these players should wear mouthguards and eye protection.[35]

A 2012 policy statement by the American Academy of Pediatrics' Council on Sports Medicine and Fitness addressed some of these concerns for baseball players between the ages of 5 and 18. The AAP calls for hitters to wear approved batting helmets with face protection. Given these injury risks, pitchers and infielders should strongly consider head and facial protection.[36]

While helmets and face shields can certainly decrease the risk of head and face injuries in baseball, it is worth pointing out one area where protective equipment has not been shown to prevent catastrophic injuries from projectiles in sports.

December 6, 2010

Thomas Adams stood behind home plate in the Blessed Sacrament school gym in Paterson, New Jersey. He played catcher during an evening practice with the Braves, his Professional Baseball Instruction League travel team. The Garfield High School sophomore missed a pitch that slammed into his chest protector.

The 16-year-old stood up and said "I can't breathe" before he collapsed. Paramedics rushed him to St. Joseph's Regional Medical Center. Adams was in cardiac arrest, and he was pronounced dead later that night.

The teen's father had dropped his son off for practice only minutes before he rushed to the hospital. "I go in the hospital, all these doctors are trying to pump him back to life. I just sat there in shock," Mr. Adams told CBS. "I mean how could this be? Thirty minutes ago he was alive and the weird thing is he had all the protection so it's . . . there's no line to the reason."[37]

Adams most likely suffered commotio cordis. This is a blunt, nonpenetrating traumatic force to the chest that causes an irregular heart rhythm. Commotio cordis often causes sudden cardiac death.

Over half of the reported cases of commotio cordis have occurred in sports. While youth baseball is most often associated with these tragic events, they can occur in any sport with projectiles traveling through the air. Hockey pucks, softballs, and soccer balls have caused these events. The occurrence of commotio cordis events is influenced by the exact time of impact during the athlete's cardiac cycle, a direct impact over his heart, and the speed and hardness of the projectile.

A registry to collect data on commotio cordis events was started in 1998. Since then 230 deaths have been attributed to commotio cordis, but that number might underestimate its true incidence. Barry J. Maron, MD, a cardiologist at the Minneapolis Heart Institute Foundation who oversees the registry, explained, "We know it's underreported because there is no mandatory reporting. We just don't know how much."[38]

Doctors can only diagnose commotio cordis after all other causes have been ruled out, but it's estimated to account for approximate 20% of sudden cardiac deaths in young athletes. It is second only to hypertrophic cardiomyopathy as a cause of sudden cardiac death in this population. Almost half of these events occurred during competitive sports.

While any sport with projectiles flying at high speeds can present a risk for commotio cordis, it is most often seen in youth baseball. Surprisingly, the baseball does not have to be traveling at top speeds to cause such an event. Pitches between 30 and 50 mph caused 25% of cases.[39]

Dr. Jordan Metzl, a primary care sports medicine physician at the Hospital for Special Surgery in New York City and author of *The Athlete's Book of Home Remedies*, observed that commotio cordis events depend largely on where on the chest the blow hits. It can occur in any sport with a fast projectile that hits a young athlete between beats at the wrong point over the heart.

Generally, more cases of commotio cordis have been reported in boys. The discrepancy might result from more boys than girls playing baseball and lacrosse, the sports most often associated with commotio cordis in the United States.[40]

Tragically, commotio cordis events are fatal in up to 90% of cases. The early use of an automated external defibrillator has been shown to improve chances for survival. When this resuscitation began within three minutes of impact, 25% of the patients survived. Only 3% survived if the resuscitation began after three minutes, according to studies by Link and Maron.[41]

Children and adolescents may be vulnerable to commotio cordis trauma because their chest walls are more pliable, and therefore susceptible, to compression forces to the chest wall.

According to witnesses of the event, Thomas Adams was wearing a chest protector.

Much of the research that has been done on commotio cordis has been funded by NOCSAE. The organization found that most of the kids who have died from a commotio cordis event were wearing chest protectors, even robust ones.

Doerer and others evaluated 85 commotio cordis cases that occurred during competitive sports. Thirty-two of the victims were wearing chest protectors. About one-quarter of the players were hit directly on the chest protector, while

78% were hit in an area not covered by the protective device. Moving the arms could have adjusted the device so that the ball struck an uncovered area over the heart.[42]

"It's not the amount of padding. It's how it manages the energy," Oliver noted. This is one of the factors NOCSAE is studying to try to develop an equipment standard for commotio cordis.[43]

"The only thing that seems to make a difference in the literature is probably the hardness of the ball," Dr. Metzl remarked. "Using a little bit of a softer ball in Little League probably makes sense for this and for some of the face injuries too."[44] The US Consumer Product Safety Commission also recommends these softer "safety" baseballs.

Despite the disappointing data on chest protectors preventing commotio cordis, the AAP still recommends their use by young catchers, but not for baseball players at other positions.

As with blows to the head or the back of the neck, like what killed Philip Hughes, the chest of a cricket player is vulnerable to commotio cordis, Dr. Brukner noted.[45] Fortunately, these events are rare in the sport.

Dr. Metzl agreed that these events, whatever the sport, are tragic.

"When it happens, it's such a shock because these are totally healthy kids who are out doing something that's supposed to be very healthy—playing baseball. One second they're totally healthy, and then 15 minutes later, they're dead."[46]

Clearly these events are tragedies. Helmets, especially those that protect the face, will prevent a large percentage of them in cricket and baseball. Padded caps might provide more protection than the traditional caps in baseball, but helmets or caps with protection that extends lower over the face and temple regions would certainly be safer.

The further the protective surface extends over the face or over the neck and back of the head, the more pitchers and batters in baseball and batsmen in cricket will likely resist using them. Even if professional organizations recommend specific helmets, it could prove very difficult to require players to wear them.

It might be better to approach changes to protective headgear by implementing them at the youth levels. In 1979 the National Hockey League (NHL) mandated the use of helmets in ice hockey, but allowed players already in the league to sign a waiver to play without a helmet. Sports and leagues could utilize a similar "grandfather" system to implement equipment use at the high school and college levels while allowing pros to opt out.

If baseball mandated helmets with or without facial protection for pitchers, or facial protection for batters, doing so at the youth level might be most effective. Major league batters eventually grew accustomed to helmets with ear flaps. If young players had to wear this equipment from the beginning of their playing days, they would be familiar with it in the pros.

When cricket adopted newer helmets, many players were reluctant to change, but they gradually accepted them.

"It's like wearing seat belts," Dr. Green claimed. "You wouldn't get in your car without it now. It just feels like part of your driving. The same thing with this, it's going to eventually feel like that's going to just be part of pitching, but it's going to take a while."[47]

Kids at young ages have not grown accustomed to traditional gear, so they could get used to helmets with face protection as youth pitchers or infielders. Young batters might learn to play with batting helmets with face shields, or helmets like those in cricket, if they used them from the start.

One strategy other than additional equipment might eliminate some of these head and facial injuries to pitchers. Parents and coaches should teach young pitchers to finish their follow-through facing the plate with the glove up. Dr. Green cited Greg Maddux as an example of this ideal technique.

Not only could a pitcher then see the ball coming screaming off the bat right at him, but his glove would be in position to protect him. Not only might he be safer, but he might become a better fielder. After all, Greg Maddux won 18 Gold Gloves.

Shortly after the death of Phillip Hughes, Australian national cricket team captain Michael Clarke announced that Hughes's Australian cricket shirt number 64 would be retired immediately.

"The world lost one of its great blokes this week and we are all poorer for it. Our promise to the Hughes family is that we will do everything we can to honour his memory," Clarke tearfully expressed in his speech.[48]

Hughes died 144 years after the last professional cricketer, George Summers, suffered a similar fate from a ball hitting him in the head. The bowler who hit Summers, John Platts, never bowled fast again.

Sean Abbott, who bowled the bouncer that tragically hit and killed Phillip Hughes, attended Hughes's funeral. Weeks later, he bowled for New South Wales against Queensland at the fateful Sydney Cricket Ground.

Abbott's fifth ball was a bouncer.[49]

5 / *MARC BUONICONTI*

Catastrophic Injuries in Football

"Marc has a great instinct going for the ball, and it's natural. He gets to the hole in a hurry. I think sometimes he gets to the hole so quick that he can't set up for the tackle."[1] Former All-Pro and Hall of Fame linebacker Nick Buoniconti spoke those words about his son Marc, an inside linebacker at The Citadel, in 1983. Those seemingly innocuous words foreshadowed a tragic event that would befall his son about two years later.

October 26, 1985

The Citadel had traveled to Johnson City, Tennessee, to take on East Tennessee State. In the second quarter, with the Citadel leading 7 -0, East Tennessee State running back Herman Jacobs took the ball on third down before being flipped in the air by a defender. "The next thing I know, the guy was flying in the air," Marc Buoniconti described to a reporter 25 years later. "I could see him doing a cartwheel with his head on the ground and his feet in the air, the number 20 jersey in the air."[2]

Later in the game, Marc Buoniconti suffered what would be a life-changing injury. Less than one year later, he described the event to Linda Marx of *People* magazine: he ran to his left as Herman Jacobs tried to get the one yard needed for the first down. Another player hit Jacobs as he dove. Buoniconti hit him on the side of his hip, describing it as a tackle he had made millions of times before.

Then he rolled on the ground, totally limp. Buoniconti knew instantly he had broken his neck. He lay on the ground for what felt like an eternity. He couldn't feel any pain, but he struggled to breathe. He couldn't talk or make any sounds.

Citadel athletic trainer Andy Clawson rushed to Buoniconti and instantly realized what was happening. Buoniconti recalled that Clawson's eyes were "as big as golf balls," as the player's legs were floppy and twisted.

People surrounded the fallen player as athletic trainers took off his helmet and cut off his uniform and shoulder pads. An ambulance arrived a half hour later. Strapped to a stretcher with sandbags on both sides of his head, Buoniconti fought to keep breathing during the 15-minute ride to a local hospital.

When he arrived in the emergency room, doctors put a tube down his throat and connected him to a ventilator.

Marc Buoniconti was paralyzed, completely dependent on that machine to keep him alive.[3]

A catastrophic cervical spine injury, by definition, is a structural disruption of the cervical spinal column that can damage the spinal cord. Over 25 years later, Buoniconti remains a quadriplegic from the catastrophic cervical spine injury he suffered on that fateful Saturday afternoon in October—a dislocation of the third and fourth cervical vertebrae.

The mechanism of most cases of catastrophic cervical spine injury in football is remarkably consistent.

Contact with the player occurs at the crown of the helmet. In most cases, the muscles on the sides of the cervical vertebrae and the intervertebral discs between these vertebrae in the neck effectively dissipate these forces.

If an athlete attempts to tackle or block his opponent with his head down, he puts his spine in a much more vulnerable position. The cervical spine normally has a concave alignment. If the player flexes his neck 30 degrees, the spine becomes a segmented column, like a stack of dimes.

With his head down and his spine in this straightened position, an impact delivered to the top of the head creates a compression force between the head and the trunk. Imagine a car in a crash test video that runs directly into a wall at top speed. The wall (head) doesn't budge. Momentum keeps the back end of the car (the body) speeding toward the wall. The front of the car (the neck) buckles and collapses.

Anatomically this mechanism of injury is best described as an axial loading of the cervical spine. With the head stopped and the trunk still moving, the intervertebral discs attempt to dissipate the compressive force. If the force exceeds what the discs can withstand, buckling and angular deformity in the bones and discs of the cervical spine result. Fractures of the bones, dislocations between the bones, or both, can occur, often driving bony fragments or disc material into the spinal canal. The bone or disc fragments can potentially cause a spinal cord injury.

In the early 1970s football experienced a spike in catastrophic cervical spine injuries. That rise coincided with the adoption of more protective football helmets. While the new helmets aimed to decrease the risk for skull fractures and other severe head injuries, they might have inadvertently increased the risk for neck injuries.

Dr. Barry Boden has studied catastrophic sports injuries extensively. "Because of this new football helmet, a lot of the players started to feel invincible. There was a real spike in the number of these quadriplegic events in the mid-1970s. What was probably happening was the athletes were starting to use their heads for tackling."[4]

Marc Buoniconti's spinal cord was crushed at the moment of impact between his head and Herman Jacob's back.

Athletic trainers from both teams rushed to his aid, but Buoniconti never moved. The process of cutting off his jersey and pads, putting a brace on his neck and lifting him into an ambulance took over half an hour. Tom Moore, coach of The Citadel, stood near Buoniconti on the field for a few minutes before he vomited behind the visitors' bench.

Nick Buoniconti, his wife Terry, and Marc's sister Gina flew from Connecticut to join Marc at the Johnson City Medical Center, where the ambulance took him later that night. Marc's brother Nick Jr., a senior linebacker at Duke, was playing in a game against Maryland. He was informed of Marc's injury in the locker room after his own team's loss.[5]

Marc was transferred by private plane to Jackson Memorial Hospital in Miami two days later. There the family met Dr. Barth Green, a prominent neurosurgeon.

Dr. Green performed surgery to stabilize Marc's cervical spine in early November. The surgery went well, with no complications. It required just over an hour, noted Jackson Memorial Hospital spokeswoman Zandra Thompkins after the procedure. The surgery would allow therapists and nurses to move Buoniconti, but it most likely would not restore his ability to walk.[6]

Over the next five months, Buoniconti lost 80 pounds, and he desperately clung to a ventilator. Under Dr. Green's guidance, Marc gradually started to increase his time off the machine—1 minute, then 5, 10, 20 minutes a day—until he could control his diaphragm.

Once off the breathing machine, Buoniconti moved to a rehab center. Multiple sessions of physical therapy and occupational therapy filled every day. Therapists stretched his muscles to keep them loose and moved the joints throughout his body to prevent contractures. They used electrical stimulation to try to get his muscles to fire.

Even after his discharge from rehab—and still to this day—Buoniconti requires assistance with eating, washing, and getting dressed.[7]

Buoniconti, who had scholarship offers from football powers like Georgia, Oklahoma, and Penn State but chose to attend the military school in Charleston, South Carolina, never played football again.

For Herman Jacobs, the player with whom Buoniconti collided, life would never be the same again either. He managed to finish his college career and attempted to play semiprofessional football. He could never really focus on football after Buoniconti's injury.[8]

Jacobs acknowledged the toll Buoniconti's condition took on him. He told the *Miami Herald* soon after the injury, "I know this wasn't my fault, but somehow I feel responsible. I hate it. I hate to see people get hurt."[9]

Jacobs now works as an assistant manager at a restaurant in Johnson City near the stadium where the devastating injury occurred.

Marc Buoniconti's cervical spine injury is certainly a tragedy. Are these catastrophic events common in football?

Dr. Boden and a team of researchers collected data from the National Center for Catastrophic Sports Injury Research. Using injuries reported between September 1989 and June 2002, they sought to determine the incidence of cervical spine injuries in high school and college football. They analyzed all catastrophic cervical spine injuries, including fatalities, nonfatal injuries that lead to permanent neurologic functional disability, and serious injuries that did not lead to permanent functional disability.

Over the 13-year period, an average of just over 15 direct catastrophic cervical spine injuries occurred in high school and college football combined each year. Since so many more athletes play high school football in the United States than college football (an estimated 1.2 million kids played high school football in the 2001–2002 academic year), the incidence rate of these injuries was much higher in college football.

Annually 4.72 college football players per 100,000 suffered these injuries, compared to 1.10 high school football players per 100,000.

Seventy-six football players suffered quadriplegia, as Marc Buoniconti did, between 1989 and 2002, or approximately six players per year. While the absolute number of players rendered quadriplegic was greater among high school players than college players, the incidence rate of quadriplegia was 1.5 times higher among college athletes.

Injuries that resulted in quadriplegia most often affected defensive backs, making up about 44% of the total. Players on special teams accounted for around 19%, followed by linebackers at approximately 17%.

The greater speed, size, and strength of college athletes could create larger forces upon collision, increasing the risk for these injuries.

The nature of the injuries largely correlated with Buoniconti's as well. Generally, football players are much more likely to suffer catastrophic cervical spine injuries during games rather than practices. Injuries that result in quadriplegia tend to occur in defensive players, especially defensive backs, special teams players, and linebackers. Almost four in five players suffer one of these devastating injuries while attempting to make a tackle.[10]

In the days after Marc Buoniconti's injury, these injuries became much less common, according to Dr. Frederick Mueller. Mueller studied these injuries during his more than 30 years serving as director of the National Center for Catastrophic Sports Injury Research at the University of North Carolina at Chapel Hill.

Dr. Mueller emphasized that statistics don't mean anything to the athlete who suffers the injury or to his family. "You know, when you look at the incidence rate for a hundred thousand or more, you might look at that and say, 'Oh, it's not too bad.' But then you see that kid in a wheelchair for the rest of his life, and it's pretty bad."[11]

The single bar face mask first appeared in 1955. Reportedly Cleveland Browns coach Paul Brown and the team's equipment manager assembled the makeshift crossbar after quarterback Otto Graham took a shot to the face during a game. They quickly put the bar on his helmet and sent Graham back into the game.[12]

With the introduction of the full face mask in 1975, more dangerous methods of tackling an opponent appeared in football. Spearing refers to a player intentionally using the crown of his helmet to strike an opponent. Face tackling refers to a player driving his face mask or the front of his helmet into the numbers or chest of a runner.

Prior to the face mask, defenders mostly used their shoulders to contact their opponents. Presumably due to the perceived protection provided by the face mask, defensive players now felt safe striking with their helmets.

Quadriplegic cervical spine injuries peaked in the mid-1970s, with about 30 occurring each year. Largely due to the efforts of Dr. Joseph Torg to identify the problem, educational efforts began to teach players to tackle properly, without using their heads.

In 1976, with the incidence of quadriplegia events at its highest-ever levels, the NCAA and the National Federation of State High School Associations barred players from intentionally using their heads to contact opponents when blocking and tackling. The American Football Coaches Association Ethics Committee soon followed suit and condemned these practices.

Data from the National Center for Catastrophic Sports Injury Research show that these rules have been somewhat effective. Catastrophic spine injuries that resulted in permanent spinal cord injury decreased from approximately 20 per year between 1971 and 1975 (just before the rules changed) to 7.2 per year from 1991 to 2001.[13]

In an attempt to decrease cervical spine injuries even further, the NCAA removed the word "intentional" from its spearing rules. This change attempted to make it easier for referees to call the penalty by removing the need to judge a player's intent.

These rule changes and the efforts to educate players and coaches at all levels about proper tackling techniques have helped decrease the incidence of catastrophic cervical spine injuries in football.

Continued education of coaches and athletes will probably decrease the number of catastrophic events even further. However, we likely will never be able to completely prevent these injuries. They can occur despite the best education, as players don't always intend to hit an opponent using their heads.

"Even if the kids are being taught properly, at the last minute they might not be too sure what they want to do. Then they drop their head. Or the running back changes direction, so they change direction, and they do have contact with the head or face," Dr. Mueller reasoned.[14]

Despite the spear tackling rule and tackling education, we have not completely eliminated the risk. Continued education and attempts to further study rule changes in football might help.

One rule change could help decrease these events. Since special teams' players suffer a large portion of these injuries, moving the kickoffs after each touchdown up five yards might protect these players. By moving them forward, more kickoffs would result in touchbacks with fewer returns. Given that the players on the kickoff team barrel down the field at 20 or 25 mph, we might see fewer quadriplegic injuries to members of the special teams in the future.

Rule changes are one way that many sports have tried to eliminate—or at least reduce—serious injuries. Dr. Gary Green, the medical director for MLB, compared the decision to remove collisions at home plate to the spear tackling rule in football.

Like football's ban on spear tackling, banning home plate collisions between a base runner and a catcher doesn't require new equipment. And it really doesn't detract from the game itself. Players just have to become aware of the rule and abide by it.

In the first few years since the rule was adopted in 2014, fewer concussions have occurred in baseball.

"It doesn't make sense to lose your catcher for two weeks for one run in the course of the season," Dr. Green rationalized.[15]

Still, as recently as 2006, approximately six catastrophic cervical spine injuries resulting in a player becoming permanently quadriplegic occurred in football every year.

"By banning spear-tackling the incidence of cervical spine injuries resulting in quadriplegia was reduced from 30 to 6 cases per year," Boden emphasized. "It may be impossible to completely eliminate the problem, but we should strive to reduce the number of injuries as much as possible. Continued surveillance is necessary, especially since the spear-tackling rule was strengthened a few years ago."[16]

In his study of catastrophic cervical spine injuries in high school and college football between 1989 and 2002, Boden cited the legal ramifications of these injuries. At least 18 of the 196 incidents led to lawsuits or insurance settlements.[17]

Marc Buoniconti sued The Citadel; the team's athletic trainer, Andy Clawson; and the team physician, E. K. Wallace. The case went to trial in 1988.

Buoniconti's attorneys claimed that the medical staff should have kept the linebacker from playing in the game due to a sprained neck that had caused him to miss practice that week. They also argued that he never should have played with a strap connecting his face mask to his shoulder pads, which aimed to prevent his head from snapping back.

Attorneys for The Citadel and Dr. Wallace blamed Buoniconti for tackling Jacobs head first. While no penalty for intentional spearing was called on the play, they asserted that Buoniconti's spearing was responsible for his quadriplegia.

The jury in the Charleston County Court of Common Pleas needed less than three hours of deliberation before exonerating Dr. Wallace. The insurance company representing The Citadel and Clawson offered Buoniconti an $800,000 settlement, which he accepted.[18]

Eight years after the settlement, the University of Miami and The Citadel wanted to honor Buoniconti at halftime in their game at the Orange Bowl. He declined.

At the time, Buoniconti expressed his resentment against The Citadel in the *Miami Herald*. "The way the Citadel treated me felt awfully cold, and it has left an everlasting impression. It was a military school, so I compare it to being shot in the battlefield. They left me there to die."[19]

Every year 12,000 people in the United States suffer a new traumatic spinal cord injury like Buoniconti's.[20] Essentially one such injury occurs every hour of every day.

While football might be one of the most visible causes of spinal cord injuries, it represents less than 1% of all spinal cord injuries. In fact, sports as a whole only comprise the fourth most common cause. Sports and recreational activities accounted for 7.93% of spinal cord injuries in the United States between September 2005 and May 2012, according to the National Spinal Cord Injury Statistical Center. Vehicular accidents, accidental falls, and acts of violence—in decreasing order—represent a larger share of spinal cord injuries.[21]

In sports, football is associated with the highest number of catastrophic cervical spine injuries, but it is by no means the only sport that exposes its athletes to this risk. Gymnastics, ice hockey, skiing, rugby, diving, pole-vaulting in track and field, cheerleading, and other sports present risks for spine injuries. In fact, the incidence of cervical spine injuries per 100,000 participants is higher in gymnastics and ice hockey than in football.[22]

Regardless of the mechanism of injury, spinal cord injuries create huge financial burdens—on top of the physical and emotional impact—on the patient and his or her family. The National Spinal Cord Injury Statistical Center in Birmingham, Alabama, estimates that the annual health-care and living expenses for a patient with a high tetraplegia injury between C1 and C4, like Marc Buoniconti suffered, average $829,843 in the first year alone. For each subsequent year, the patient faces almost $150,000 of expenses. The lifetime cost of an injury like Buoniconti suffered, for a 25-year-old patient, is approximately $3.27 million.[23]

"If you're one of these six athletes who sustain a cervical spine injury with quadriplegia, it's a real tragedy," Dr. Boden remarked. "The rest of your life is going to be extremely difficult, not to mention the huge financial costs. The burdens are extremely high."[24]

Marc Buoniconti was 19 years old at the time he became a quadriplegic.

Buoniconti said that his medical expenses exceed $500,000 each year. Fortunately, a catastrophic insurance policy his dad Nick obtained as president of US Tobacco pays those bills.[25]

Looking at Marc's daily schedule, it is not surprising that his injury is so costly. He requires around-the-clock nursing assistance. Just starting his day is quite an ordeal. He wakes up around 8:00 a.m. His nurses catheterize him, help him take a shower, stretch his muscles and joints, check his blood pressure and other vital signs, administer his medications, and help with his physical therapy.

"If I'm lucky, I'm in the chair by 11 or 12," Buoniconti told Erik Brady of USA Today. "And then I go face the day."[26]

Fortunately for the roughly 300,000 Americans living with a spinal cord injury, Marc Buoniconti does face each day with determination and passion. He has spent over 25 years since his injury trying to find a cure for the paralysis that afflicts so many people.

When Marc was transferred to the University of Miami/Jackson Memorial Medical Center in October 1985, he and his family met neurosurgeon Dr. Barth Green. Green was cofounder and chairman of The Miami Project to Cure Paralysis.

The campaign, which aims to cure paralysis, strokes, Alzheimer's disease, Parkinson's disease, and other neurological disorders, has assembled a team of hundreds of scientists and researchers. It had just launched earlier that year and had yet to raise much money. After Marc's injury, he and his father worked tirelessly to raise awareness for the campaign. Within three months, The Miami Project had raised $800,000.[27]

Now Marc, who went on to obtain a degree in psychology from the University of Miami, serves as president of The Miami Project to Cure Paralysis and president of the Buoniconti Fund. This fund-raising arm of The Miami Project has amassed over $350 million since his injury in its efforts to find a cure for paralysis.[28]

Through Dr. Green and his team of neurosurgeons and scientists, The Miami Project has become a leader in spinal cord research. In 2013 researchers published findings from a six-year study using hypothermia as a treatment for acute spinal cord injury. By using cool IV fluids to bring a patient's core body temperature down to 33°C, 43% of patients obtained better neurological outcomes.[29]

Also in 2013, surgeons with The Miami Project performed the first Food and Drug Administration (FDA)–approved Schwann cell transplantation in a patient with a new spinal cord injury. Schwann cells insulate individual nerve fibers in the peripheral nervous system. Surgeons take a biopsy of a sensory nerve in the leg in order to replicate the Schwann cells in the lab. They then transplant the Schwann cells into the spinal cord injury site between 26 and 42 days after the initial injury.[30]

It is unlikely The Miami Project will find a cure for paralysis in time to heal the project's inspiration, Marc Buoniconti. Buoniconti's relationship with The Citadel, though, has finally healed.

On September 30, 2006, The Citadel retired Buoniconti's number 59 at halftime of the game against Chattanooga. The school even framed the white road jersey that the medical staff had cut off him on the field 20 years earlier.

"It's like a dam has opened up after all these years," Buoniconti told USA Today's Erik Brady before the event. "My emotions are going to flow. A void in my heart has been filled. Time heals."[31]

The message for young football players, and for the parents and coaches who teach them, is simple. Do not tackle with your head down. Always keep your head up. Players should always see the play and see the field. If they keep their heads up, they have a great chance of avoiding a serious injury.

Despite rules to eliminate spear tackling and abundant education of tackling techniques for coaches and players, we will probably never rid football of catastrophic cervical spine injuries. Hopefully Buoniconti, Green, and their team can heal future generations of players who suffer these tragic injuries.

6 / SARAH BURKE

The Dangers of Extreme Sports

January 10, 2012

Sarah Burke, a six-time medalist at the Winter X Games, attempted a routine flat spin 540 at the bottom of the 22-foot Eagle Superpipe at Park City Mountain Resort in Park City, Utah. The energy drink company Monster, which sponsored Burke, had rented out the halfpipe so that Burke could train for the Winter X Games, set to take place in Aspen later that month.

The 540 was a move the champion freestyle skier had landed thousands of times. Burke, after all, was the first female to ever successfully land a 720, 900, and 1080 in a competition.

She had also fallen thousands of times, as she did on this jump. As she landed, Burke over-rotated, whipped forward, and hit her head.

For a short time, no one on the course seemed to notice.

When a fellow skier called Sarah's name with no response, many athletes rushed to her aid. Minutes later, paramedics called for helicopter transport.

Sarah Burke was in cardiac arrest.

In an article she wrote days later for ESPNW, champion snowboarder Gretchen Bleiler suggested, as many would in the coming days, that it did not appear to be a serious crash. "So why is she in the hospital after a fall that looked like it shouldn't have even caused a concussion?"[1]

In an unfortunate coincidence, Burke was now fighting for her life after falling on the same Superpipe where snowboarder Kevin Pearce had suffered a traumatic brain injury just over two years earlier.[2]

Arguably the most influential and successful athlete in women's halfpipe, Burke had suffered injuries throughout her career: a broken thumb, broken ribs, a dislocated shoulder, and even a fractured vertebra in her lower back suffered at the 2009 X Games. She persevered and returned to the top of her sport.

"I've been doing this for [a] long time, 11 years," she explained in a 2010 interview. "I've been very lucky with the injuries I've had. It's part of the game. Everybody gets hurt. Looking back on it, I'd probably do the exact same thing again."[3]

Sarah Burke was born in Barrie, Ontario, on September 3, 1982. She started skiing at five years old. At an early age, she dreamed of competing in the Olympics.

Freestyle skiing was in its infancy as Burke began skiing. With a love of skiing and jumping in the woods, freestyle skiing came naturally to her. By high school, she entered a big air competition in the Canadian Nationals, although no women or junior boys had entered.

Sarah competed against 23 men, many of whom were professional skiers, that day in Québec City. She finished fourth.[4]

She won most halfpipe events she entered. Unfortunately, women's events either didn't exist on the professional tour at the time, or they paid much less prize money to female winners than to males. Sarah could have fought to win what little prize money there was in women's halfpipe, but instead she fought to grow the sport. She found girls who were interested in freestyle skiing in online chat rooms and encouraged them to join her halfpipe clinics.

Eventually the X Games added women's freestyle halfpipe and slopestyle, as well as awarding equal prize money to the women.

Just as Sarah fought for opportunities for women on the slopes, she fought to overcome the damage those events inflicted on her body. She competed in slopestyle in the 2009 X Games, not because it was her best event, but because she fought for its inclusion in the competition. She broke a bone in her lower back in that event.[5]

In the documentary *Winter Sessions: Rory Bushfield and Sarah Burke*, she described her resilience in overcoming injuries. "Being that I've been skiing for a really long time now, I've definitely had a fair share of injuries. It's part of the job. It's what comes with the territory. I guess I'm really good at crashing. I paid for it."

"I think you should scare yourself every day," Burke explained in the documentary. "I'm a firm believer in getting your heart going and trying something different or new and overcoming it."[6]

But now, lying on the snow in the Superpipe at Park City, her heart was not going.

"Sarah is a very strong woman and she will most certainly fight to recover," Rory Bushfield, Burke's husband, said in a statement released hours after his wife's injury.[7]

Canadian Freestyle Ski Association CEO Peter Judge would later observe that the fall was "nothing out of the norm, nothing on the extreme end of the spectrum,"[8] Moments after her fall, Sarah Burke was treated by ski patrol and then transported to base patrol, where she was airlifted to the University of Utah. There she remained intubated and sedated while doctors evaluated her injuries.

Soon doctors found that Burke had a tear in her vertebral artery. The vertebral arteries are blood vessels that travel within the bones of the cervical spine and carry blood and oxygen to the brain. They are essentially tethered in relation to the head and can be injured in a whiplash-type injury. Interruptions in the blood flow in these vessels can result in brain injury that may run the gamut from minimal to life threatening.

Tears, or dissections, of the vertebral artery can cause severe headaches, confusion, and weakness. If the bleeding is severe, the patient can wind up in a coma or die. Since these injuries can be fatal, surgeons usually repair the artery urgently. Fortunately, many patients can recover completely in weeks to months.

In Burke's case, Dr. William T. Couldwell, the chair of neurosurgery at the University of Utah, operated on Burke to repair the tear in her vertebral artery. Dr. Couldwell and other doctors at the University of Utah would follow the course of her brain recovery before they could determine if she would recover completely.

Burke's injury rocked the skiing community. Fans and fellow athletes waited anxiously for any news on her condition. They took to social media to urge their hero to fight to recover. Hashtags like #believeinsarah and #prayingforsarah-burke flooded Twitter.

On January 19, 2012, at 9:22 a.m., she lost that fight. After Burke passed away, her organs were donated, as she had wished. In a statement her publicist, Nicole Wool, said that Sarah had suffered "irreversible damage to her brain due to lack of oxygen and blood after cardiac arrest."[9]

Sarah Burke was 29 years old.

Freestyle skiing is a relatively new sport, so little data exist on injuries in the sport.

In 1982 a study published by Patrick A. Dowling, MD, in the *American Journal of Sports Medicine* collected data from the United States Ski Association's freestyle competitions over four seasons between 1976 and 1980, well before the advent of halfpipe competitions. Dowling found an incidence rate of 2.8

injuries per 1,000 skier-days. He did note that over half of the injuries in all freestyle competitions involved aerials, and he warned that these competitions be increasingly scrutinized due to the inherent risks of catastrophic injuries.[10]

At the World Cup level, halfpipe became one of the five freestyle events. In halfpipe competitions, competitors each ski down a 100- to 140-meter-long pipe with walls ranging from 3 to 4.5 meters high. Each athlete performs a series of flips and turns as she skis off the wall, into the air, and back onto the pipe again.

Authors of a 2010 study in the *British Journal of Sports Medicine* gathered data from World Cup skiers over three seasons: 2006–2007, 2007–2008, and 2008–2009. The researchers identified all acute injuries that occurred during competitions in those competitive seasons.

Among the 662 total World Cup freestyle skiers, 291 acute injuries occurred. Almost one third (32%) were classified as severe injuries, meaning the athlete missed more than 28 days of training and competitions. Looking at all freestyle disciplines, the knee was the most frequently injured body part, as 27% of injuries involved the knee; 13% of freestyle injuries involved the head.[11]

Another study, also published in the *British Journal of Sports Medicine*, further examined head injuries in World Cup competitions. Not only did the authors look at freestyle skiers, but they also included Alpine skiers and snowboarders. They collected data over seven consecutive seasons through 2013. They found that concussions comprised the majority of head and face injuries. About one-fourth of all of these injuries were severe. Freestyle skiing had the highest rate of head injuries compared to Alpine skiing and snowboarding, and women had a higher injury rate than men.[12]

Dr. Tom Hackett, an orthopaedic surgeon at the Steadman Clinic in Vail, Colorado, and physician for the US Ski and Snowboard teams, argued that injuries in these sports aren't more common than in traditional sports like football, basketball, and soccer in terms of sheer numbers. The problem is the morbidity. When an injury does occur, it can often be much worse.[13]

December 31, 2009

Sarah Burke was not the first star athlete to be critically injured on Park City's Superpipe.

Snowboarder Kevin Pearce had recently entered a sponsorship agreement with Nike, and the company built the halfpipe in Park City for his training. Nike felt that he could soon surpass Shaun White and reach the top of the sport. In less than two months, Pearce was supposed to compete for gold at the Vancouver Olympics.

On New Year's Eve morning, with his close friends watching, Pearce tried to land a trick that could guarantee him an Olympic medal if he successfully landed it in competition. This time, he didn't. He missed the landing and crashed onto his head. He was taken off the course on a stretcher and quickly moved to the University of Utah hospital.[14]

Kevin Pearce had ascended in the sport quickly, after entering the pro ranks at only 18 years of age. He won the quarterpipe event in the Oakley Arctic Challenge in 2007 and 2008, and he became the Ticket to Ride champion after the 2008 season. After he won the silver medal in Superpipe in the 2009 Winter X Games in Aspen, Pearce was seen as a credible threat for a gold medal in Vancouver.

His crash in Park City ended his Olympic dreams. Pearce suffered a traumatic brain injury and was in a coma for a week. As shown in the documentary *The Crash Reel*, Pearce battled numerous problems after that crash—memory loss, visual impairment, loss of fine motor skills, and bad judgment.

Through years of rehab, Kevin Pearce worked to overcome his brain injury, learning basic motor skills again, improving his memory, and eventually returning to his daily activities.

Pearce wanted to compete in snowboarding again, but doctors warned him that it was too risky. One fall and one blow to the head could kill him. He did finally get back on a snowboard on December 13, 2011, but he never competed again.

Kevin Pearce is still active in the snowboarding community, often serving as a commentator. He works as an advocate for research and education on traumatic brain injuries and the use of helmets.

February 20, 2014

The Olympic Games for which Pearce trained in hopes of winning a medal in 2010 was the same competition Sarah Burke wanted to win in Sochi in 2014. The only problem was that women's freestyle skiing halfpipe was not an Olympic sport.

Getting the halfpipe into the Olympics was very important to Burke. She lobbied the International Olympic Committee (IOC) for years, enlisting her fellow athletes to join the cause. Bushfield said Burke almost succeeded in getting the sport added to the Vancouver Olympics. Instead of protesting the decision, she fully supported the snowboard halfpipe. And she helped get the freestyle skiing halfpipe into the games in Sochi.

French skier Marie Martinod came out of retirement to return to World Cup competition at Burke's request. "[Sarah] had this contest in La Plagne [France] next to my place and after the contest she passed by," Martinod told NBC Sports. "She said, 'Marie I just want you to know that I'm working [getting halfpipe] into the Olympics. It's going to happen, for sure, and you should think about coming back.' That was the last time that I saw her."[15]

The IOC finally added freestyle halfpipe in April 2011. Had she not crashed in Park City, Burke likely would have entered that first Olympic competition at the age of 31.

Twenty-year-old American Maddie Bowman won the first gold medal in the women's freestyle skiing halfpipe. Marie Martinod finished second for the silver.

As the medalists took the podium, they pointed to the sky out of respect for the woman who had given them their chance to compete.

Like many young female skiers, Bowman idolized Burke when she was just beginning in the sport. Now an Olympic champion, Bowman pointed to her fallen hero. "Sarah Burke is watching over us tonight, and we just want to honor her as much as we can."[16]

Without question, Sarah Burke was one of the most dominant women in action sports. Her accomplishments are staggering. She was a six-time Winter X Games medalist, including four gold medals in women's Ski Superpipe. She won events on the FIS World Cup, the Association of Freeskiing Professionals AFP World Tour, and the Winter Dew Tour. In 2007 Burke became the first skier to win an ESPY Award for Female Action Sports Athlete of the Year.

She was arguably even more impressive off the slopes.

Burke earned cover appearances on magazines, including making the FHM list of 100 sexiest women. She had endorsement deals with companies like Helly Hansen, Monster, Salomon, Roxy, and Smith. She even visited military troops in Iraq.

Perhaps it was that success—both in the halfpipe and in business—that surprised so many people when she was injured in Utah. When news spread quickly that Burke's family faced financial ruin from dealing with the crippling costs of her medical care, people started questioning why a professional skier with a multitude of corporate sponsors would not be covered by health insurance.

Had Burke crashed in Whistler, British Columbia, where she and her husband lived, Canada's public health insurance would have covered 100% of her medical expenses, according to the Ministry of Health in British Columbia.

Burke also carried a $5 million insurance policy provided by the Canadian Freestyle Ski Association. That policy covered competitors in sanctioned events and training where Canadian Association coaches were present. The event in Utah was a privately sponsored one, and no Canadian Association coaches attended it.

Many events require competitors to prove that they have health insurance. Burke, though, was injured in a training session, not an actual competition.

The sponsor of that event, Monster Beverage Company, makes the popular energy drinks championed by competitors and young fans alike. A spokesman for Monster told NBC News that Burke did not receive insurance through the company.

"Sponsors in general do not provide insurance for the athletes, who are independent contractors. In many contracts if not most, the athletes sign an agreement saying they understand that it is a dangerous sport and that they are responsible for their own well-being. That is fairly standard throughout the industry."[17]

Bushfield acknowledged that this is a difficult problem. He pointed out that while professional football and basketball are dangerous sports as well, there is a lot more money in those sports than in these winter sports.[18]

Hours before she passed, Burke's agent appealed to her fans for help. Michael Spencer started a fund-raising website to help Sarah's family pay a fraction of her medical expenses, expected to top $200,000. Spencer hoped the site could raise $15,000.

Sarah Burke had touched many people through her camps, interviews, and achievements, and they came through for her and her family. The site raised over $300,000.[19]

Still, the question remains that if one of action sports' biggest stars cannot pay medical expenses, what should happen to the sports themselves and the thousands of up-and-coming athletes across the world?

After all, the Winter X Games were becoming a phenomenon. After ESPN debuted the X Games in Big Bear Lake, California, in 1997, they became wildly popular. Television ratings soared.

The 2012 Winter X Games, held weeks after Burke's death, drew a total of 35.4

million viewers in the United States, including live and repeat telecasts. The target demographic, males aged 18 to 34, increased by 16%.[20]

ESPN started a global series of events to capitalize on the popularity of these sports and the increased exposure of the athletes all over the world. Sponsors lined up to pay for that exposure to millions of athletes and fans.

Part of what made these competitions so popular—both for the competitors and for the fans who watched in person or on TV—were the amazing stunts the competitors were trying. Forget the Olympic motto "faster, higher, stronger"; the X Games ushered in aerial maneuvers that were truly death defying. And fans loved them.

The sports evolved quickly. Event organizers and course designers created larger halfpipes as the athletes wanted to perform more acrobatic maneuvers. While the sponsors and the public loved the stunts, the athletes chose to push the envelope.

While watching some of the competitions and crashes in the 2013 Winter X Games, *Deadspin* writer Brent Rose published an article titled "It's Only a Matter of Time before Someone Dies at the X Games." He was a longtime fan of these sports, but this event was the first he attended in person.

In his article, Rose noted his amazement that no one had died performing one of these stunts in the X Games. "As I watched these athletes fly over my head, it really hit home just how miraculous the zero-casualty rate was. 'Maybe it's safer than it looks,' I thought for a brief moment. And then they started dropping like planes over Midway," he wrote.[21]

Caleb Moore would die later that day.

January 24, 2013

Texas-born snowmobiler Caleb Moore attempted to land a backflip in the snowmobile freestyle contest in the 2013 Winter X Games in Aspen. While certainly daring, a backflip was nothing new to Moore. Moore had successfully landed backflips hundreds of times in his short career.

This backflip was different. Moore under-rotated, and the skis of his machine caught the lip of the landing platform. He flew over the handlebars. His 450-pound Polaris snowmobile barreled into him, briefly knocking him unconscious.

Caleb soon roused and asked his brother Colten what had happened. He walked out of the stadium before being taken by ambulance to Aspen Valley Hospital with a concussion.[22]

Caleb and Colten Moore grew up in Krum, Texas, racing all-terrain vehicles. They used their skills jumping ATVs and transferred their focus to flipping snowmobiles. They constructed a foam pit in their backyard and taught themselves how to flip the snow machines.

Caleb won a bronze medal in the 2010 Winter X Games snowmobile freestyle competition after only 30 days of practice. The following year, he won a bronze again. He won a silver medal in the best trick contest in 2012 despite suffering a pelvic fracture in practice the day before the event. His brother Colten won the gold medal.[23]

Only 30 minutes after his brother Caleb crashed and his snowmobile slammed into him at the 2013 Winter X Games, Colten also crashed, leading to a separated pelvis.

Doctors at Aspen Valley Hospital treated Caleb Moore for a concussion before they found bleeding around his heart. A helicopter took him to St. Mary's Hospital in Grand Junction, Colorado.

About six hours passed between Caleb's crash and his arrival in Grand Junction. He underwent advanced cardiac life support during transport, and the medical providers performed a pericardiocentesis to try to draw blood from the sac around his heart.[24]

With blunt thoracic injuries, blood can collect within the pericardial sac around the heart. That fluid can decrease the blood entering the heart and weaken the heart's ability to pump blood. That condition, called cardiac tamponade, is a medical emergency.

A surgeon or cardiologist can draw this blood out from the pericardial sac by inserting a needle through the chest. Cardiac ultrasound guidance can help direct the needle into the fluid collection. The procedure can help stabilize the patient and allow doctors time to treat the underlying injuries.

The pericardiocentesis helped Caleb's heartbeat and blood pressure return, according to the autopsy performed later, but it might have been too late. The cardiopulmonary arrest during the transport led to anoxic encephalopathy, or lack of oxygen to the brain.[25]

Caleb underwent emergency heart surgery the next morning, and he remained in the intensive care unit. A spokeswoman for the family told reporters in the coming days that "a secondary complication involving his brain"—likely the lack of oxygen—had resulted from the cardiac injury.[26]

Caleb Moore died one week after his crash, at 9:30 a.m. on January 31. His death was the first in the 18-year history of the X Games. According to the autopsy report, Moore died from "blunt force chest injury and complications thereof." The injuries found by Robert A. Kurtzman included a cardiac contusion, contusion of the chest wall, rib fractures, and a mild brain injury.[27]

Snowmobiling is a popular winter sport. As one might expect with vehicles that weigh hundreds of pounds and are capable of traveling at high speeds, injuries can occur. Add in inexperienced drivers, reckless behavior, and alcohol, and catastrophic injuries and deaths can result.

In fact, a 2003 study showed that snowmobile accidents result in roughly 200 deaths and 14,000 injuries annually.[28]

Authors of a 2014 study collected data from patient injuries caused by snowmobile accidents that presented to the University of Rochester Medical Center in Rochester, New York, between 2004 and 2012. They found that one-third of the injuries resulted from the rider being thrown from the snowmobile or the vehicle rolling or flipping over, 27% involved striking a stationary object, 9% resulted from being struck by the snowmobile, and 9% percent involved the patients' being injured by the snowmobile itself.

Head injuries occurred in 35% of patients. Thoracic trauma, like the injuries Caleb Moore suffered, also negatively impacted the victims.[29]

Snowmobile competitors in the X Games are far from inexperienced, though. Unlike recreational drivers, these extreme athletes launch the vehicles 60 or more feet in the air, flip them over, and even separate from the machines before rejoining them before landing.

Maybe spectators should wonder how no one had died before Caleb Moore did.

Moore might have been the only competitor to die in the 2013 X Games, but he certainly was not the only one seriously injured. In addition to Colten's pelvic injury, New Zealand skier Rose Battersby suffered a fracture of her lumbar spine in practice, requiring surgery. Slopestyle skier Ashley Battersby broke her leg. Jackson Strong, another snowmobile competitor, failed to regrab his machine after a backflip, and the vehicle sailed into the crowd. Amazingly, no one was injured.[30]

After Moore passed away, X Games organizer ESPN promised to "conduct a thorough review of this discipline and adopt any appropriate changes to future X Games."

In an interview on *Outside the Lines*, Scott Guglielmino, ESPN's senior vice president of programming and global X events, reiterated that the organizers would work with course designers and the athletes to eliminate as much risk as possible from freestyle snowmobiling.[31]

Particularly concerning, though, was the athletes' increasing performance of stunts in which they leave the machine, spin in the air, and remount the vehicle. "We are certainly interested in when they become separated from the snowmobile and they go downhill after that—such as Caleb's crash," Guglielmino said on *Outside the Lines*. "We do not want to see snowmobiles landing on athletes, so that is something that is going to be very much the focus of our review in this instance."[32]

Subsequently, ESPN eliminated the Moto X Best Trick and Snowmobile Best Trick events at the X Games.

News of Caleb Moore's death stunned the extreme sports world. Caleb, though, would not have called snowmobile freestyle extreme but "a lifestyle," according to his agent.[33]

The risk-taking behavior exhibited by Burke, Moore, and thousands of other competitors begs a fundamental question: Can any effort on the part of organizers, course designers, equipment manufacturers, and doctors actually make these sports safe?

One potential improvement would be to hire the best course designers. There can be significant variability in the courses at the Olympic level, the Mountain Dew tour, and the X Games. In fact, Dr. Hackett lobbied the IOC to insist that course designers not be selected much like political appointees but because they make the best, safest courses.

"There are different engineers out there that have an interest in this, that do research in this, that say, 'The approach angle should be 18 degrees and the lift of the jump should be 30 meters long and angled at 70 meters at the top and there should be a jump gap distance of this.' They really nerd out on the intricacies of the engineering approach, the actual science of these jumps. The guys that do this, they all totally disagree with each other," Hackett explained.

"There's a total lack of consistency in the construction of a lot of these venues," he asserted.[34]

If an athlete knew the designer who built a particular course, he would probably have a higher degree of comfort and trust in pushing the envelope than if he didn't know what to expect from the course.

Still, even with the best course design, athletes can suffer injuries while performing acrobatic tricks.

At the top of the halfpipe in Park City, where Sarah Burke and Kevin Pearce suffered their catastrophic injuries, an enormous warning sign serves as a last attempt to caution athletes about the risk of injuries.

Entering the halfpipe, the sign asserts, "exposes you to the risk of serious injury or death. Inverted aerials are not recommended."[35]

Terrain parks generally, even ones not associated with injuries to such famous athletes, present real risks. A 2010 study published in the journal *Injury Prevention* showed that compared to injuries sustained on the slopes, injuries suffered in terrain parks were more likely to involve the head, face, and back; were more likely to result from high falls; and were more likely to require hospital transport.[36] These risks apply not only to X Games competitors, but also to the young athletes who emulate them.

To learn these tricks, athletes take risks. Sure, using airbags, trampolines, and foam pits can make it safer. In an interview on TSN Radio shortly before her death, Burke explained that she had suffered numerous injuries despite trying to protect her safety. "But it is a sport that's trial and error, and you have to try it on snow sometimes and it's not always going to go right."[37]

At the end of the day, extreme sports like snowboarding, freestyle skiing, and snowmobiling—and their warm-weather counterparts like skateboarding and motocross—rely on athletes regulating themselves.

Former snowmobile racing star Paul Thacker explained this dilemma to Jason Blevins of the *Denver Post* in the days after Caleb Moore's accident. "We've all accepted the risk, and we know what playing the game means," Thacker acknowledged.[38]

Thacker should understand the risks. While training for the 2011 X Games, he landed wrong, and his snowmobile's handlebars hit him in the chest. He injured vertebrae in his back and was rendered paraplegic.

Thacker returned to the 2013 X Games and competed in adaptive snowmobile racing. Of the eight competitors in that race, seven had been disabled in snowmobile or motorcycle accidents.

Despite these injuries, very little has changed to make the sports appreciably safer. And rarely does anyone call for a fundamental change to any of these sports. To event organizers and the athletes who compete in them, these are simply accidents.

Ask Devin Logan, a freestyle skier who won a Winter X Games silver medal in slopestyle at the age of 18. "These accidents that have happened are unfortunate and terrible," he argued to Billy Witz of FOX Sports. "But they're accidents. It's as safe as it can be. It's an extreme sport."[39]

Rory Bushfield insisted that the athletes understand the risks. "If you're out there doing what you love, then you're assuming the risks, and that's your decision. At the end of the day, nobody put a gun to anybody's head to do anything."[40]

The athletes recognize that injuries are part of the sport, and many ignore the seriousness of these injuries. Snowboarding star Gretchen Bleiler fractured her eye socket and nose and suffered a concussion—her fourth or fifth concussion, she guessed—while practicing a flip.

"It's a bit I wouldn't say blasé, but it comes with the territory," she noted to Rachel George of USA Today when discussing the attitudes many competitors have about concussions and other injuries.[41]

After all, if they do get hurt performing a 1080 in a halfpipe or a backflip on the snowmobile, at least it will have been worth it. Maddie Bowman, who later won the Olympic freestyle halfpipe gold medal in Sochi, made that argument.

"I think we love the adrenaline rush, and you just kind of go, 'Well, if I'm gonna get hurt—knock on wood—I'm going to do it doing something really cool.' That's what we love to do."[42]

Sarah Burke knew her sport was dangerous, but that was partly why she loved it, according to Bushfield. "She knew the risks, and she was out doing what she loved to do. A lot of people are going to die doing things that they don't love doing. It's almost a blessing in itself to be able to do what you love freely, and have that be all it is."[43]

The day before Caleb Moore finally passed away, *Washington Post* writer Cindy Boren wrote a column questioning these extreme sports. The title of her column asks an important question: "When Is Enough Enough?"[44]

Despite Sarah Burke's and Caleb Moore's deaths, these sports are as popular as ever. In fact, ESPN reinstated snowmobile freestyle for the 2014 X Games, and Colten took home the gold medal, a win he dedicated to his brother.

Every year the athletes raise the bar higher and higher. They invent new tricks and exceed the limits with the old tricks. And with that drive to push the limits of what can be achieved comes an even greater risk of injury.

Gretchen Bleiler described the fine line professional athletes walk in these sports in an article she penned for ESPNW in the days after Burke's crash:

Our job as pros is to walk a very fine line; be the best but stay healthy so you can continue to progress and be at the top. You can't push the sport and yourself if you're always hurt. Being at the top means never being satisfied with what you're comfortable with—comfortable means you've stopped pushing and you're either going to get passed or you already have been. But if you're constantly pushing yourself, then you're exposing yourself to falls and injuries. And that is the fine line I speak of.[45]

That "fine line" is razor thin.

On top of the pressure athletes place on themselves to push the boundaries of what is humanly possible is the pressure from corporate sponsors. These companies pay top dollar to the athletes in the hopes that their performances will impress young fans. Even if it's just implied, those companies need these stars to try more amazing and yet more dangerous stunts.

Even if the event organizers and corporate sponsors radically change these events in the hope of avoiding catastrophic injuries among their pro competitors, it might not have much effect on the kids performing these tricks all over the world.

After all, the roughly 35 million television viewers of the 2012 X Games likely pale in comparison to the number of kids watching stunts like Burke and Moore performed on YouTube.

In the age of the GoPro camera, anyone can become famous on the Internet. A kid can mount a camera on his helmet and try a dangerous stunt. The more dangerous or radical his trick or the nastier the crash, the more views he gets.

There is an unsanctioned competition taking place among athletes of all ages and skill levels all over the world, playing out over the Internet, with rapidly escalating stakes.

"Some people get out there, and they get above their skill level," Bushfield explained, noting that he coaches young athletes at summer camps. "Still, you get out in the element, and people are doing crazy things, and you want to do it too, but you're not ready."[46]

Dr. Hackett noted the same problem. "You've got this other branch of more amateur guys, the guys that are watching YouTube videos and then trying to emulate the guys who are really good at these sports. I think there is a population of athletes out there that are more beginners that may not be quite as careful in their approach."[47]

Parents of kids who do want to participate in these sports should approach them as they would more traditional sports like football, baseball, and soccer. Instead of kids watching YouTube and learning these tricks through trial and error, they should work with a qualified coach. The coach can teach them the necessary skills. The kids can slowly advance in the difficulty of their stunts as the coach ensures that their skills have progressed appropriately. Working with a qualified coach and not trying maneuvers beyond their skill level can help prevent many catastrophic injuries among young athletes.

As for the top competitors, we can hope the athletes will hold themselves back, but it probably will never happen. These are elite athletes who love their sports. They want to be the best, and that drive pushes them to soar through the air, twisting and turning faster and higher. They know they can get hurt. They know they probably will get hurt, and possibly very badly. But they love what they do, and they will keep doing it.

Several years have passed since Burke's death. Rory Bushfield recalled how Sarah lived life to the fullest. He hoped people remember Sarah Burke not for her death in the halfpipe, but for the wonderful life skiing gave her.

"She would never want anybody to be scared to ski the halfpipe. She would want people to embrace what's there. If they loved doing it, she would want them to do it."[48]

7 / DAVE DUERSON

Long-Term Brain Damage in Football

February 17, 2011

Sunny Isles Beach was about as far from Soldier Field—both geographically and figuratively—as a football fan could imagine. Yet that warm, relaxed Florida locale—not the stadium where Dave Duerson was feared by offenses as a famed defensive back for the Chicago Bears—is where the injury that could change the sport forever occurred.

His condo in Sunny Isles Beach is where Duerson chose to commit suicide.

According to Dan Pompei of the *Chicago Tribune*, Duerson's ex-wife Alicia received a text message at 3:00 that morning. "I love you. I always loved you. I love our kids," Duerson texted. Three days earlier, Duerson had talked to his three sons and one daughter for the last time. He wished them a happy Valentine's Day and told them, as he told Alicia, that he loved them.

After Alicia tried to call him several times with no answer, she received a final text from Dave Duerson. "Please, see that my brain is given to the N.F.L.'s brain bank."[1]

To understand why the four-time Pro Bowl safety would make such a request, we must look back at his football career.

Despite being a four-year starter at Notre Dame, team captain, and all-American selection, Duerson fell to the third round in the 1983 NFL draft. Talk of the Fighting Irish star's future legal and political ambitions might have played a role, but defensive teammate Dan Hampton had a different view.

In an interview with Paul Solotaroff in *Men's Journal*, Hampton recounted how Duerson initially seemed too soft to defensive coordinator Buddy Ryan. "Buddy didn't care if you were black, white, or green: He wanted smashmouth, and Duerson wouldn't nail guys. In practice, Buddy'd yell, 'That shit ain't cuttin' it! You dive on the ground again, I'm firing you!'"[2]

Duerson grew to accept Ryan's charge, and he became known as one of the fiercest hitters in the sport. In only his second season as a starter on that famed Bears defense, Duerson recorded seven sacks. Those seven sacks were the most by a defensive back ever in a season, a record that would not fall for almost 20 years.

In hindsight, it's probably easy to see that those hits took as much of a toll on Duerson as they probably did on the recipient. Alicia recalled that the blows did little to deter her ex-husband.

"Dave would get concussed on the first or second series and play the whole way through, or get a dinger in the second half and be back at practice Wednesday morning," she recounted to Solotaroff.[3]

Did Dave Duerson's suicide result from damage related to those concussions?

"I don't want to say that was the reason," Alicia Duerson told the *Chicago Tribune*. "I don't want to give a reason because I don't know. I only know what he told me—'Get my brain to the NFL. I think there is something wrong with the left side of my brain.'"[4]

Dan Pompei of the *Chicago Tribune* provided an account of Duerson's careful planning of his final act. At 2:30 p.m., Duerson's fiancée, Antoinette Sykes, called Ron Ben-David, the general manager of Ocean One, the condominium where the former Bears star now lived. She asked Ben-David to check on Duerson because she had not heard from him.

Ben-David knocked on the door and got no response. Minutes later, two security guards reported that Duerson's SUV was parked in his spot. Sykes granted Ben-David the right to enter the condo.

He and the guards tried to use a key to enter, but the door wouldn't open. Ben-David called 911 at 2:51 p.m. Fourteen minutes later paramedics arrived, followed shortly by police officers. They pushed through a chair that was keeping the door from opening.

The officers found Duerson lying under a sheet in a pool of blood.

In one of the notes he left, Duerson described his family issues, his financial trouble, and his growing mental issues. And as he expressed to his ex-wife, he stressed that he wanted to donate his brain to science.[5]

By shooting himself in the chest, Dave Duerson gave researchers the ability to study his brain.

Roughly 150 times each year a brain arrives at the Brain Bank at the Bedford Veterans' Administration Medical Center in Bedford, Massachusetts, where Dave Duerson's arrived in 2011. In its cold morgue, a noted neuropathologist spends much of her time each day studying these brains.

Dr. Ann McKee is the chief neuropathologist there, responsible for intensely scrutinizing the tissue of every brain her team receives. These are the brains of former soldiers—soldiers of war and soldiers on the football field.

And time after time, McKee finds evidence of trauma in these brains. She sees brains that have atrophied to a size and weight much smaller than what the brain of a football player should be. She sees abnormal accumulation of a particular protein in specific regions of the brains.

This brain damage now has a name—a diagnosis well known outside of medicine thanks in large part to Dr. McKee and her team: chronic traumatic encephalopathy (CTE).

McKee serves as the neuropathologist for the Center for the Study of Traumatic Encephalopathy. Among the other members of CSTE are Dr. Robert Stern, the director of Boston University's Alzheimer's Disease Clinical and Research Program; Chris Nowinski, founder of the Sports Legacy Institute; and Dr. Robert Cantu, a clinical professor of neurosurgery at Boston University.

The CSTE aims to collect brains of fallen athletes with early cognitive issues. Over 500 athletes have promised to have their brains delivered to the center for analysis after they die.

The CSTE maintains a patient registry, and the team interviews the families of the deceased athletes, obtaining information such as the sport and position played, the number of concussions suffered, and the presence of symptoms.

Dr. McKee takes the brains and studies them.

Dr. Cantu stressed the importance of this registry. "Out of that registry will come a lot of people that died without symptoms, and we'll start to get a better idea of the incidence and prevalence of this problem. Right now, it is very, very rare that we receive the brain of anyone who was asymptomatic."[6]

As of July 2015, the CSTE had analyzed the brains of 91 NFL players. Dr. McKee found evidence of CTE in 87 of them, including Dave Duerson's.[7]

Dave Duerson was born in Muncie, Indiana, the youngest of the four children of Julia and Arthur Duerson Jr. From an early age, young Dave quickly became a star in basketball and baseball, but he was dominant in football.

Unlike most future NFL stars, Duerson was arguably just as successful off the field. He made the National Honor Society in high school. He learned to play the trumpet and the tuba. He served internships at a law firm and with Sen. Richard Lugar. He earned a bachelor's degree in economics and openly dreamed about owning factories and running for the US Senate.

Duerson's football days earned him two Super Bowl rings. He won one with the 1986 Chicago Bears on the famed "Monsters of the Midway" defense. He won another in 1991 with the New York Giants.

As Duerson's days in football came to a close, members of both the Republican and Democratic Parties courted him to run for office. Ultimately he chose to enter the business world instead.

After opening a McDonald's franchise in Louisville, Kentucky, Duerson became a principal owner of a meat processing plant near his hometown of Chicago. In little time, Duerson's plant generated revenues of over $60 million per year.

Soon he had a mansion in Highland Park and expensive cars. He hosted sports talk shows and traveled to Europe to meet with presidents of foreign companies. His postfootball future looked to be even brighter than his stellar playing days.[8]

What happened, then, to bring a man so successful on and off the field to commit suicide two decades later?

To answer that question, we need to look within his brain to understand CTE.

Chronic traumatic encephalopathy is a progressive, degenerative brain disease. While it has received the most media attention after being found in former athletes, anyone with a history of repetitive head trauma, such as soldiers exposed to blasts, can develop it.

Doctors can only conclusively diagnose CTE in former athletes after they die. On autopsy, a neuropathologist finds characteristic accumulations of a certain protein, tau. Tau exists normally within the cells of the brain. This protein normally supports the microtubules that interconnect the brain cells.

For many possible reasons, including genetic mutations and repeated blows to the brain, the tau protein can become hyperphosphorylated. The cells can break down, and the tau protein can build up in clumps called neurofibrillary tangles.

Early in the course of the disease, the abnormal tau can collect in isolated spots in the cortex of the brain. As it progresses and the brain undergoes more degeneration, tau begins to accumulate around blood vessels and deep within the cortical sulci of the brain. It can affect the hippocampus, the region of the brain associated with memory and learning. It can build up in the amygdala, a region tasked with decision making and emotions.

The degeneration of the brain affected by CTE occurs slowly. Symptoms usually do not manifest for years after the brain trauma. In some cases, it can take a decade or longer. Symptoms generally progress as tau buildup spreads and more brain tissue degenerates.

Dr. Robert Cantu is a clinical professor of neurosurgery and codirector of the Center for the Study of Traumatic Encephalopathy at the Boston University School of Medicine. Cantu described three clusters of symptoms in CTE, which are difficult to distinguish from Alzheimer's disease.[9]

There is a mental cluster of symptoms that often starts with memory impairment. It can progress to more profound alterations in memory, insight, and judgment, which Cantu called "executive function impairment." Frank dementia can occasionally develop in later stages.

Lack of impulse control, marked by irritability and physically and verbally abusive behavior, comprises the second cluster of symptoms.

The third clinical part of the triad relates to emotional problems, especially depression. Anxiety and panic attacks often develop.

When attempting to make the diagnosis of CTE, a doctor must factor in the patient's exposure to brain trauma. If the player had a high exposure, such as thousands of subconcussive blows to the head from football or boxing, then developed these symptoms, the physician will likely find CTE. Unfortunately, the only way to make a definitive diagnosis is by examining the brain after the player dies.

In 2012 Dr. McKee and her team at the Boston University School of Medicine and the Center for the Study of Traumatic Encephalopathy published their findings from 85 patients—64 were athletes—found to have CTE by autopsy. Combined with a case history, they attempted to correlate each patient's symptoms with the brain findings to describe the spectrum of disease in CTE.

In stage I CTE, the brain usually remains about the normal weight, and limited tau tangles exist in the superior and dorsolateral frontal cortices. Clinical symptoms include headaches, difficulty with concentration, and short-term memory loss. Depression and aggression can start to appear.

In stage II CTE, the ventricles appear enlarged. Tau protein and neurofibrillary tangles can collect in multiple discrete areas of the cerebral cortex. Depression and mood swings more commonly accompany memory loss and headaches. Impulsivity, exclusivity, mood swings, and even suicide begin to manifest.

As the disease advances to stage III, the brain starts to atrophy and the ventricles dilate further. Neurofibrillary tangles are found diffusely throughout multiple areas of the brain. Cognitive decline is more apparent as memory loss, trouble with attention and concentration, mood swings, aggression, depression, and apathy worsen.

Stage IV CTE represents the most severe brain degeneration. The brain's weight is significantly less than normal ones or even brains with less advanced CTE. Tau protein buildup is noted diffusely throughout the cerebrum, brain stem, and spinal cord. Severe memory loss and dementia, paranoia, aggression, explosivity, and language problems are notable. In McKee's study 31% of the patients with stage IV CTE were suicidal at some point in their course.[10]

What is important to note about the disease's progression is that the brain degenerates slowly. Memory loss, confusion, bad judgment, impulse control struggles, depression, and dementia might show up months after brain trauma. Or it might take many years for the disease to bring down a former star athlete.

It is difficult to know when Duerson's decline began, but it was a dramatic fall from the multi-million-dollar plant, fancy house and cars, and trips to Europe.

According to Paul Solotaroff in *Men's Journal*, in 2002 Duerson sold his controlling stake in the meat processing plant after troubles with his business partner began. Duerson opened his own plant, which featured high-tech freezers he had bought from a Dutch company. Those freezers were unreliable, and Duerson's company struggled to supply Burger King and Olive Garden chains. His company quickly floundered, and he was forced to borrow money, then had to close the plant.

Through the struggles, his employees and family began noticing that he was angrier and treating people badly. Ex-wife Alicia noticed a sudden onset of temper, wild mood swings, and even violent tendencies. The husband she had fallen in love with, she told Solotaroff, "would never do that; he never showed violence toward me. It was the changes."[11]

Those behavioral changes manifested most vividly in an incident at Notre Dame in 2005. Late one February night, Dave and Alicia argued in their hotel room. Duerson threw Alicia out of the hotel room into the hall in what he later called "a three-second snap." Alicia went to a local emergency room with dizziness and cuts to her head. Duerson later pled guilty to domestic battery and resigned from the board of trustees at Notre Dame.

In the next few years, Duerson realized something more than regular aging was happening. His memory increasingly failed, so he often wrote notes to remember dates and locations. He couldn't sleep well. He complained of headaches and blurry vision.

After his divorce from Alicia in 2009, he moved into the Ocean One condo in Sunny Isles Beach, where he was rarely seen. Even there, he did his best to hide his financial desperation and symptoms.

Even his fiancée, Antoinette Sykes, whom Duerson met less than a year before he took his life, did not understand the gravity of his issues. "I knew he had headaches and—and a lump on his skull that he was worried about," Sykes told Solotaroff. "Maybe he wanted to shield me, but he seemed so excited about spending the rest of our lives together. On our last night, Valentine's, he joked that I owed him 29 more because we'd committed to 30 years of wedded bliss. And then I flew home to pack my things to move down there."[12]

On the morning of February 17, 2011, Duerson texted Sykes, "My dear Angel, I love you so much and I'm sorry for my past, but I think this knot on my head is the real deal."[13]

When authorities found his body approximately 12 hours after he shot himself in the chest, the rest of the condo was immaculate. Despite Duerson's failing brain, which had led to his memory and mood struggles, the detectives noted that they had never observed a suicide so meticulously executed and planned.

Dr. Cantu sees this progressive decline in patients later diagnosed with CTE.

"There are horrible life changes in terms of memory, emotion, and lack of impulse control, which heaps gobs of negativity on them, divorce, addiction, businesses that fail," Cantu explained to Jane Leavy of *Grantland*. "It's a vicious cycle, a perfect storm. The final event for those that die young is not the brain damage per se but what the brain damage has led them to do, which is what caused Dave Duerson to put a gun to his chest."[14]

As he wished, Dave Duerson's brain was sent to Boston University's Center for the Study of Traumatic Encephalopathy. McKee examined Duerson's brain and "found indisputable evidence of C.T.E. in the tissue samples, with 'no evidence of any other disorder,'" according to Alan Schwarz in the *New York Times*.

"It's tragic that Dave Duerson took his own life, but it's very meaningful that he recognized the symptoms of the disorder—it validates this condition," McKee claimed.[15]

Dr. McKee showed Leavy the slides of Duerson's brain for her 2012 *Grantland* interview. "You see all those little spots of damage?" Dr. McKee asked Leavy. "And he doesn't even have the worst case of this. This is really substantial disease, especially since he's only 50."[16]

Dave Duerson had stage III CTE.

Ex-wife Alicia and their four children attended the Boston press conference at which McKee's team announced the findings of Duerson's CTE. One of the children, Tregg, who had also suffered a concussion playing football, spoke his wish that his father's death would help future generations of football players: "It is our hope that through this research questions that go beyond our interest may be answered—questions that lead to a safer game of football from professionals to Pop Warner."[17]

Progressive neurologic deterioration had been described in boxers in 1928. That form of brain disease, also related to repetitive head trauma, became known as dementia pugilistica.

In 2005 Dr. Bennet Omalu studied the brain of former Pittsburgh Steelers center Mike Webster. Dr. Omalu was the medical examiner for Pittsburgh, and since Webster had died in his jurisdiction, he had the task of performing the autopsy.

Omalu expected to find a brain with signs of Alzheimer's disease, but he saw very different features. He found abnormal proteins and neurofibrillary tangles inconsistent with Alzheimer's disease.

Two years later, another ex-Steeler died in his area. Dr. Omalu was not working when Terry Long died, but the pathologist who performed the autopsy saved the brain for him. He spoke to Long's wife to confirm that Long had tried to commit suicide several times, as Mike Webster had.

Now Omalu had two cases of CTE—in two former professional football players.

He published his findings on Mike Webster in the journal *Neurosurgery*. In that paper, "Chronic Traumatic Encephalopathy in a National Football League Player," Omalu described the degenerative changes seen in the brain, which he proposed resulted from long-term repetitive blows to the brain, possibly from football.

After the paper was published, Drs. Ira Casson and Elliot Pellman from the NFL's Mild Traumatic Brain Injury (MTBI) Committee, involved in guiding the NFL's concussion policies, asked the journal to retract that paper.

"We have demonstrated that Omalu et al.'s case does not meet the clinical or neuropathological criteria of chronic traumatic encephalopathy. We, therefore, urge the authors to retract their paper or sufficiently revise it and its title after more detailed investigation of this case," they wrote in a letter to the editor published in the journal in 2006.[18]

In response to that letter, Kenneth C. Kutner, an assistant professor of neuro-psychology at Weill Cornell Medical College and one of the reviewers of Omalu's study prior to its publication, called it a "seminal study in the field." In contesting Casson's opinion, he wrote, "Specifically, they took an extreme stand in actually urging the authors to retract the article. Their stand is quite excessive and, in my opinion, inappropriate. Articles should be considered for retraction if they contain fabricated data, contamination of data, or allegation of misconduct. It is my opinion that there is no justification for retracting this article."[19]

The now-defunct MTBI Committee published one of its 16 studies in the journal *Neurosurgery* in December 2005. "Professional football players do not sustain frequent repetitive blows to the brain on a regular basis," members of that committee asserted in the paper. They also claimed that chronic damage "has never been reported in American football players."[20]

Omalu's paper, however, did report CTE in a professional football player, Mike Webster. Earlier that year, a federal court had come to a similar conclusion.

Webster had filed a disability claim in 1999 with the NFL retirement board. The board concluded that repeated blows to the head rendered Webster "totally and permanently disabled." In documents obtained by *Outside the Lines* and *Frontline*, the director of the NFL's retirement plan, Sarah E. Gaunt, wrote on May 8, 2000, "The Retirement Board determined that Mr. Webster's disability arose while he was an Active Player." She concluded that Webster's medical reports "indicate that his disability is the result of head injuries he suffered as a football player with the Pittsburgh Steelers and Kansas City Chiefs."[21]

Dr. Edward Westbrook, a neurologist who performed an independent examination of Webster for the retirement board, told Steve Fainaru and Mark Fainaru-Wada that he was certain "multiple hits" from football had caused Webster's problems.

Webster won partial benefits from the board—over $8,000 per month—but was denied full compensation because the board believed he did not become fully disabled until his playing days were over. After Webster's death, his estate sued the retirement board.

On April 26, 2005, the same year members of the MTBI Committee tried to force retraction of Omalu's CTE paper about Webster, the federal court ruled in favor of Webster's estate, awarding $1.8 million.[22]

The NFL would not acknowledge a link between repeated concussions and long-term brain injuries until December 2009.

Dr. McKee and Chris Nowinski held a press conference to discuss football and CTE at the 2009 Super Bowl to educate the public about CTE and the concussions and subconcussive blows in football that they felt led to the disease. The NFL's MTBI Committee asked McKee to present her cases to the committee. The committee was resistant to her findings.

"We've seen this time and time again in medicine, when there's a shift in our thinking, and someone says that there's something different," McKee explained. "We all resist change. I think the more invested you are in the procedure or the activity, the more likely you are to resist any change. The NFL clearly is very invested in protecting the sport that is the center of their livelihood, and they're going to be resistant to the suggestion of change just out of basic human nature."[23]

Critics often claim McKee is trying to bring down football, but she insisted, "I know I don't think about football. Honestly, I think about the health and well-being of these families. I think about the health and well-being of these people, these athletes, and also military veterans. Frankly, that's where my concern lies, just in trying to prevent this from happening to other individuals. I would say that my focus is not on a sport. It's not on an activity. It's really on health and maintaining brain wellness."[24]

As more and more cases of CTE have been found and more studies have confirmed these brain changes, more awareness—and acceptance—have followed.

In April 2010 the NFL gave the Center for the Study of Traumatic Encephalopathy $1 million to help with its research.

More and more research has led most neurologic experts to conclude that CTE is associated with repetitive brain trauma. It could result from repetitive subconcussive blows. These mild blows to the head—such as those experienced by offensive and defensive linemen when they collide at the start of each play—are likely more a factor than diagnosed concussions.

"There's this one thing that we do know about CTE. Every individual who has had a neuropathologically-confirmed diagnosis of CTE has had one thing in common, and that is a history of repetitive hits to the head," Dr. Robert Stern observed.[25]

The challenge in establishing links between playing football and developing CTE is the distinction between correlation and causation. Essentially, repeated trauma to the brain is required for a former athlete to develop CTE, but it alone does not necessarily cause CTE. We don't know how many hits are necessary to start the brain's degeneration. We don't know what kinds of hits cause these changes. And we don't know what other factors are involved.

Since CTE can only be confirmed by autopsy after a player's death, currently we don't have a good method to calculate the incidence of CTE. Given the huge number of kids that play youth football, some of whom eventually play at higher levels, why don't we hear of far more cases of CTE?

After all, when factoring in professional, nonprofessional, college, and high school football, approximately 1.8 million athletes played football in 2009. Even if the symptoms don't appear for years after athletes retire from football, one might expect more athletes to develop CTE.

Genetic factors could influence the risk for CTE. For example, people who carry the apolipoprotein E (APOE) gene's ε4 allele might be more susceptible to developing CTE. APOE ε4 has also been associated with longer recovery time and more severe cognitive deficits following single traumatic brain injuries in professional football players and boxers. APOE ε4 carriers are believed to have worse outcomes both in the short term and the long term following head injuries.

Although CTE does have some correlation to the APOE ε4 allele, it isn't a one-to-one correlation, Dr. Cantu observed. The majority of cases don't have it, but some of the cases with the greatest amount of dementia do. Much more research into genetic links such as APOE and other risk factors is needed.[26]

Other factors probably exist as well, given that not all players exposed to the same amount of head trauma wind up developing CTE. Nutritional and environmental factors that we haven't found yet likely play a role in who develops CTE.

Mike Oliver, the executive director of NOCSAE, made that same point regarding the role of football helmets in brain injury. A variety of factors that could have nothing to do with protective equipment could influence the development of concussive events. The underlying health of the athlete, his blood pressure, hydration, electrolyte imbalances, and other factors could be involved.[27]

Until tests can detect CTE brain changes in living patients, we will never truly know the incidence of CTE among football players.

In July 2015 Dr. McKee's group compiled their data on the cases of CTE they had diagnosed in former football players: 87 of 91 NFL players studied showed brain evidence of CTE.

Perhaps more worrisome were the group's findings about players at different ages and skill levels. Seven of nine semiprofessional players, twenty-six of thirty-two college players, and seven of twenty-four high school players examined had CTE.[28]

Since these were cases in which athletes had symptoms, and the athletes or their families wanted the brains studied, one could argue that these data are flawed by selection bias. Certainly this is at least somewhat true, Dr. McKee admitted. Although 87 of the 91 brains might have had CTE, that by no means suggests that 87 of every 91 football players will develop these changes.

> Very select sample, no question about it. Here's what I would say to that. It's not been difficult for us to collect cases of CTE. We don't know what the exact incidence and prevalence of this disease is. That's probably going to require being able to diagnose it in living people to come up with a real number. One thing that it does say to us is that this is not uncommon because it's been quite easy for us to collect these cases over the last seven years, and really just beginning in earnest about four years ago. They're out there.
>
> We only recruit for exposure to this sport. We don't ask for symptoms, but of course families usually donate only if they're interested in finding out why a person behaved in the way they did, or maybe they committed suicide. There's usually some reason why a family wants to donate, and that skews it much more towards people that are symptomatic and have the disease. Even that said, we've been remarkably successful at finding it.[29]

Dr. Cantu agreed that the numbers might be skewed because they mainly receive brains from athletes whose families noticed symptoms before the players died.[30]

The bottom line, however, is that if even a small percentage of the 1.8 million athletes who play football each year develops CTE, we have a big problem.

Diagnosing these former athletes after death helps us learn more about CTE, but it doesn't help those athletes. We need to identify them while they are still playing football, or at least while they are still alive and healthy.

Research into tests to identify brain changes in living patients is under way. A 2013 study published in the *American Journal of Geriatric Psychiatry* by Gary W. Small and other researchers used a certain type of scan—FDDNP-PET—to identify tau deposits in the brain. They administered that test to five retired NFL players with mood and cognitive symptoms. They identified tau deposits in characteristic regions of the brain not present in five control subjects they tested.

The researchers admitted that they cannot confirm CTE in these ex-players until autopsy. More research and more patients are needed to see if this test will help doctors in future years.[31]

Ira R. Casson, MD, and several other researchers used MRI studies as well as neurological and neuropsychological tests to evaluate 45 retired NFL players. In their study, published in the September–October 2014 issue of *Sports Health*, they concluded: "MRI lesions and neuropsychological impairments were found in some players; however, the majority of retired NFL players had no clinical signs of chronic brain damage."[32]

In an editorial in the opening pages of that issue entitled "Better News," *Sports Health* editor in chief Edward M. Wojtys, MD, claimed that Casson's study painted "a more optimistic picture than recent studies and press reports."

"Most important, this study appears to refute the current belief, held by many, that the cumulative effect of concussion in NFL players results in chronic brain injury. While 13% showed objective evidence of brain trauma, 87% did not, despite the use of very sensitive techniques for detecting injured brain tissue," Dr. Wojtys wrote.[33]

Still, is a study of former NFL players showing chronic brain damage in 13% of them really better news for football? That's essentially one in seven players. Of the 11 offensive players and 11 defensive players on the field at one time, three would develop chronic brain injury.

No wonder many retired NFL players fear they could wind up like Dave Duerson one day.

Today many current and recently retired NFL players think it's only a matter of time before their brains start to fail. A *Sporting News* survey of 125 former NFL players found that 68%—more than two in three—worry that they will decline mentally or believe that they have already started doing so.[34]

Actuarial data given to a federal court by the NFL as part of a settlement of the class-action lawsuit brought by over 4,500 former players gives players good reason to worry. The league recognized that up to one-third of all retired NFL players could eventually develop long-term cognitive dysfunction. For some players, the risk could be up to 35 times greater than it is for the general population.[35]

Certainly suffering concussions on the gridiron presents at least some risk. Retired players who suffered three or more concussions during their playing days were three times more likely to be later diagnosed with depression.[36] They were five times more likely to be diagnosed with mild cognitive impairment, according to studies published by Kevin Guskiewicz and his team.[37]

Authors of a 2012 study published in the journal *Neurology* looked at data on more than 3,000 former NFL players who had spent at least five years in the league. They found that those players were four times more likely to die of brain diseases like Alzheimer's disease or amyotrophic lateral sclerosis (ALS, better known as Lou Gehrig's disease) than the average American adult.[38]

Available research seems to indicate that the length of exposure to football, especially at a high level, affects a player's risk of developing CTE.

Dr. Stern aims to learn why one person might be prone to developing CTE while another person isn't. Knowing that the brains of boys go through a critical window of development between the ages of 10 and 12, he and others in his lab published two studies in 2015 looking at the age of first exposure to tackle football and its effect on the brain and cognitive function.

In the first study, published in the journal *Neurology*, they studied matched pairs of former NFL players between the ages of 40 and 69 who played football for at least 12 years and at least two seasons in the NFL.

They found that former NFL players who started playing tackle football before age 12 performed significantly worse on tests of memory, problem solving, and estimated verbal intelligence than those who started playing at 12 or older.

The research team then looked at a specific part of the brain that undergoes a tremendous amount of maturation between ages 10 and 12, the corpus callosum. This is a bundle of nerve fiber tracts that carry information between the two hemispheres of the brain. They determined that the former NFL players who started playing tackle football before age 12 had significantly worse alterations of the integrity of these brain structures than those who started playing at age 12 or older.

Dr. Stern warned that these studies must be interpreted with caution. The participants were a very select group of people: those who went on to play professional football. The studies cannot be generalized to people who only played up to high school or only played up to college. They can't be generalized to people who are playing the sport now, because it is a different era in how this sport is played, for better or worse.

This information does start to offer insight into the problem, though. "What it does say in my mind is it begins to answer our hypothesis, which is if you expose the developing brain to repetitive head impacts during a potential critical window of vulnerability, there may be later life consequences."[39]

Clearly not every football player will develop CTE. This research, though, does seem to suggest that kids who start playing tackle football at an early age, especially before age 12, could be at risk. The longer they expose themselves to brain trauma in the form of concussive and subconcussive blows, the greater their chances could be of developing the disease.

The challenge is knowing when and how much brain trauma is too much. It's hard to argue that today's players, at least in the NFL, understand the risk. But is it possible for them to play for years and get out of the sport before any long-term damage occurs?

Even with documented concussions, it can be difficult for players to know when to stop and when a doctor should advise them to retire. No threshold number of concussions has been shown, so we can't know exactly how many is too many.

Symptom duration is one possible factor. An athlete with a history of multiple concussions, especially where the degree of impact decreases with increasing numbers of concussions or the symptoms last longer each time, is a candidate for retirement. Likewise, an athlete with only one concussion but one that was severe enough to cause symptoms to last for months might consider retirement as well.

Dave Duerson was one of those former players who understood that his brain function was deteriorating. Interestingly he never sought compensation from the NFL retirement board, which Mike Webster and other players turned to for help with their brain injuries.

Perhaps more surprisingly, Duerson sat on that very committee. This was the same former player who had testified as a plaintiff for the players against the NFL in trials that led to free agency and other rights for players, including the creation of a board to hear the disability claims of former and current players.

Former Minnesota Vikings guard Brent Boyd recalled to Paul Solotaroff that the board routinely denied the disability claims of former players with cognitive impairment. Suffering from depression he felt was related to brain injuries in football, Boyd claimed, "They made it real clear that they'd fight me to the death, like they did with Mike Webster. They were supposed to push for us, but were in the owners' pockets. You had to live in a wheelchair to collect."[40]

Duerson was appointed to the board in 2006 and often berated former players. He openly questioned Boyd's claim that football had caused his issues in front of a Senate committee. At a congressional hearing, Duerson became involved in an altercation with two former players who were speaking out for injured veterans. And he called a radio talk show to call Brian DeMarco a liar after DeMarco openly discussed his rejection by the board.

Boyd later argued that Duerson was part of the problem. "He caused more suffering personally than all the other board members combined," he asserted.[41]

John Hogan, an attorney who helped retired players with their disability claims, told Solotaroff that Duerson should have discussed his own struggles to help himself and others fighting the same battles. "He really could've changed the story for vets, and done it from the inside without saying mea culpa. He didn't have to indict the system. All he had to do was say, publicly, 'I'm sick, and I need help like these other guys.'"[42]

After his suicide in 2011, Duerson's family did speak up. They filed a wrongful death suit against the NFL. They claimed that the league did not do enough to prevent or treat the 10 or more concussions Duerson reportedly suffered during his career. They argued that those injuries led to his brain damage and ultimately cost him his life.

"If they knowingly failed to inform and implement proper safety concussion procedures, then their indifference was the epitome of injustice," Tregg Duerson remarked in a press conference announcing the family's lawsuit against the league. "The inactions of the past inevitably led to the demise and death of my father."[43]

Eventually the case brought by Duerson's family against the NFL was rolled into a class-action lawsuit involving about 5,000 former players and their families.

Just before the start of the 2013 season, attorneys for the NFL and former players announced a proposed settlement. The agreement would reportedly cover all former players—approximately 18,000 of them—and their beneficiaries.

As part of the $765 million settlement, the league would set aside $675 million for damages. This fund would include payments up to $5 million for a retired player diagnosed with Lou Gehrig's disease, up to $4 million for a player's death due to a traumatic brain injury, and as much as $3 million for a player suffering from dementia.

The settlement also reportedly proposed $75 million for medical exams for retired players and $10 million for concussion education and research.

As part of the settlement between the NFL and retired players, the league would not be obligated to acknowledge that it had withheld information about the dangers of blows to the head from football.

District Court Judge Anita Brody initially rejected the proposed settlement, citing concerns that $675 million would fail to compensate every athlete who might one day need financial assistance. Brody granted preliminary approval to the settlement once the NFL agreed to remove the cap on damages.

"A class action settlement that offers prompt relief is superior to the likely alternative—years of expensive, difficult, and uncertain litigation, with no assurance of recovery, while retired players' physical and mental conditions continue to deteriorate," Brody argued.[44]

On April 18, 2016, the US Third Circuit Court of Appeals upheld a district court's approval of the settlement.[45] Duerson's family had filed an objection to the settlement, calling the agreement unfair for limiting payments to families of players who develop CTE.

Bill Gibbs, the attorney for the family, passionately condemned the settlement. "Duerson did not kill himself for CTE to be forever eviscerated from the NFL's lexicon."[46]

Whether or not the NFL knew the dangers of concussions and repetitive subconcussive blows and hid them from players, media attention to the problem has dominated coverage of the sport over the last few years. Clearly efforts to make pro football safer are underway, but it is difficult to tell if they are working.

The NFL announced that concussions dropped 13% between 2010 and 2011. Some credited moving kickoffs from the 30-yard line to the 35 and increased awareness of head injuries for the decrease.

According to a report from ESPN's *Outside the Lines* and PBS's FRONTLINE, these numbers might not tell the entire story. Mark Fainaru-Wada and Steve Fainaru pointed out that concussion numbers from the postseason, practices, and bye weeks likely were not included in the data. The concussion total might actually be about 50 higher.

According to a Concussion Watch database created by *Outside the Lines* and FRONTLINE, the number of players listed in team injury reports averaged 5.4 per week in 2009, 7.6 in 2010, and 8.4 in 2011.[47]

Increased awareness of concussions might have led to more cautious management of these injuries by NFL medical staffs. In a study published in a 2010 issue of *Sports Health*, Ira Casson provided data comparing concussion treatment between the periods 1996–2001 and 2002–2007. In the second period, the number of players held out of play for more than seven days doubled compared to the first period. The percentage of players held out for more than 14 days increased from 1.8% to 5.9%. The mean number of days that players missed due to a concussion increased from 1.92 to 4.73. The authors of the study believed that more understanding and caution among the players, coaches, athletic trainers, and doctors existed after 2002.[48]

Many former NFL players, journalists, and even physicians have claimed that the media have sensationalized the topic of CTE and unnecessarily scared parents. Dr. McKee disagrees:

> I think the media has been very helpful. This is a problem that needs urgent recognition. It's a crisis that needs immediate attention. We need to get ahead of this problem because this is something that's affecting athletes at the prime of their life. Yes, there's been some sensationalism about this disorder, but this is a problem that the public needs to address and needs to get ahead of as soon as possible. I think the media has played a very important role in keeping this in the public awareness, keeping it at the top of our minds because there's a tendency for us to become complacent and just roll over and forget about the importance of this disease.[49]

Ultimately the decision by professional athletes to play football comes down to risk. If everyone involved—professional athletes, youth players, parents, and coaches— knows the risks involved in playing football, then they can make a rational decision.

Even President Barack Obama, when asked by David Remnick of the *New Yorker* if he would allow his kids to play football, admitted that players today know what they're getting into. "At this point, there's a little bit of caveat emptor," Obama remarked. "These guys, they know what they're doing. They know what they're buying into. It is no longer a secret. It's sort of the feeling I have about smokers, you know?"[50]

Despite many fearing for their future health, today's pro players—unlike those in Dave Duerson's days—largely understand the risks of repeated blows to the head, and yet they choose to keep playing. Despite doctors recognizing the dangers of concussions, much of the diagnosis and treatment of athletes' injuries still relies on the players telling someone they got hurt.

That is a huge challenge for the medical staffs of football teams. Athletic trainers and team doctors stand on the sidelines and try to watch every player on the field. It's almost impossible to see every hit from the sidelines, and it is easy to miss a player appearing dazed for a few seconds. The NFL and college conferences have attempted to remedy this problem by placing concussion "spotters" in the press boxes. These observers could call down to the athletic trainers or team doctors if they see athletes who appear to be concussed. Still, we have heard many professional athletes admit that they don't always tell the medical staffs that they have suffered an injury.

Despite our knowledge of the health risks, a majority of players would play with a concussion. A 2012 *Sporting News* survey of 103 players from 27 teams found that 56% of players admitted that they would hide concussion symptoms to keep playing.[51]

Surely these numbers are scary, and the media attention to concussions and CTE has cast a negative light on the game. The question, then, is what effect knowledge of these risks is having on younger players.

ESPN *the Magazine* surveyed 300 prep players about concussions in 2010, before Dave Duerson committed suicide and the players' concussion lawsuits against the NFL began. In the survey, 45% of prep players said that they would risk permanent brain damage for a chance to play in the NFL. Over half of them—54.1%—would want a star teammate who suffered a concussion during a hypothetical state title game to stay in the game.[52]

Many people have likened the risk of developing CTE from professional football to cigarette smokers developing lung and other cancers. Understanding the risk and avoiding that risk by not doing it plays at least some role in both cigarette smoking and banging heads in the NFL.

Parents and young athletes must understand that the risk of long-term brain injury is not limited to NFL players. High school football players might have an even higher risk for brain injuries than college athletes. A 2013 study by the Institute of Medicine and the National Research Council found that high school players suffer 11.2 concussions for every 10,000 games and practices, compared to 6.3 among college players.[53] In addition, concern exists that concussion symptoms last longer in younger athletes.

It is unknown how likely it is that those concussions lead to chronic brain disease in high school athletes, so parents might dismiss the risks for their children.

The brain of a young athlete under the age of 14 is more vulnerable than those of older, more mature athletes. Myelin is the protective coating of the nerve fibers. It adds strength and aids in the transmission of the nerve fibers. Unmyelinated nerve fibers are more easily damaged by violent shaking of the brain.

Most of the circuitry between different regions of the brain develops from the ages of 10 to 12. By injuring the brain during these years, a player might set himself up for intellectual or emotional problems or issues with impulse control.

While young football players aren't exposed to tackles with the same impact that NFL players deliver, they also don't have the same neck strength to help withstand those forces. Their disproportionately larger heads and weak necks create what Dr. Cantu called a bobblehead doll effect.

"This bobblehead doll effect means you don't have to hit a youngster's head very hard or even another part of their body and you whiplash the brain. You shake it quite violently."[54]

Perhaps it is no surprise that Dr. Cantu now advocates that children avoid tackle football until they are 14 years old.

Dr. Stern also questioned the head trauma to which parents expose their kids:

When I take my scientist hat off and put my normal person hat on, I have to ask, "Does it make sense to expose our children to repetitive hits to their head during a time when we know their brains are developing in an extensive fashion?" We do everything else to protect our kids, to make sure they are safe in all ways. It's amazing all the things we do in our society to improve the safety of our children and to make sure they have the very best health and are injury free and have the best possible outcomes in life. And yet, as a society, we condone dropping kids off at a field where they then hit their heads over and over again, in a sanctioned fashion.[55]

It is important to point out that sports other than football also present a risk for brain trauma. Dr. Cantu stated that young soccer players should not be allowed to head the ball under age 14. Ice hockey players should be restricted from total body checking under age 14 as well.

Dr. Cantu's concerns about soccer heading stem somewhat from concerns about repeated blows to the head. More, though, he worried that most of the traumatic events occur during the act of heading. Young players go to head the ball, and they collide heads with an opponent, take elbows to the head, or fall and hit their heads.[56]

Brandi Chastain, a member of the 1999 US Women's National Team that won the Women's World Cup, acknowledged her worries about the risks of heading in soccer for young players. She and teammates Cindy Parlow Cone and Joy Fawcett teamed up with the Sports Legacy Institute and the Santa Clara Institute of Sports Law and Ethics to start a campaign called Parents and Pros for Safer Soccer.

The campaign calls for the sport to eliminate heading the ball for athletes under age 14.

Chastain wants to leave soccer in a better place than it was when she and her teammates started playing. She believes that the campaign can make a difference not only for young players who still suffer symptoms from concussions and can't play, but also for the sport and the next generation of kids who will play soccer.

"I honestly think there are more people coming to grips with the fact that concussion and concussion syndrome, this CTE, this is the real deal," Chastain explained. "This is not kids being weak or being lazy or not being tough enough. This is real. We don't know enough about the brain. I sure don't. I'm not a scientist. What I have heard and what I have seen in studies is alarming. As a parent and as a coach, I have to be responsible and educated. If I can't say for sure that what I'm asking these kids to do is safe, then there is no reason for me to have them do it."[57]

The US Soccer Federation announced in late 2015 that it was implementing several safety initiatives aimed at decreasing head injuries in soccer. In particular, players under the age of 10 will be prohibited from heading the ball. Heading will be limited in practice for players between the ages of 11 to 13.

These guidelines will apply to all youth national teams and academies under US Soccer as well as the Major League Soccer youth club teams. For other leagues, these guidelines would only serve as recommendations.

If a young athlete does want to play football, though, what can a parent do to minimize the risk of brain trauma? Much like in boxing, these impacts are probably impossible to completely avoid. Since the brain is more vulnerable at a young age, a mother could restrict her child to playing flag football until he is 14. He could learn the techniques and skills of his position and concentrate on strategies in the game. Then, when he is older and his brain is more developed, he could play tackle football.

As he starts tackle football in high school, the young athlete's risk of brain trauma does not disappear. Therefore, he and his team can practice without some of the activities that produce repetitive brain trauma. Although NFL teams practice throughout the season and frequently in the offseason, running drills and practicing plays, they have a limited number of practices over the course of a season in which players wear full pads, hit each other, and take players to the ground.

"As parents, let's not get paranoid about it," Dr. Cantu reasoned. "All of our kids are going to have head trauma as they grow up. We have a pretty good protective system for occasional head trauma, but no head trauma is good for the brain. You cannot condition the brain to take head trauma."[58]

In a February 13, 2012, article in *Grantland*, economists Kevin Grier and Tyler Cowen presented a possible scenario that could bring about the end of football. Other notable thinkers have made similar arguments, including Malcolm Gladwell, George Will, and Buzz Bissinger. While seemingly too big and popular to disappear, football could suffer a gradual death brought about by numerous events.

First, Grier and Cowen point to lawsuits over concussions and CTE. Multi-million-dollar lawsuits could scare volunteer coaches, referees, and doctors away from high school football. Insurance companies fearful of these lawsuits slowly stop insuring schools and teams. When helmets and other technological approaches fail to decrease concussion rates, high schools and colleges shut down football programs. Sponsors start to shy away from the sport, and football becomes less profitable.

The most telling—and likely—point the economists make is that the pool of talented players slowly dries up. Parents become increasingly wary of the health risks in the sport and steer their kids to other activities.[59]

Many diehard football fans believe such a scenario is impossible, but we are already starting to see cracks in the resolve of parents.

An Associated Press poll of 1,044 adults found that 44% of parents are uncomfortable with their children playing football.[60] Worse, a recent *Outside the Lines* survey of 1,000 parents conducted by ESPN Research and the Global Strategy Group found that 57% say the increased attention to concussions in football has made them less likely to allow their sons to play football.[61]

These fears aren't shared just by the average mom and dad across America, either. Notable ex-NFL stars such as Troy Aikman, Kurt Warner, and Terry Bradshaw have expressed reservations about encouraging their sons to play football. Even President Obama admitted that if he had a son, he would "have to think long and hard" before letting him play football, he told the *New Republic*.[62]

There is evidence that parents' concerns are actually leading to a drop in youth football participation.

Pop Warner, the largest youth football program in the United States, recently experienced a drop in participation for the first time in decades. Despite growing every year through 2010, the organization saw a drop in participation of 9.5% over the two-year period from 2010 to 2012.

The chief medical officer for Pop Warner, neurosurgeon Dr. Julian Bailes, acknowledged that the concerns over brain injuries were "the No. 1 cause."[63]

The National Sporting Goods Association has reported a similar trend, finding a 13% decrease in participation in tackle football between 2011 and 2012, especially among kids aged 7 to 11.[64]

The NFL recognizes this trend and notes its efforts to make the game safer. In an ESPN article by Paula Lavigne presenting the data from the *Outside the Lines* survey of parental concerns, NFL spokesman Greg Aiello emphasized the league's role in promoting concussion education and safety. Among its strategies, the NFL has lobbied states in support of the Lystedt Law, a law in Washington State that requires any athlete who suffers an injury that appears to be a concussion to be removed from the practice or game and kept out until cleared by a medical professional. Similar laws now exist in all 50 states.[65]

Each year a small but growing number of parents decide that football is not worth the risk. On the other hand, many parents and fans love the game despite the research studies and media reports.

Is there a middle ground where we can make the sport safer?

Removing any player suspected of having a concussion from a game or practice is a good start. Whether there is a law about it or not, coaches, athletic trainers, and doctors must recognize the signs and symptoms of concussions and pull the player out. The risk of a much more serious injury increases dramatically as the concussed player returns before his brain has fully healed.

Ideally the parents of the concussed athlete would have the child fully evaluated by a neurologist or neuropsychologist familiar with concussions and concussion evaluation. Physicians could use cognitive and psychological tests to fully evaluate the brain function rather than relying on the athlete admitting symptoms.

Teams and schools should use baseline concussion tests before each season so that the neurologists have an accurate assessment of the cognitive function of each child when healthy. And physicians could readminister the test as the player heals from his brain injury.

Parents and coaches should stress to the athletes that they must tell someone that they have suffered a head injury. The player needs to understand the symptoms—whether headaches, dizziness, sensitivity to light, blurry vision, nausea, or any others—and tell the coach. He can tell the team doctor or athletic trainer. We have seen how athletes at all levels of football, from the NFL to high school, deny symptoms to stay in the game. That attitude must change.

Ironically, despite suffering numerous concussions in his career, Dave Duerson took these injuries seriously when his son Tregg played. In a high school game, Tregg got up from a tackle and staggered off the field. Duerson charged down from the stands to the sidelines and grabbed his son's helmet so he couldn't return to the game. At halftime, Duerson took Tregg to the hospital for evaluation. Duerson kept his son from playing for three games.[66]

One of the popular ideas to stem the concussion problem is to have parents buy state-of-the-art helmets. Unfortunately, while these newer helmets might absorb some of the impact from a big blow, they can't control rotational forces to the head or the whiplash-like blows to the brain when it collides with the skull from a hit to the chest. Even these high-tech helmets can't prevent all concussions.

Mike Oliver of NOCSAE points out the difference between two types of brain injuries: "There are those that occur from a focal injury, so if you hit somebody in the head with a hammer, for example, and break the skull, you get an injury to the brain."

Helmets probably protect athletes from those impacts fairly well. For the other type of impact, in which the brain rattles around within the skull, helmets probably provide little benefit.

"The analogy would be to the egg inside an egg shell," Oliver stated. "I can protect that egg shell. I can wrap it up in all kinds of things and drop it off a 10-story building. The egg won't crack. It will survive, but the stuff inside the egg, that yolk is going to be scrambled. Asking a helmet to prevent that yolk inside the egg, if you will, from moving around or folding in on itself or twisting, there's just so much that the helmet can do."[67]

When we specifically look at helmet technology, Oliver offered some discouraging data. Despite analyses showing that newer helmets might resist impacts 15% or 20% better than helmets bought 10 or 15 years ago, researchers haven't seen any benefit in terms of concussions. Studies have found no association between the brand or the age of a helmet and the likelihood of concussion.

A soon-to-be released study looked not only at the age and brand of the helmet, but also specifically at the model of helmet and its Virginia Tech star ratings. At the high school level, the researchers found no correlation between the likelihood of a concussion and what model of helmet an athlete wore or what its star rating was.

Parents often want the newest, most expensive technology, thinking that these helmets are the most protective. "So far, the data in the field doesn't suggest that that's the case," Oliver lamented.[68]

One challenge is predicting which head impacts will cause a concussion. Oliver knows that for every 90 G impact that causes an athlete to suffer a concussion, there can be hundreds that don't. That observation could pose one challenge to an idea that has become more popular: putting sensors into helmets.

Research looking into placing sensors in helmets seems promising. In theory, a sensor would send an alert to an athletic trainer or other person on the sidelines whenever an athlete absorbs a head impact above a certain level. Then the athletic trainer could pull the player out to fully evaluate him.

These sensors could create a challenge for a team's medical staff. An athletic trainer might have to pull a kid out of a game to evaluate him every time the sensor records an impact above a certain level, say 90 Gs. Most of the time, the athlete won't have a concussion. And the sensor wouldn't alert the athletic trainer to a blow of 50 or 60 Gs, even though serious concussions can occur at that level of impact.[69]

It's not that helmets aren't important. Athletes should wear new or reconditioned helmets if possible. The helmets should fit properly, and they shouldn't be altered to make them fit. The helmet, though, cannot prevent every head injury.

Efforts to tweak the rules will continue, and some might be incrementally effective at lowering concussion rates. Moving kickoffs up five yards might help. Eliminating kickoffs would probably help more. Removing targeting—a player launching himself to hit an opponent in the head—would help. With the size and speed of today's players, would we have to eliminate tackling—or at least the tackling of certain players, like quarterbacks—to really make it safe?

What about the numerous subconcussive blows to the head players take?

Steven P. Broglio, PhD, ATC, and others at the University of Michigan studied head impacts absorbed by high school football players. They found that the typical high school player took an average of 774 head impacts over the course of the season, or about 50 per week. Linemen sustained the largest number of impacts, averaging over 1,000 per season.

The Michigan researchers then looked at whether eliminating contact between players at practice could decrease those numbers. They calculated the impacts to the head from games, contact practices, and noncontact sessions. If teams limited contact practices to just one session per week—at the high school level, many teams have daily contact practices—head impacts would drop 18% over the course of the season. Removing all contact from practices would reduce head impacts 39% for the average player.[70]

"I think the number one problem with football is the subconcussive hits, and unfortunately at this point, it's an intrinsic feature of the sport," Dr. McKee acknowledged. "There's subconcussive traumatic exposure for the players on virtually every play of the game. That's the real danger of football, and I think that's going to be the hurdle of making it safer. How do you get that out of the game?"[71]

That's where the dilemma arises for parents. Can we truly make football a safe sport for kids to play? Or can we just make marginal improvements? To truly make the game safer, we could need to tweak the rules so much that football barely resembles the sport millions of fans watch each week.

And what about the schools? Can high schools really afford to spend tens of thousands of dollars on·sensors and helmets? And what about the youth football leagues? Can these teams, or the parents of the kids on these teams, afford that kind of money?

The question will increasingly become whether all of these ideas, these changes, the equipment and personnel, are feasible for the schools and the teams, from the NFL down to Pop Warner. And are they sustainable? Or will parents decide that football is too violent and not worth the risk?

Michael Timothy Duerson is the brother of Dave Duerson. About a year after Dave's suicide, the people of Muncie, Indiana, wanted to hold a life appreciation event in honor of Dave. At the event, people started donating money, although Michael was not seeking donations. He had to decide what to do with the money.

Michael started the Dave Duerson Athletic Safety Fund. All of the money went to help kids in the Muncie school system. They have enough money to provide baseline ImPACT testing for all athletes from the 5th through 12th grades. The fund pays for postconcussion tests for players. It even pays the doctor's bills for any student-athlete whose parents don't have health insurance.

The fund also provides each school in Muncie with two pairs of concussion goggles. Kids put on these goggles, causing them to experience the symptoms of a concussion. Duerson says the goggles have been very popular. He hopes that with repeated exposure to the goggles and the educational curriculum his group provides through the schools, players will be more likely to tell a coach, parent, or medical provider that they are hurt.

Duerson is now working to implement the same programs in every public school in Chicago, where his brother played professional football.

Michael Duerson knows the dangers of concussions, not just from living through Dave's experience, but also through suffering a brain injury himself.

He played basketball at IUPUI in Indianapolis, Indiana. Mike was cocaptain of the team. He recalls taking a charge during a game in a winter tournament in St. Cloud, Minnesota. His opponent ran into him. Duerson's feet went into the air as he landed on his head.

Due to a blizzard, it took his team four days to drive back home. Duerson was not diagnosed with a concussion or treated for one until he got home. His cousin noticed blood coming out of both his ears.

Michael Duerson developed paralysis on the left side of his body that persisted for six months. He still has memory loss. He explained that he takes about 20 pills a day, having been diagnosed with every psychological illness except Tourette's. "I think that's because God doesn't want me cussing people out."[72]

Michael Duerson is part of the Sports Legacy Institute. He has agreed to donate his brain and spinal cord to be studied after his death.

This chapter could have focused on Mike Webster as the first ex-NFL player to be diagnosed with CTE. Dave Duerson seemed to be the better choice, because he represents the dilemma parents face—and that we all face—about football.

Duerson played through concussions his entire career, but he had his son evaluated in the hospital and held him out for weeks. He was a man whose brain failed him, leading to financial and personal disaster, but he had the foresight to commit suicide in a way that preserved his brain for research.

Finally, Dave Duerson denied numerous former players any help while he sat on the NFL retirement board, but he also might have been a martyr for dying and having his brain studied so that future players could avoid the same fate.

Parents are becoming increasingly conflicted about letting their kids play football. Many of them have even played the sport themselves. At some point, one wonders if we will see more people conflicted about even watching football.

Parents must weigh the evidence and make the decision that is best for them and their children. Yes, we clearly need much more research into the risk factors for CTE to help us understand which players might be more at risk. However, it makes logical sense that we need to reduce overall brain trauma to young athletes, especially the repetitive impacts. For some parents, that choice might be letting the child play tackle football once he enters high school. Others might choose to push their children away from the sport entirely, trying to avoid potential issues later in life.

"I think it's important that everyone be able to make their own decision," Dr. McKee concluded. "They need to weigh the evidence. It's not perfect. We certainly don't know all the answers. I think they should be concerned, especially when, speaking as a parent, you want your child to grow and develop to their full potential. I think most parents wouldn't want to do anything or encourage their child to do anything that may limit their potential in life. Right now, I think you have to be very cautious about letting your son or daughter play football because of the inherent risk of the sport."[73]

In the coming years everyone—parents, coaches, doctors, school athletic directors, and yes, the athletes themselves—will have to decide what to do about football.

Medical Evaluation and Clearance
of Athletes to Play

June 19, 1984

"Portland selects Sam Bowie. University of Kentucky."

Commissioner David Stern's announcement of the second pick in the 1984 NBA draft surprised few people. After all, Bowie had arrived at Madison Square Garden carrying a Portland Trail Blazers jacket.

"Sam Bowie, the young man who came back from a stress fracture injury of the left shin bone. He was out for two seasons, redshirted, and he has come back. He has returned strong with Kentucky. And he's now the second pick in the draft."[1]

Those words, spoken by USA Network commentator Al Albert, were followed by an analysis by Lou Carnesecca. The former St. John's coach complimented Bowie's quickness, his ability to block and pass, and his ability to run up and down the floor.

"I think he's gonna make a great, great pro," Carnesecca proclaimed.

In reference to Bowie's two-year injury layoff, Carnesecca remarked, "Well, I think it shows the type of perseverance he has. That he was able to withstand all that misery and come back and perform, and look where he is now."

Moments later, after Bowie had shaken hands with the NBA commissioner, he answered questions from USA's Eddie Doucette about the evaluation performed by his new team. "Well I went up to Portland, and they gave me about a seven-hour physical. They didn't let anything out. I don't know if that's referring back to the Bill Walton situation. I know he had a stress fracture, but as far as I'm concerned, I'm 100% sound."

Sam Bowie's selection as the second pick in the 1984 NBA draft is widely considered to be the worst pick in NBA history. It wasn't that he followed University of Houston center Akeem (now Hakeem) Olajuwon, as much as the player who was taken after him.

The Chicago Bulls selected Michael Jordan with the third pick.

Years later, in an ESPNU documentary about his injury-plagued career called

Going Big, Bowie denied that there was controversy over the Trail Blazers passing on Jordan at the time. "No one batted their eye. No one said, 'Do you believe Portland took Bowie before Jordan?'"[2]

The Portland Trail Blazers entered the draft looking for a big man. In the prior draft, the team had selected small forward Clyde Drexler, an athletic shooter and future Hall of Famer. They also had Jim Paxson and Kiki Vandeweghe. They needed a center.

In 1977 the Trail Blazers won an NBA championship led by center Bill Walton, but chronic foot injuries limited his effectiveness. Walton left the team in 1979. General manager Stu Inman looked to find a center to guide the team back to the playoffs. Inman had two players in mind to fill the void in the middle.

Entering a coin flip that would determine if Portland or Houston would obtain the first pick, the Trail Blazers planned to pick Olajuwon if they won the coin toss and Bowie if they didn't win it.

Larry Weinberg, owner of the Portland Trail Blazers from 1975 to 1988, called that coin toss—unsuccessfully. "I don't kid ya. I would have been ecstatic if we had won. I'm thrilled that we'll be having the opportunity to draft the second best player in the college draft."[3]

Word spread around the NBA that the Blazers would select Bowie. The team flew him to Portland for a medical evaluation with team physician Dr. Robert Cook. The center discussed the team's motion offense and how he could play Walton's former role with head coach Jack Ramsey. Bowie felt confident he was headed to the Pacific Northwest.

Not everyone was convinced that Bowie was the best choice, though. University of North Carolina head coach Dean Smith called Inman to lobby for Jordan. Indiana coach Bob Knight, who had coached Jordan in the 1984 Olympics, also implored Inman to draft Jordan. According to ESPN's Tom Friend, Knight loved Michael's killer instinct.

"But, Bob, I need a center," Inman argued.

"Then play Jordan at center," Knight responded.[4]

Even current Blazers Clyde Drexler and Mychal Thompson pushed for the team to pick Jordan, arguing that Drexler and Jordan could become "the greatest backcourt in history."[5]

Portland took the center out of Kentucky.

After the ESPNU documentary aired in 2012, Harry Glickman, who had served as the Trail Blazers team president in 1984, addressed the controversy that has followed that selection in the three decades since the team made it. In an interview with the *Oregonian*, Glickman claimed that Jordan was never a real consideration.

"If you look back at the draft, if we hadn't selected [Bowie], we wouldn't have selected Jordan. We probably would have gone with Charles Barkley."[6]

The Chicago Bulls were excited that the Blazers took Bowie, but not solely because it gave them the chance to pick a player who would become arguably the greatest NBA player of all time.

Rod Thorn, the Bulls general manager, looked more at the risk Sam Bowie presented. In *Going Big*, he recalled, "I was thinking, 'Please don't take Jordan,' but for an entirely different reason. We had come to the conclusion that we would not take Bowie because of his injury."[7]

Sam Bowie grew up in Lebanon, Pennsylvania, where basketball proved to be a stabilizing influence in his tumultuous childhood. His father, who once played for the Harlem Magicians, became an alcoholic and later divorced Sam's mother. On one occasion, Sam rode with friends who stole a car and robbed a house. His family lived in a 660-square-foot home with especially low ceilings, a problem for a teenager approaching seven feet tall.

While his height would help him as he entered high school, it threatened to halt his basketball career before it got started. In fourth and fifth grade, Bowie couldn't play because he was taller than the league's five-foot-six height limit.

"My second year of playing basketball, I was not allowed to play anymore because I was too tall. So my first experience with basketball was a bad taste because I thought it was a negative being the size that I am. My father said that they would regret the day that they turned his son down from participating in their program. . . . It was almost like it was a challenge to me to show the rest of the world that I'm going to be a basketball player regardless of my physical size," Bowie explained in the documentary.[8]

Sam Bowie became one of the top prospects in the country in a class that included Ralph Sampson, James Worthy, Isiah Thomas, and Dominique Wilkins. He often referred to himself as the "million dollar kid," dreaming of the day he would make the NBA and take care of his family. He chose to attend the University of Kentucky for his college ball.

As a freshman, Bowie averaged 12.9 points per game and 8.1 rebounds per game. Coaches voted him a first-team all-SEC selection.

Bowie was selected to the 1980 Olympics team that ultimately did not travel to Moscow because of President Jimmy Carter's decision to boycott the games. Instead the team played games against NBA players. Bowie held his own and gained tremendous confidence heading into his sophomore season.

Kentucky's coach, Joe B. Hall, noted Bowie's progress early in that sophomore season. "His second year, we could just see he was going to be one of the most dominating players to ever play the game."

"The game was coming easy to me," Bowie recalled in the ESPNU documentary. "I was putting up some good numbers, maybe 18 points a game. It was a mortal lock that I was going [to] the pros as soon as this next month of college basketball is over."[9]

February 21, 1981

In a home game against conference rival Vanderbilt, Bowie's career changed forever, only no one knew it at the time.

After blocking a shot under his own basket, the center ran down the court and raised his hand to call for the ball. Dick Minniefield lobbed an alley-oop pass that Bowie slammed home. A Commodore player undercut him, causing Bowie to land awkwardly with all of his weight on his left leg.

Bowie played the rest of that season, but he knew something was wrong with his leg.

"After my second year of playing, I developed a little discomfort in my tibia," Bowie described. "They took regular x-rays and nothing showed up, but I continuously had some swelling and discomfort. Then they finally did a bone scan, and the bone scan indicated what they called a stress reaction."[10]

A stress reaction can often be a precursor to a stress fracture. In the tibia it could represent a potential problem for an athlete in a running and jumping sport like basketball.

While some tibial stress fractures heal uneventfully, others can be problematic for athletes. Stress fractures located on the anterior aspect of the tibia face tension forces that tend to pull the ends of the stress fracture apart. Stress fractures in this location often require long periods of nonoperative treatment, compared to stress fractures along the posterior and medial border of the bone. These anterior tibial stress fractures present a real risk for not healing at all.

Sam Bowie's stress fracture would prove to be one of those challenging cases.

Bowie recalled how doctors placed him in a long-leg cast. Every six weeks he would undergo X-rays so that his doctor could monitor the healing of the bone, which was minimal. He developed significant muscle atrophy in that leg over the 46 weeks he was in a cast. He even saw different orthopaedic surgeons for advice on how to get the fracture to heal.[11]

Coach Hall noted that the team and team doctors tried everything they could to get Bowie's shin to heal. Repeating cast treatments, electrical stimulation, and trips to see orthopaedic surgeons across the country all failed to help the stress fracture heal.[12]

In the fall of 1982 Bowie decided to undergo an operation. Dr. Rocco Caland-ruccio, an orthopaedic surgeon at the Campbell Clinic in Memphis, Tennessee, performed a surgery that involved placing a bone graft in the fracture site to help it heal, Bowie explained. That operation essentially eliminated yet another year of basketball. Now, assuming the surgery would finally help the bone heal, Bowie just hoped to play one final season.[13]

Bowie ultimately missed 61 games over the two years and seven months it took his injury to heal.

Bowie did not play like the future star he had resembled early at Kentucky, but he played respectably. He averaged 10.5 points, 9.2 rebounds, and 1.9 blocks for the Wildcats that season. He even pulled down 17 rebounds in a midseason battle with Houston and the Cougars star center Akeem Olajuwon.

He never felt that he returned to his preinjury level of play at Kentucky, but he did guide his team to the Final Four before the Wildcats ultimately lost to Georgetown and the 1985 number one draft pick, Patrick Ewing.

Bowie lamented: "[L]ooking back on it now, when I took off for that last alley-oop, that was the last time I was 100% sound physically. It's been a nightmare ever since that play."[14]

January 10, 1986

While Sam Bowie's career will always be remembered for his being drafted ahead of Michael Jordan despite realistic injury concerns, it was actually Jordan who suffered a serious injury first as a pro. As discussed in the next chapter, Jordan suffered a fracture of the navicular in his foot and missed 64 games during his second season with the Bulls.

Somewhat ironically, Bowie recalled that the draft debate was actually reversed then, as Jordan faced a possibly career-ending injury. "And the comment that I heard was, 'I'm glad we drafted Bowie instead of Jordan.'"[15]

Less than three months after Jordan went down, Portland's center followed. In a road game against Milwaukee, Trail Blazers small forward Jerome Kersey jumped for a rebound and stumbled, falling on Bowie, injuring the same leg that had kept him off the court for two seasons. Sam Bowie was carried off the Bucks' court on a stretcher.

After playing his entire rookie season relatively injury free, his second season was now over. Doctors diagnosed him with a cortical defect in that same tibia that previously had the stress fracture. This injury would cost him 44 games. It took 37 weeks to heal.

Early in his third season, Bowie spun toward the baseline to shoot a hook shot in a home game against the Dallas Mavericks. He landed awkwardly, but on his opposite right leg. He fell and immediately started pounding the floor with his fist. The obvious deformity in the middle of his leg portended an ominous injury.

In that November 7, 1986, game, Bowie had fractured his right tibia.

Surgery soon followed, and a surgeon fixed the fracture with a plate and screws. Bowie lost yet another season. His recovery took 51 weeks, causing him to sit out 77 games.

When he finally returned for what would be his fourth season, Bowie was excited to help his team and reward the Portland fans who were counting on him. Unfortunately, fate seemed to be against him once again. In the warm-ups for an October 1987 exhibition game against the Cleveland Cavaliers, Bowie felt a familiar pain in his right leg.

Blazers team physician Dr. Robert Cook explained what Bowie had done in *Going Big*. "He developed a very unusual stress fracture. It was so rare, there were only 35 reported worldwide. The majority of them were in male ballet dancers. He just had an anatomical and physiologic predisposition to that injury."[16]

Another surgery followed. The maligned center from Lebanon, Pennsylvania, played in only 20 games that season.

What was worse for Bowie was hearing the talk about Michael Jordan. When Jordan came to Portland, he seemed to play with a fire that suggested he wanted to make the Trail Blazers management regret drafting Bowie instead of him.

Bowie knew what fans were thinking. "He was on a mission when he played Portland. I had to sit there and watch it and hear the oohs and ahs. I know what was behind those oohs and ahs, that we've got this dud on the bench with two legs that nobody would want."[17]

June 28, 2007

Thirteen years later Portland faced another critical draft decision.

The Trail Blazers entered the 2007 NBA draft with the first overall pick. That year, two players stood out.

Greg Oden was a seven-foot, 280-pound center with a seven-foot-two wing-span who left college after one year at Ohio State. Kevin Durant was a dynamic scorer from the University of Texas. Comparisons to the Bowie-Jordan debate were inevitable.

Sports pundits spent weeks weighing the pros and cons of both players. Most of the debate centered around on-court variables. On paper, Oden seemed to be a can't-miss prospect. After all, he had guided his high school team, Lawrence North High School, to three straight Indiana Class 4A basketball championships. In his one season at Ohio State, he averaged 15.7 points and 9.6 rebounds and took them to the national championship game. In that loss to Florida, Oden scored 25 points and grabbed 12 rebounds.

Like Bowie, Oden did bring some medical concerns, even though Oden only missed two games compared to Bowie's two full seasons. Oden suffered an injury to his wrist and had ligament repair surgery after high school. If his injury came up for discussion among sportswriters, though, it was to point out how well he could tolerate pain and play with one good hand.

By the time David Stern stepped up to the podium at Madison Square Garden, Portland had already sold 3,000 season tickets in anticipation of the Blazers' future. An enormous Oden jersey billboard already hung from the Rose Garden Arena.

"With the first pick in the 2007 NBA Draft, the Portland Trail Blazers select Greg Oden from Ohio State University."

Unfortunately, Portland fans received bad news about their presumed team savior even earlier in his career than had been the case with Sam Bowie.

September 13, 2007

Less than three months after the NBA draft, Greg Oden underwent arthroscopic surgery on his right knee and woke up to the news that he would miss the 2007–2008 season.

Team physician Dr. Don Roberts performed the exploratory surgery. After-ward, he discussed his operative findings and expectations.

Dr. Roberts found an area of articular cartilage damage approximately the size of a fingertip in Oden's knee. Based on that finding, Roberts decided to perform a microfracture procedure.[18] In a microfracture, the surgeon takes a small pick to poke holes three to five millimeters apart to try to stimulate blood flow into the cartilage defect. The blood and subsequent inflammatory process theoretically create fibrocartilage. Fibrocartilage is more brittle and less durable than the hyaline cartilage, but provides more shock-absorbing capability than exposed bone.

While Dr. Roberts expressed optimism about Oden's future because of his youth and otherwise normal knee outside of the single area of cartilage damage, the team announced that its future center would be on crutches for about eight weeks. Full recovery would take 6 to 12 months.

Trail Blazers general manager Kevin Pritchard described Oden's reaction to the findings of surgery, noting that Oden felt bad for the team and the fans. "Greg looked at me as he was coming out of his surgery, and he and his mom Zoe probably said 'sorry' 20 times. I could feel the weight of the world on his shoulders. And as a leader and as leaders of this organization, my first thought was how lucky we were to have a guy that cares about the organization that much."

Pritchard emphatically stood by the team's decision to draft the former Buckeyes star. "We picked the right kid; he cares about his organization. And I can't [overemphasize] how bad he felt, and not because he had to go through the rehab and all that, but because he felt like he let us down. And he hasn't let us down at all."[19]

Given the seriousness of a season-ending injury and cartilage damage in the knee, questions immediately surfaced about the surprising news. Pritchard claimed that the Blazers had performed MRIs on Oden's knees before the draft. Those MRIs reportedly showed his knees to be "absolutely pristine."[20]

When Oden developed swelling in his knee days before surgery, the team repeated an MRI and found the articular cartilage damage. According to an ESPN report, Pritchard also noted that microfracture was a known option heading into surgery. He claimed that the team sent Oden's MRI to several orthopaedic surgeons. One prominent surgeon who largely championed the microfracture surgery—Dr. Richard Steadman—felt that Oden would need the procedure. Other surgeons could not make a definitive recommendation, so the team planned an exploratory arthroscopy.[21]

Now the Trail Blazers faced the prospect of a year without their number one pick. That injury and missed year began the start of the comparisons of Greg Oden to Sam Bowie.

In his first season playing in the NBA, Greg Oden showed signs of the potential that made him the number one pick in 2007. Unfortunately, that season revealed his potential for suffering injuries as well.

Only 13 minutes into his first game, Oden exited with a foot injury and missed several weeks. In February he knocked knees with Golden State's Corey Maggette, causing him to miss another month. He played only 61 games due to injuries but averaged 8.85 points and 6.95 rebounds.

Oden barely made it into December the following season before getting hurt. In a game against the Houston Rockets on December 5, Oden attempted to block a shot by Aaron Brooks and fell to the floor. Oden fractured his left patella. He underwent season-ending surgery to fix the fracture.

Almost one year later, in November 2010, Oden underwent microfracture surgery, this time in his left knee. Another season finished before it started.

By the 2011–2012 season, the Blazers were cautiously optimistic that Oden could contribute. Unfortunately, his rehab was not progressing as the team hoped. By February 2012 the big man had arthroscopic surgery on both knees within a few weeks. The second of those procedures was expected to be a cleanup operation on his left knee, but his orthopaedic surgeon found more articular cartilage damage and performed a second microfracture on that left knee and third microfracture surgery overall.

By now, Oden had not played in well over two years. In the five seasons Oden was expected to play since being drafted ahead of NBA superstar Kevin Durant, he had played in only 82 games—the equivalent of one full regular season.

Blazers president Larry Miller and head coach Nate McMillan shared the frustrations that Greg Oden clearly had. "It's hard to put into words the heartbreak for everyone involved, but especially for Greg," Miller told reporters after Oden's third microfracture surgery. "He's a young man who has experienced a great number of physical challenges in his playing career and today is yet another significant setback for him," Trail Blazers president Larry Miller said in a prepared statement. "We have a lot of empathy for Greg and his family during this difficult time."[22]

"I'm sure he's saying, 'Why Me?' Sometimes in life, things like that happen, and you wonder why it's happening to you."[23]

The Portland Trail Blazers released Greg Oden in May 2012.

Oden's love for basketball pushed him to attempt a return. He underwent the experimental treatment Orthokine in May 2012 and sat out the 2012–2013 season to try to rehab his knee. After his 2012 microfracture, his surgeon advised him to retire.[24] Instead of struggling through pain and rehab, he could have gone on with a normal life outside of basketball.

Instead, he fought back onto the court. He signed with the Miami Heat for the 2013–2014 season. On March 24, 2014, Oden made his fifth start for the Heat, playing 15 minutes against his original team. Although he made it back to play, Greg Oden was a shell of the player he was or could have become.

June 28, 2006

Oden never fulfilled his promise due to degenerative changes in his knees brought about by damage to the articular cartilage and the subsequent microfracture surgeries. Those issues manifested shortly after his NBA draft, not before he was selected.

One year before drafting Oden, the Portland Trail Blazers had acquired a player, Brandon Roy, who did have knee concerns before entering the NBA. Roy did not initially seem to be a bust, as he won Rookie of the Year honors and gained 127 of 128 votes for that award in the process.

Concerns about the Seattle native's health had appeared years earlier and possibly foreshadowed a quick decline.

Roy became a college prospect by his junior year of high school. He declared his intention to sign with the University of Washington that season. An injury to the meniscus in his left knee also occurred in that junior season. Roy would later injure the meniscus in that same knee during his rookie season with Portland.

After a brief flirtation with the idea of going to the pros straight out of high school, Roy ultimately became a member of the Huskies. By his sophomore season, he was starting every game, helping the team make the NCAA tournament. He planned to return for his junior season and then declare for the NBA draft.

In only the third game of his junior year, in November 2004, a knee injury hindered his game, but this time it was his right knee. Roy tore the lateral meniscus in that right knee in a game against Oklahoma. Surgery and a month on the sidelines followed. While he did return to play 23 games that season, he only averaged about 24 minutes a game.

Projected as a late first-round or early second-round pick, Roy chose to return to Washington. Managing to stay healthy, the six-foot-six guard won Pac-10 Player of the Year and first-team all-American awards.

Entering the 2006 NBA draft, Roy was widely projected to be a top six pick. He worked out for five teams, including Portland and Minnesota.

Most scouting reports glowed, featuring Roy's various basketball strengths: his jumping ability, quickness, and creativity. Concerns about his knees simmered just below the surface, though.

Portland entered the 2006 NBA draft coveting two players: Roy and Texas forward LaMarcus Aldridge. Holding only the number four pick in the draft, Kevin Pritchard worked several draft day trades, first acquiring the number seven pick from Boston. He exchanged the player the Blazers had drafted at number four, LSU forward Tyrus Thomas, for Aldridge and another veteran. Portland concluded the draft by swapping the player he had drafted at number seven—Villanova's Randy Foye—with the guard Minnesota had picked at number six—Brandon Roy.

That draft seemed like an enormous success for the Trail Blazers. Roy won Rookie of the Year, and the team had exciting prospects in Aldridge and Spanish point guard Sergio Rodriguez. Fans hoped the draft marked the beginning of a rebuilding process to overcome many draft disappointments.

Perhaps it was the apparent success of the team's draft in 2006 that made Greg Oden's injuries and struggles after the draft only a year later so painful.

Like Oden, though, Brandon Roy's knees would not hold up long. Repeated knee injuries and operation after operation, including arthroscopic surgery on each knee in 2011, led to the development of significant arthritis in both knees. He retired after only five seasons with the Trail Blazers, citing pain from a lack of cartilage in those knees. In a statement released by the Trail Blazers organization, Roy said that his family, his health, and his quality of life had led him to choose to quit playing basketball.[25]

Eventually Roy decided to attempt a comeback. After sitting out the 2011–2012 season, he signed a two-year, $10.4 million contract with the Timberwolves. Only nine games into the 2012 season, Roy underwent an operation to "clean out" debris after his knee collided with a Milwaukee Bucks player. That surgery marked his seventh knee surgery since his junior year of high school. He now admitted that his knees had grade III arthritis, telling Jason Quick of the *Oregonian*, "Level IV is when you get a knee replacement."[26]

Brandon Roy's professional career might simply be the story of a player whose body failed to withstand the demands of a grueling sport. In fact, had Sam Bowie and other Blazers draft picks not failed to reach their potential due to injuries, no one may have questioned Roy's selection in the 2006 draft lottery despite prior injuries to both knees.

Perhaps the most painful disappointment for the franchise came with the physical struggles of another number one pick, Bill Walton.

Bill Walton was a winner from the early days of his basketball career. He led his Helix High School team in San Diego to two California Interscholastic Federal High School titles. He chose to attend UCLA to play with legendary coach John Wooden. In his three seasons on the UCLA varsity basketball team, UCLA won 86 games and lost only four. The Bruins won the NCAA title in 1972 and 1973, and Walton was named NCAA Tournament MVP both times.

Bill Walton started playing basketball when he was eight years old, unaware that he had structural congenital defects in his feet. "I just thought everybody's feet hurt all the time," he remembered.[27]

Walton suffered a serious knee injury at age 14, requiring his first orthopaedic surgery. In college, he suffered a fracture in his back.

"I had a bad foundation with bad feet. I had a crooked, bent and non-functioning knee, and then I broke my spine when I was 21. All of that working together, working against each other, and the fact that I continued to play basketball and remained very active, that just led to all kinds of long-term problems."[28]

After being chosen by Portland with the number one pick, the redheaded center played in only 35 of the team's 82 games in that first season. Injuries limited him to 51 games in his second season, but he still averaged 16 points and 13 rebounds per game.

Walton did get healthier in the next two seasons, which were arguably his best and the best for the team. He played in 65 games in the 1976–1977 season, winning the NBA MVP award and guiding Portland to its only NBA championship. The following season, he posted career-high averages for points and assists before injuries started to slow him again.

Walton missed the entire 1978–1979 season because of a foot injury. He became so frustrated with the medical care of the Trail Blazers medical staff that he filed a malpractice suit. He left the team the following season, signing a seven-year contract with the San Diego Clippers. Foot injuries hampered him again, as he played in only 14 games over the next three seasons.[29]

Walton played sporadically for the Clippers from 1982 to 1985 and was traded to the Boston Celtics. The former UCLA star served as the backup to center Robert Parrish and earned the NBA's Sixth Man award. He helped the Celtics win the NBA title that season.

In the 1986–1987 season, he only played 10 games because of stress fractures in his foot. Deciding that his foot pain was too great, he ultimately retired in 1987.

Like Brandon Roy, Walton considered making a comeback in 1990. One day he stood up to walk and felt excruciating pain in his foot and ankle. Doctors found a partially dislocated ankle with degenerative bones grinding on each other. Bill Walton needed an ankle fusion to treat the pain.

In 2008 another injury from his playing days—a back injury—started causing him so much pain that he contemplated suicide. He told Howard Beck of the *New York Times* in 2010, "I had a life that was not worth living. I was on the floor and unable to move. The closest that I can come to describe it is, visualize yourself being submerged in a vat of scalding acid, with an electrifying current running through it. And there's no way to ever get out."[30]

That back injury happened at UCLA when he was 21 years old. He told Beck that he was "low-bridged" by an opponent. He missed two weeks and wore a corset with steel rods while he played.

The spine surgery to treat his back, performed almost two decades after his initial injury, took eight and one-half hours, four incisions, two titanium rods, and four bolts.

Walton claimed he has now undergone 37 orthopaedic surgeries, including his back, his two fused ankles, and multiple other joints.[31]

Bill Walton was ultimately inducted into the Hall of Fame. Although he led Portland to one NBA title and won another as a backup in Boston, most NBA analysts feel that he never achieved the heights expected of him after his brilliant college career. His body simply did not hold up.

> The two variables that you can never predict with certainty—one, how hard a
> player will work, how motivated he'll stay, and two, his health.
> —Bill Walton

The medical evaluation of players entering professional sports has become critical as sports have grown in popularity and exploded financially. It is one problem for a team to simply choose players who don't turn out to be very good. Portland fans might lament missing out on future NBA legends Bob McAdoo in

1972, Larry Bird in 1978, and Michael Jordan in 1984 when they drafted LaRue Martin, Mychal Thompson, and Sam Bowie in those years.

It can be difficult to project which players will excel at the professional level, though. What frustrates Trail Blazers fans, though, is when their team selects top prospects only to see those players barely play due to injuries. That is where many point to Portland as having the worst draft luck of any professional sports franchise.

Is it really luck that previously uninjured players stay healthy, or bad luck if they don't? Should a team be able to predict which injuries will become big problems in the coming years and which are anomalies that will have no adverse impact on players' later careers?

With championships at stake and millions of dollars owed to the players, teams rely on their medical staffs and increasingly sophisticated tests to predict the future. These evaluations have come a long way since the college days of Bill Walton.

"When I played, the physical was basically, 'Can you play?' If I said yes, then I passed the physical. If I said I couldn't play, then I didn't pass," Walton recalled.[32]

The NBA utilizes a combine similar to the NFL Draft Combine. Part of the combine involves the medical evaluation of prospects. A bad evaluation could have a dramatic impact on a player's stock.

For example, in 2012 Ohio State forward Jared Sullinger was given a medical record flag over concerns about a back problem. Sullinger fell from a likely top five pick to the 21st pick by Boston. Sullinger later missed much of his rookie season after undergoing back surgery.

Los Angeles Lakers team physician Dr. Stephen Lombardo described the evaluation process. While he pointed out that the screening process has become much more sophisticated since the days of Bill Walton and Sam Bowie, there are some important indicators that don't rely on MRIs or echocardiograms.

Dr. Lombardo teaches his orthopaedic surgery fellows to ask athletes two important questions during these evaluations. Has the player had any problems, like specific injuries or lingering pain? Has the player missed any games in high school and college?

He explained that if the answers to those two questions are "No," then the prognosis for the player is good.[33]

The medical evaluation process of the NFL Draft Combine is thorough, to say the least. Players go to multiple medical stations, where team doctors analyze every aspect of their health.

At the internal medicine evaluation, teams' internal medicine doctors check the players' heart, lungs, kidneys, and so forth by physical examination and laboratory tests. A player with a history of any medical condition or who exhibits any abnormal findings might undergo further testing, such as a cardiac stress test.

A player also undergoes multiple orthopaedic examinations, as each orthopaedic station has athletic trainers and orthopaedic surgeons from multiple NFL teams. Team doctors ask the players about any and all injuries (even those from many years earlier) and obtain X-rays and MRIs of those body parts. They examine the player from head to toe and check the motion, stability, and strength of every body part the player has previously injured, whether or not he had surgery. Hand, foot and ankle, and spine surgeons often examine players for those specific areas in addition to the review by sports medicine orthopaedic surgeons.

"This is the best physical examination most of these young men ever get," Dr. Matt Matava, head team physician for the St. Louis Rams and the former president of the NFL Physicians Society, noted.[34]

All of this medical information is compiled into a report available to all NFL teams. Each team's medical staff assigns each player a medical grade. Some teams use letter grades, like A through F, while others might use numerical scores.

Before the draft, the coaches and general manager meet with the team's medical staff. Dr. Matava indicated that the team might really like a player despite knee arthritis or some other musculoskeletal problem.

"I tell the team's management, 'If you like the player, based on his football talent, then draft him. I can give him an A, a C, an F or whatever. If you're set on drafting him because of his ability, and you want to disregard some of his medical issues, then that's your right to do. I'm just trying to provide you with an assessment of his medical risk, his ability to play at the start of the season, and whether his medical issues will likely allow him to play one year, three years, five years, etc.'"[35]

These medical assessments are largely subjective. For example, there could be one player who has had an ACL reconstruction but has fully recovered. Another player might have never suffered a really serious injury but has dealt with a number of smaller injuries. The team's medical staff might rate the player with the multiple lesser injuries lower, predicting that he will always be in the training room getting treated for nagging injuries.

One significant difference between football and professional basketball, baseball, and hockey, though, is that NFL contracts are not guaranteed. If a player can't stay on the field due to injuries or medical problems, the team can release him. Still, pro teams don't want to miss a red flag and essentially waste a draft pick on an athlete who can't play.

Professional teams want to determine which injuries turn out to be worse in terms of declines in on-field performance or career length. While predicting performance metrics after injuries is challenging in the NFL due to players playing different positions with very different activities and responsibilities, studies published in sports medicine journals are beginning to help teams with this information.

For example, a study out of the University of Pennsylvania looked at the performance of NFL running backs and wide receivers after ACL reconstruction. The researchers didn't examine any medical outcomes, such as knee stability tests or subjective outcome scores. They only looked at football statistics, calculating a power rating based on yearly total yards and touchdowns.

They found that more than one-fifth of the players never returned to an NFL game after undergoing ACL reconstruction. For the running backs and wide receivers who did return to play, their player performance dropped by one-third.[36]

A study performed by Robert H. Brophy, MD, looked at the career length of players after an ACL injury and those who underwent an ACL reconstruction combined with a partial meniscectomy. Injuries that cause ACL tears often result in simultaneous meniscus tears. He found that players who had isolated ACL reconstructions did not have shorter careers, but players with combined ACL and meniscus surgeries did.[37]

Having a partial meniscectomy, like Brandon Roy had during his career, therefore might shorten an athlete's overall career.

The question then becomes how successfully team doctors predict an athlete's medical future based on his past injuries and his present exam and tests.

In 2008 Dr. Brophy and others associated with one NFL team published a study reviewing the orthopaedic ratings they had given players at the NFL Combine from 1987 to 2000. They wanted to see how well the ratings predicted the likelihood of playing in the NFL and the duration of a player's career. They compared the orthopaedic grade assigned to each player by the head team doctor, Russell F. Warren, MD, to data collected from the Elias Sports Bureau. The data included information on each player's round drafted, the number of seasons he played, and the number of games he played.

The team's medical staff assigned ratings as follows. An athlete received a high passing grade if he had no history of surgery and only minor injuries that did not limit playing time in college and would not likely limit his ability to play in the NFL.

An athlete received a low passing grade if he was currently healthy but had a history of injury or surgery that limited his playing time in college or might limit him in the pros. If he had sustained an injury at the end of his college career and was not currently healthy but most likely would be completely healed soon, he also received a low pass.

An athlete with a history of significant injury or surgery that was likely to limit his time in the NFL or was a current problem received a failing grade.

Between 1987 and 2000, the NFL team's medical staff gave 3,536 players a high pass, 1,227 a low pass, and 284 failing orthopaedic grades.

The authors of that study found that 58% of the players who received a high pass played at least one game in the NFL, and 55% of players who received the low pass did so. Only 36% of the players who received a failing grade, however, ever played in the NFL. Players with a high grade ultimately played a mean of 41.5 career games, compared to 34.2 games for players with a low grade and 19.0 games for athletes with a failing grade.[38]

It would be difficult to know exactly what ratings Sam Bowie, Greg Oden, Brandon Roy, and Bill Walton would have received without being involved in the evaluations of each player. From what is known from media reports of their prior injuries alone, though, Greg Oden would have likely received the highest orthopaedic grade. His wrist injury did require surgery and caused him to miss time during his single season in college, so he probably would have been a low pass.

Brandon Roy might have been a low pass given his bilateral knee surgeries but healthy senior college season. On the other hand, having had injuries to the meniscus in each knee could have caused some teams more concern.

Bill Walton's history of injuries dating back to college might have dropped him to a low pass. Sam Bowie would likely have earned a low pass at best, assuming that the tibial stress fracture that caused him to miss two seasons was truly healed. The Chicago Bulls pulled him off their draft board, and other teams might have given him a failing grade under such a system.

Dr. Matava pointed out an interesting aspect of the medical combine and these evaluation processes:

> One thing the NFL Combine reveals is that football at a high level is a very
> Darwinian process. It really does tend to eliminate the weaker from the stronger

players as they progress from high school to college and on to the professional level. A high school player who tears his ACL, then dislocates his shoulder, then breaks his ankle, tends not to make it to the Division-I college level. Similarly, players who play Division-I football and have multiple injuries, often do not make it to the NFL Combine. If they do make it to the Combine, their medical grade may preclude being drafted very high. It's not just a player's ability that dictates their draft status. They may be good college players, but don't have whatever physical attributes it takes to make it to the higher level. Alternatively, we tend to see this same phenomenon with most of the first-round draft picks, as well. There is just something about their anatomy and physiology that allows them to play at a very high level without experiencing multiple, significant injuries.[39]

Certainly medical evaluations have become much more sophisticated in the last few decades. Echocardiograms, stress tests, and MRIs are utilized now to try to obtain as much information as possible. The MRI was just beginning to be used in orthopaedic practices in the early 1980s when the Trail Blazers evaluated Sam Bowie.

Sam Bowie remarked that he went through a very thorough medical evaluation at the combine. He said the Trail Blazers specifically did additional tests of the injured tibia and the opposite one. He underwent X-rays and scans with dye injected in his veins. Bowie ran on a treadmill and jumped up and down on that injured left leg. Dr. Cook even tapped on the tibia where the fracture had occurred.[40]

That aspect of his exam has earned the most scrutiny. In the ESPNU documentary *Going Big*, Bowie described his discomfort during the test.

> I can still remember them taking a little mallet, and when they would hit me on my left tibia, and "I don't feel anything," I would tell 'em. But deep down inside, it was hurting. If what I did was lying and what I did was wrong, at the end of the day, when you have loved ones that have some needs, I did what any of us would have done.[41]

Multiple outlets reported that quote from the documentary as Bowie lying to the Trail Blazers to get drafted. Bowie explained it differently.

"When you go as a draftee, you're selling yourself. It's a job interview. As an athlete, you always have some discomfort somewhere, but you're not going to sit there and say, 'I wouldn't draft Sam Bowie because his shoulder hurts.' With my situation, they had done numerous exams and physicals. They made me do all kind of physical tests to see if I was healthy enough to be drafted. It is a huge process."[42]

This controversy brings up an important question about these medical evaluations. Clearly the tests are more sophisticated now, so doctors will catch more abnormal findings than they did back in 1984. But these X-rays and MRIs just show the structural integrity of bones, tendons, ligaments, and cartilage. They don't show pain. Unless a player tells the doctor that an exam test hurts, that doctor might not realize the extent of an injury or that there is a problem at all.

Along the same lines, what should happen if an athlete doesn't want to undergo a medical test out of fear the team will find something wrong?

March 30, 2005

During a game against Charlotte, Chicago Bulls center Eddy Curry's heart skipped a beat or two. That irregular heartbeat led to appointments with cardiologists across the United States as the Bulls searched for answers. Was this episode simply a benign arrhythmia, or did it suggest an underlying condition called hypertrophic cardiomyopathy, which could kill him instantly?

Chicago general manager John Paxson offered Curry a one-year, $5 million contract, but he insisted that Curry submit to DNA testing.

Curry had seen Dr. Barry Maron, the director of the Hypertrophic Cardiomyopathy Center at the Minneapolis Heart Institute Foundation. Dr. Maron recommended that Curry undergo a DNA test. He told Howard Beck of the *New York Times* that a DNA test could help make the diagnosis. "It can only prove you have it, but not prove you don't."[43]

Dr. David Cannom, a Los Angeles cardiologist, declared Curry's heart to be structurally sound and cleared the big man to play.

After Curry refused to take the DNA test, Paxson traded Eddy Curry to the New York Knicks. This debate led not only to questions of financial liability and a player missing games but much more catastrophic potential outcomes. Paxson feared Curry could drop dead on the court. Hypertrophic cardiomyopathy, after all, is the most common cause of sudden cardiac death in athletes.

"In my heart, I would never put anyone in jeopardy," Paxson explained to reporters. "If this were a child of mine, I would have done the same thing."[44]

Timothy Epstein runs the sports law practice for Duggan Bertsch, LLC, in Chicago. He said that professional teams have a contractual right to test players medically and psychologically within the collective bargaining agreements. They can perform comprehensive physical examinations of the athletes and claim that a player is not medically cleared to participate.

"Generally, if you're going to be a physical specimen as an athlete participating in a physical game that requires physical exertion, you're paid money to do that," Epstein explained. "Those people paying you that money have the right to make sure that what they've invested in is actually going to produce at the level they think it will, and it's going to produce for the time that they hope it will. For them to be able to do that, they need to and have the right to be able to test you."[45]

Without question, the medical evaluation process for prospective athletes is becoming more sophisticated. In some ways, it will become more complicated as well, as questions continue to arise about what tests teams can order and how forthright players are.

It is almost certain that teams will occasionally take calculated risks on players with histories of injuries. Every few years, one of those decisions will be wrong, and the team will waste a pick on a player fans will call a bust.

Sam Bowie is often called the biggest bust in the history of the NBA draft. Even rapper Jay-Z references Bowie being picked ahead of the Bulls' pick of Michael Jordan at number three, in the song "Hola' Hovito":

> I ball for real, y'all niggaz is Sam Bowie
> And with the third pick—I made the earth sick
> M.J., hem Jay, fade away perfect.[46]

Bowie, for one, rejects the notion that he is a bust. After all, he played 511 of 820 games over 10 years in the NBA on two broken legs. Sure, he wasn't an All-Star, but he might have been if he had never landed badly against Vanderbilt.

In *Going Big*, Bowie recalls how he sat with other members of that famous 1984 draft class in Madison Square Garden waiting for his name to be called.

"When I was joking with Olajuwon and when I was cutting up with Charles Barkley, I knew deep down inside that I physically wasn't what those guys were. I wasn't the player that I wanted to be from my first day in the NBA."[47]

9 / *MICHAEL JORDAN*
Return-to-Play Decisions in Sports

October 29, 1985

In only his second year in the league, Michael Jordan was already earning praise. Bob Sakamoto of the *Chicago Tribune* called the former University of North Carolina star "the heart and soul of this up-and-coming franchise."[1] Tribune columnist Bernie Lincicome argued that Jordan was "maybe the greatest natural basketball talent, inch for inch, in this young decade."[2]

The Chicago Bulls star's success derived not only from freakish physical ability but also arguably the best work ethic ever seen in sports. Described by Pulitzer Prize–winning author David Halberstam as "the hardest working NBA practice player . . . ever seen,"[3] Jordan always showed up first for practice and left the gym last.

Perhaps it was this work ethic that contributed to the only major injury of his legendary career.

The 1985–1986 season started well for Jordan's Bulls. The team won all eight preseason games. He scored 29 points in the team's regular season-opener against the Cleveland Cavaliers, including scoring three late baskets that helped lead the Bulls to a one-point overtime victory.

In the second game against Detroit, Jordan withstood a brutal blow by Pistons center Bill Laimbeer and guided the team to a 121–118 win.

The Bulls' third win of the season, though, came at a great cost.

With 45 seconds remaining in a game against the Golden State Warriors, Jordan jumped to grab a rebound. As he landed, his left foot jammed into the court.

X-rays of his foot taken immediately after the injury did not reveal a fracture or other injury. Jordan struggled with starting and stopping due to his foot pain, so the team kept him out of the lineup for the next two games. The Bulls lost both contests.

Perhaps it was seeing his team flounder without him that pushed Jordan to return quickly. "It seemed better; it felt like I was progressing," Jordan told Sakamoto. "I was jumping off the floor during the shooting drill, and it felt pretty natural. Maybe I was so anxious to get back, I didn't feel the pain."[4]

As always, Jordan was the first player on the court at the Bulls' practice facility when they returned home, going through exercises with the team's athletic trainer and taking part in a shooting drill. This was his first opportunity to see how his foot would respond to basketball before he went to the hospital for evaluation of his foot.

The results of that evaluation were devastating to the team and its star player. A CT scan showed that Michael Jordan had a fracture of the navicular, a small bone in the midfoot.

"When I heard it was cracked, that really hurt me," Jordan explained. "What do I do from here? Six weeks of nothing? All I could think of was I would lay up, and do nothing.

"I don't feel too well. I've never gone through anything like this before, and I don't know how to deal with it. Right now, I can cry all night and wake up tomorrow and find out what it's all about."[5]

The team announced that it would place the shooting guard on the injured list. He would be out at least six weeks. At the time, Jordan was expected to miss 22 to 25 games.

"The way I feel now, I want to go off and hide somewhere and get better," Jordan said. "This is a time I have to take it within myself and think about things. Think about why this is happening to me.

"Something good has got to come out of this. I just can't see it right now."[6]

Stress fractures commonly afflict athletes. They occur with repetitive load applied to a bone. The repetitive forces cause microscopic fractures that don't heal due to either excessive bone resorption or inadequate bone formation.

Stress fractures of the foot and ankle are particularly common in runners, military recruits, and athletes in jumping sports like basketball. Basically, any stress applied to a part of the body over and over creates a risk for a stress fracture.

Michael Jordan's competitive demeanor on the court during games and practices certainly carries such a risk.

The navicular is particularly vulnerable to a stress fracture. This midfoot bone is located on the medial side of the foot—the side of the great toe—at the top of the arch of the foot. The central part of the bone not only faces tremendous shear stresses with running and jumping, but it is an area with poor blood supply. Navicular stress fractures today are classified as high-risk stress fractures of the foot and ankle.

Towne and others first described a navicular stress fracture in a human patient as a case study in 1970.[7] In the following years, doctors believed that stress fractures of this bone were rare. As imaging techniques evolved and physicians' understanding of these injuries increased, the incidence of navicular stress fractures rose.

A 2012 study by Alissa J. Burge and others reported that navicular stress fractures account for about one-fifth of all stress fractures of the lower extremities, making them the third most common stress fracture of the lower body.[8] In 1985, however, sports medicine doctors had little experience diagnosing and treating them.

In his book *Playing for Keeps*, David Halberstam recounts Michael Jordan's struggles with being separated from basketball. Jordan was particularly frustrated not only with being on crutches and in a cast, but also with not knowing how long these restrictions would be necessary.

Initially the team hoped Jordan's fracture would heal in six to eight weeks, but soon concern set in that the Bulls star would miss the entire season.

Bulls team physician Dr. John Hefferon recalled his visits with Jordan as they tried to determine if the stress fracture was healing, a slow process he compared to watching grass grow. Possibly because the use of CT scans to follow stress fractures for healing was relatively new, Hefferon took a cautious approach and kept Jordan in a cast.

Jordan spent much of his time away from Chicago in Chapel Hill, where he had played college ball, helping the Tar Heels win the national championship four years earlier. As his pain decreased, he practiced shooting drills. He grew increasingly convinced that his foot had healed enough to play.

Still, by February and March, several months after that fateful game against the Warriors, Hefferon opposed any thoughts of letting Jordan return to play. The player brought a sneaker to each doctor's visit with the hope that he could walk out without a cast. In one of the later visits, Jordan refused to go back in a cast, until Hefferon finally persuaded him.

Jordan's case for removing the cast and returning to the court was simple. He knew his body better than anyone, including doctors. And he knew he wasn't hurting and believed that he was ready to play.[9]

Navicular stress fractures are considered high risk for athletes due to a significant risk of nonunion. The shear forces imparted by running and jumping on the central aspect of the bone, coupled with a relatively poor blood supply to this region, create a higher-than-normal risk for a serious injury in an NBA player.

Athletic trainer Jeff Stotts, an injury analyst for Rotowire.com and founder of InStreetClothes.com, discussed the trouble NBA players in particular have if they suffer a navicular stress fracture.

Stotts has kept a database of every injury for all NBA players in the league since the 2005–2006 season. He observed that of the more than 900 players with injuries in his database, only seven had suffered a navicular stress fracture. Three of those seven players—Zydrunas Ilgauskas, Curtis Borchardt, and Yao Ming—either suffered a recurrent fracture or needed additional surgery.[10]

Decades earlier, though, NBA doctors and teams knew far less about stress fractures of the feet and why their athletes suffered them. In 1987 New York Knicks team physician Dr. Norman Scott told *Sports Illustrated* that at least one-third of NBA players had suffered some form of foot fracture.[11]

The NBA and its team doctors decided to study stress fractures to better diagnose, treat, and prevent them. They began analyzing players from teams in Chicago, Boston, Phoenix, Philadelphia, Portland, Sacramento, and Washington. Using high-speed cameras, researchers would assess stress on the players' feet with cutting and stopping quickly. They would also look at other basketball-related variables, such as the type of shoe worn, court surface, high arches, and flat feet.[12]

Another doctor determined to find the underlying causes of and risks for navicular stress fractures was Dr. Stan James of the Slocum Center for Orthopedics and Sports Medicine in Eugene, Oregon. His team wanted to understand the mechanics of the foot in order to predict which athletes are at risk for these fractures—and thus try to prevent them from occurring.[13]

His interest in navicular stress fractures was understandable. Dr. James was one of two orthopaedic surgeons who evaluated Michael Jordan to help Dr. Hefferon and the Chicago Bulls decide when to clear him to play basketball.

In 1981, less than five years before Jordan became the most famous athlete to ever suffer this injury, Letha Y. Hunter, MD, of the University of Washington published a study with two case reports of these stress fractures. The title of her article asks the same question that NBA teams started asking later that decade: "Stress Fracture of the Tarsal Navicular: More Frequent Than We Realize?"[14]

One year later, Dr. Joseph S. Torg and researchers at multiple institutions published the first study reporting the outcomes for athletes with navicular stress fractures. They studied the effectiveness of different treatments for young male athletes with navicular stress fractures. The researchers compared immobilization of the athlete in a cast and making him completely non-weight-bearing to simply limiting activity but allowing weight bearing or allowing weight bearing in a cast.

Torg and his group found that all 10 of the fractures treated with non-weight-bearing casts healed uneventfully, usually in six to eight weeks. Four of the nine patients who were allowed to continue weight bearing were unable to return to aggressive physical activity. These patients developed a recurrence of the fracture, the fracture was slow to heal, or it didn't heal at all.[15]

In 1992 Karim Khan and other Australian researchers similarly showed how dangerous these stress fractures are. Compared to 86% of athletes treated in a cast and made strictly non-weight-bearing, only 26% of athletes allowed to bear weight with only decreased activity successfully returned to play sports.[16]

Multiple studies have confirmed fairly good rates for return to play in athletes with navicular stress fractures treated in cast immobilization with strict restrictions on weight bearing for six to eight weeks.

The challenge with this treatment, as Michael Jordan demonstrated, is that it can be hard to convince an elite athlete to accept it. Athletes often worry about stiffness developing in the foot and ankle from being immobilized for so long. They also worry about the loss of muscle strength in the leg.

Most of all, they want a treatment that gets them back on the court as soon as possible.

In recent years, surgery to compress the fracture with screws placed across the bone has become more common. Often surgeons resorted to surgery if a navicular stress fracture did not heal. These were often salvage operations that required surgeons to take bone from other parts of the body and place it in the fracture site. Now more surgeons make the diagnosis of navicular stress fracture and offer early surgical treatment to potentially decrease the risk of nonunion and speed return to play.

More research is needed to determine if early surgery proves to be a more reliable treatment option than casting and non-weight-bearing for elite athletes.

Michael Jordan clearly was one of those athletes who grew impatient with the time it was taking before he was cleared to play.

Due to the risky nature of this injury in a player so critical to the future of the organization, team physician Dr. Hefferon consulted two orthopaedic surgeons to help guide the decision. Jordan saw Dr. John Bergfeld of the Cleveland Clinic. He also visited the previously mentioned Dr. Stan James in Eugene, Oregon.

Dr. James told United Press International that he examined Jordan in February and March that year. Given that he had most of his professional career in front of him, he advised Jordan not to return to the court until the navicular had completely healed.

"When I looked at him in February, it looked like he was doing well," Dr. James recalled. "I couldn't detect any difference in his running and jumping. He had no pain and, as far as we could tell, his muscle strength and endurance at that time were of excellent condition."[17]

While James acknowledged that Jordan believed he could play, he feared the Bulls star could hurt his foot again, and worse. "I told Michael last March that I felt there was about a 20 percent risk of reinjury if he started playing on it. As a doctor, as a professional, I expressed the opinion that I thought the risk was too high for him to resume playing."[18]

Halberstam recounts how Michael Jordan eventually convinced Dr. Hefferon, Dr. Bergfeld, Dr. James, team vice president for basketball operations Jerry Krause, and Bulls owner Jerry Reinsdorf that he could return to play. That meeting took over an hour.

Despite the team's reluctance to allow him to play, Jordan had secretly been testing his foot. In Chapel Hill, Jordan started to play in five-on-five pickup games without pain. As Jordan said to Hefferon, no one knew his body better than he did, and he knew that he was ready to play.[19]

In the month after his return to the court, Jordan himself explained his reasoning for pushing the doctors to clear him.

> I think people were just being conservative. The doctors say that the bone hasn't completely healed, but to wait for that would mean a year, maybe a year and a half.
>
> I would have listened to the doctors. I would have sat out if—and only if—they could have showed me a player with an injury comparable to mine, if there had been a player with my injury who came back and reinjured the same area.[20]

Fortunately for the Bulls—and the NBA—Michael Jordan never suffered a reinjury of the fracture or any lingering foot problem.

Four and one-half months after Michael Jordan broke a bone in his foot, the Chicago Bulls activated its franchise player. After missing 64 games, Jordan returned on March 15 in a game against the Milwaukee Bucks. Shortly after entering to a standing ovation, he dunked over the Bucks' seven-foot-three center, Randy Breuer.

The team did not simply turn him loose, though. They still took a cautious approach. Jerry Reinsdorf only allowed him to practice two hours each day. Jerry Krause instructed head coach Stan Albeck to limit Jordan's playing time to only six minutes per half.

Halberstam recounts an episode in one game early in Jordan's return when Jordan played five seconds more than what Krause wanted. By the NBA's accounting, those five seconds counted as a full minute played for official records. The next day Krause fired an angry call to Albeck criticizing him for playing Jordan seven minutes.

Soon Reinsdorf increased Jordan's game playing time to 10 minutes per half and later 28 minutes a game. Heeding management's wishes, Albeck removed Jordan from an April game against the Indiana Pacers with 30 seconds left and the Bulls down by one point. Jordan had reached his playing limit.

As the end of the season approached, the Bulls were closing in on the final playoff spot. Reinsdorf removed the playing limit, and Jordan guided the team to a clinching win over Washington.

Of course, earning the bottom seed meant Jordan's Bulls would face the team with the NBA's best record, the Boston Celtics. The Celtics, led by Larry Bird, swept the Bulls in three games.

Jordan demonstrated his future greatness in that series. In game 2 at the Boston Garden, Jordan played 53 minutes in the double-overtime loss, including the last 39 minutes without a break. In the process, he scored 63 points and broke the NBA single-game playoff scoring record.

Larry Bird, a future Hall of Famer himself, told sportswriters after the game, "That was God disguised as Michael Jordan."[21]

Michael Jordan went on to have a storied NBA career. His Bulls teams won six NBA championships. He was named league MVP five times and NBA Finals MVP six times. He was a 14-time All-Star. He won the league scoring title 10 times, and he won the NBA Slam Dunk Contest twice.

He is widely considered the greatest basketball player of all time.

Owner Jerry Reinsdorf likely understood Jordan's potential greatness and his impact on the team's success—both in terms of wins and titles as well as revenues from ticket sales and merchandise—when the second-year guard was found to have a navicular stress fracture.

Soon after the All-Star Game that season, which Jordan attended as the player with the most votes despite playing in only three games so far that season, Reinsdorf announced that the All-Star would sit out as long as necessary and possibly the rest of the season.

"His future career is much more important to us than winning games now," Reinsdorf told reporters.[22]

With his competitive fire, Jordan did not accept the team's decision and thus tried to talk the owner and club vice president out of it.

In *Playing for Keeps*, David Halberstam explains two points of contention between the team and player that did not sit well with Jordan as he tried to overcome his foot injury.[23]

Jordan believed, as did many others around the league, that by having him sit out the rest of the season, Krause and Reinsdorf accepted losing. In fact, he felt that they wanted to lose.

Chicago won its first three regular-season games with Jordan guiding the team. Without him in the lineup, the Bulls lost eight of their next nine games. Of the 64 games he ultimately missed, the team only won 21.

Without Michael Jordan, the Bulls almost certainly would have missed the playoffs. Jordan certainly believed that's what the team's management wanted.

By not making the playoffs, the Bulls would enter the NBA draft lottery. They would clearly have the chance to select a better college player than they could if they made the playoffs. It would also give the team a small chance at one of the two stars soon to enter that draft: University of North Carolina's Brad Daugherty and Maryland's Len Bias.

Jordan believed that if he was allowed to play, he could help the team win games and get them into the playoffs. Refusing to allow him to play made Jordan believe that the team was not committed to winning—at least in the short term.

The other issue bothering Michael Jordan about the team keeping him from playing after his fracture, according to Halberstam, resulted from an exchange between the player and management. When Jordan was pleading his case, Jerry Krause, the club vice president, reportedly told him that he and Reinsdorf would make the decision about when he could play because he was "their property."

According to Halberstam, "it was a statement that Michael Jordan never forgot and never forgave."[24]

It might have been an unfortunate choice of words, but it does represent the complex relationship between the players and the front office of professional sports teams. The team doctors are often caught in the middle of this relationship.

When a player is safe to return to play is not always a straightforward decision, as Michael Jordan's injury-shortened second season shows. Is it best to rush players back on the court or field as quickly as possible? Or should doctors hold the players out for longer periods of time—and maybe longer than absolutely necessary—in order to preserve their long-term health?

It is interesting in Jordan's case that the question of return to play now versus later is essentially reversed from what we often hear about in pro sports. Pro athletes often believe that owners, general managers, and coaches want to rush players back to play as quickly as possible. Basically the team wants to win at all costs, even if it isn't in the players' best interests. Playing through pain or injury now, the thinking goes, is more important than fewer seasons at the end of the players' careers.

In addition, keeping star athletes on the court, or on the field, keeps fans buying tickets and merchandise. Star players sitting on the bench can cost a team financially.

It seems plausible that pressure from owners and the desire to win factor into the decision. Fans want to see these players on the court, since they pay a lot of money for tickets.

Players also feel that responsibility. They feel responsible to their teammates and to the fans. Legendary NBA and college center Bill Walton feels that someone, though, must keep the best interests of the athletes in mind.

"Because you as the player, you feel this tremendous responsibility, you love that responsibility. You're on a team, and you're going to help the team win. Maybe the team can't win without you, and you know that, and they know that. Somebody has to always think big picture, and it can't just be today. These horrific stories that we hear on a constant basis of the ground up skeletons, there's just no joints left, the broken bones and the broken bodies which lead to the broken spirits and the broken lives. Sports, athletics—they're supposed to make you better. It's not supposed to ruin them."[25]

So on whose side is the team doctor supposed to be? Does he work for the team and essentially rush a player back from injury the minute he is relatively safe to do so? (Or does the doctor hold him out for longer, in Jordan's case?) Or does the doctor make a decision that's in the best interest of the player's short-term or long-term health?

Dr. Matt Matava is the head team physician for the St. Louis Rams and former president of the NFL Physicians Society. He claimed that coaches rarely try to influence medical decisions about an athlete's return to play.

"I say, 'With all due respect, coach, I don't tell you when to throw the ball on third and one. Please don't tell me when a player is going to be ready to play.' They have always respected that boundary when put in those terms. In fact, they often laugh when I say that."[26]

Managing expectations can often be important. For example, if a player has an injury that usually takes six to eight weeks to heal, a team physician might tell the coach to expect it to be eight weeks before the player is back on the field. If the player does return in six weeks, the doctors and athletic trainers look good for getting him back early, and the player looks good for working hard. On the other hand, if everyone expects a six-week timeline, and the player ends up requiring eight weeks, fans often think the player is lazy and the athletic trainers and doctors are wrong or don't know what they're doing.

Coaches do want the medical staff to be as aggressive as possible to diagnose and treat players. They don't want to risk reinjury, however, and turn an injury that should have healed quickly into a problem that lingers all season.

In recent years, the players' agents have asserted more influence in these decisions. Often the agents advise their clients to stay out longer and heal completely in order to avoid doing further damage.

The relationship among athletes, teams, and team physicians is complex. Many professional athletes feel that the doctors work for the teams. In this capacity, the team doctors would look to maintain their good standing with the teams' owners and management at the expense of doing what's right for the players.

Just before Super Bowl XLVII, the *Washington Post* reported a survey administered by the NFL Players' Association (NFLPA). According to the article, NFL players largely didn't trust their team doctors. The survey asked players to rate "how little they trust their team's medical staff" on a scale of 1 to 5. Of the players who responded, 78% chose 5, essentially saying that they didn't trust the medical staff at all; 15% responded with 4, and only 3% answered with 1 or 2.

The NFLPA told the *Washington Post* that the study covered all 32 teams but would not reveal how many players completed the survey.

The executive director of the NFLPA, DeMaurice Smith, was quoted about this survey in the article: "The results of the survey show that our focus should be on a much broader field that includes the physicians' ethical obligation and the duties that doctors have to treat their individuals as patients first."[27]

Dr. Matava stated that he and other team physicians took issue with this report. He explained that the league surveys players every 5 or 10 years about how they perceive their health care as part of the collective bargaining agreement. The last such survey indicated that the players were happy with their care. The team doctors knew of no new survey.

The NFL asked the NFLPA for a copy of its survey, but the study was never produced. Team doctors asked some of their players about the survey. None of the players had seen the survey or ever heard about it.

Dr. Matava spoke with the league's attorneys, who contacted people in the NFLPA and concluded that a survey had not been done, or that only a few players had been asked, which meant it wasn't a valid survey.

Dr. Matava said that the "survey" and its widespread coverage created collateral damage for the team physicians. "A patient of mine has asked me, 'You say I need surgery, but I read that the NFL players don't trust you. Why should I trust you if they don't?'"

Matava made that case to the NFLPA. "I said, you may not realize this is happening, but this sort of unsubstantiated statement does significant collateral damage to the NFL physicians who can't defend themselves in a public forum. Team physicians tend not to have significant access to the media, nor do they feel comfortable resolving conflicts in a public setting."[28]

In addition, the NFL and the coaches and management of the 32 teams wouldn't want doctors that the players don't trust. "If it was true that 78% of the NFL players didn't trust their doctors, as quoted by NFLPA's Executive Director, DeMaurice Smith, the teams would make significant changes to their medical staffs," Dr. Matava argued. "They don't want to have over three-quarters of their players unhappy with how they're being treated medically."[29]

Whether or not this highly publicized player survey was real, it does demonstrate the difficult relationships between athletes and the team physicians. Add in marketing relationships between the sports franchises and hospital systems, which pay into the millions of dollars for marketing packages, and this question of who makes the decisions gets even muddier.

The NFL has worked to separate the teams' medical staffs from marketing arrangements in order to prove the quality of medical care and to minimize public perception that medical care is bought by the highest bidder. An independent medical group reviews all of the board certifications of the NFL team physicians. It reviews each team's medical staff to ensure that it has the required number of specialists—internal medicine, cardiology, neurology, and so forth—

and that each health-care provider is in good standing with his or her national society.

The marketing contracts can complicate the relationships between professional teams and prospective health-care organizations. For example, if a city has two qualified health-care organizations, one of which offers a lot of money while the other doesn't, it could be understandable that the team will pick the one that offers more money. Matava said that he has heard Dallas Cowboys owner Jerry Jones make that argument.[30]

The bigger problem would be a professional team picking an inferior medical group over a much more qualified group solely because the inferior group offered more money.

One could clearly argue that it would make little sense for an NFL or NBA team to choose a medical provider solely based on a marketing agreement. A hospital or medical practice might be willing to pay six figures, or maybe even seven figures, to advertise that it is the "official medical provider" of that franchise. That amount barely equals the rookie contract of a single player on the team. It would be a poor investment to choose inferior physicians solely for that small amount of money.

Regardless, there is a perception among many athletes, and certainly many fans of pro sports, that team physicians largely make decisions that are in the best interests of the team owners and management. The argument then follows that a doctor would rush a player back too quickly and risk reinjury or even the player's long-term health in order to maintain favor with the coaches and front office.

However, team physicians ultimately make decisions regarding injuries and return to play after injuries or surgeries based on when it is safe for the athlete. We make a decision for the current season but keep an eye on long-term player health. Wins, losses, and championships are not the primary concern of team physicians.

"I think the important point is that we still keep the players' health as our number one priority, and not the team's performance," Dr. Matava emphasized. "These players are our patients first and foremost. Whether the team wins or loses is irrelevant to us as NFL team physicians. People have said to me, 'Well, since your job is predicated on the team's wins and losses, you're going to do whatever it takes to keep the players on the field.' I say, 'Listen, I've survived 1–15, 2–14, and 3–13 seasons. My job is not predicated on the team winning, because if it was, I would have been fired a long time ago.' When you put it in that perspective, I think the general public and the media can understand that we are doing this job primarily for the health of the players, and that we will not do anything that will get them back on the field prematurely before they are medically ready."[31]

Should Michael Jordan have been able to dictate when he could return to play basketball? Or was he basically an employee whose medical decisions were dictated by team management? And what should the team doctor have done?

Ultimately Dr. Hefferon, the consulting surgeons, and Bulls VP Jerry Krause and owner Jerry Reinsdorf reluctantly agreed to let Jordan play. Whether or not they held him out for four and one-half months to protect his foot for the rest of his career or they did it to get a prime draft pick by losing, it's hard for fans to argue that it worked out in the long run.

Even without the complicated relationships between team physicians and professional organizations, the balance between short-term and long-term health is crucial. Playing in the NBA takes a tremendous toll on the bodies of the players. Traumatic events and injuries obviously occur. Most of the damage, though, comes from running up and down the floor and wrestling with 250- to 300-pound opponents for 82 games, season after season.

These physical demands can shorten the careers of professional athletes.

"I'll always have some aches and pains and some discomfort that come from the demanding schedule and the competition," Sam Bowie acknowledged. "The average civilian doesn't realize the preparation and what goes in before the ball is actually thrown up. A lot of times the people think you turn the TV on, they throw the ball up and the game begins, but there's so much preparation prior to the actual game. There's a reason why the career expectancy in all professional sports are low in numbers. You read about Magic Johnson and Larry Bird and Michael Jordan and Barkley playing 15, 16 years, but the vast majority of players who come through there never get to see that type of career."[32]

Team physicians can advocate for players to take as long as necessary to fully recover from injuries. The culture of the team itself plays a large role in the overall health of the athletes as well. One of the best examples of a franchise that takes steps to maximize the health and longevity of its players is the San Antonio Spurs. Led by head coach Gregg Popovich, but stressed throughout the organization, the team rests certain players during road trips or back-to-back games. Popovich limits the minutes played for many of the older players almost every night, allowing the players to stay fresh late in the season. Those efforts probably have helped extend the careers of star Spurs players Tim Duncan, Tony Parker, and Manu Ginobili. And the Spurs have won five NBA titles with that approach.

This wear and tear affects football players colliding over and over in each game, baseball players who play 162 games plus spring training and postseason games over eight months, and many other top athletes.

These physical demands in basketball—and really all sports—now start sooner than ever before. With the Amateur Athletic Union (AAU) circuit and youth teams playing year-round, young players enter college basketball and the NBA with much more wear on their bodies.

Young soccer players often start playing on travel teams as early as seven or eight years old. They play all year with few breaks, traveling for tournaments most weekends after grueling practices each weekday. Youth football, baseball, and many other sports inflict a similar long-term physical toll on the athletes.

Athletes put a lot of pressure on themselves to fight through pain in order to play and win. That same drive is largely what makes them successful in their sports. They spend hours every day practicing jump shots, curveballs, and all of their skills. They have passion for their sports. They want to spend as much time as possible training and competing.

Athletes from the pros down to the youth and high school levels are competitive by nature. Maybe they aren't as competitive as Michael Jordan, but they would consider returning from an injury quickly in order to play and help their teams win.

No injury is minor, though. "You never rank, rate or compare injuries," Bill Walton stressed. "Every injury is unique in and of itself. When the injury is your injury, it's the worst injury of all. Minor surgery is what they do on somebody else."[33]

It could be a college football player trying to get back on the field only six months out from an ACL reconstruction even though his knee doesn't yet feel normal. It could be a 10-year-old baseball pitcher battling Little Leaguer's shoulder facing the prospect of sitting out four or six weeks and missing a regional tournament. It might be a high school cross-country runner trying to overcome pain in her leg while she and her team challenge for a state championship.

All of these scenarios require an athlete—and his or her parents, coaches, and doctors—to take all pain and injuries seriously. Athletes should not push through pain and try to return to sports too quickly.

This advice even applies to adults who don't play team sports. It could be a 35-year-old jogger who wants to run her first marathon. She ramps up her mileage to train for the race. Six weeks before the event, she might notice pain in her foot. Fearing that she might have a stress fracture, she might resist consulting an orthopaedic surgeon. Or if she goes and learns that she does have a stress reaction or stress fracture, she might decide to try to push through the injury anyway and try to compete.

While she isn't a professional athlete earning a large salary from training every day, she loves running. She must remember that even though she might miss that one marathon, she has 30 or 40 more years to run. Recovering fully now might allow her to run without pain for years down the road.

"Listen to your body," Walton implored. "The body is a most remarkable organism. When it hurts, when your body hurts, it's telling you to stop. You have to listen to your body. You're doing yourself, your family, your team, community, you're doing everybody a disservice when you don't listen."[34]

Late in the 2010 MLB season, Boston Red Sox second baseman Dustin Pedroia was diagnosed with a navicular fracture. The team sent the studies of Pedroia's foot to other surgeons for advice on the best treatment option.

The Red Sox manager that season was Terry Francona, manager of the Birmingham Barons in 1994. Michael Jordan played on that Barons team. Francona described how he reached out to Jordan for advice on Pedroia's navicular fracture.

"I don't call Michael very much just because I know how much people bug him. But because of Pedey, I knew that Michael would enjoy talking to him, and he did. He was almost fatherly in his advice. He was like, 'I went through this, it's tough, you got to listen.' Pedey was all ears and that was good. When guys like Michael Jordan talk, people are apt to listen more."[35]

Obviously Jordan returned to a Hall of Fame career after this tough injury, and Pedroia has fared well since his injury. But Jordan's advice, "It's tough, you got to listen" can apply to many of these difficult injury decisions, especially when parties with different interests are involved.

10 / HANK GATHERS

Sudden Cardiac Deaths and Universal Screening

March 4, 1990

It was a dunk that college basketball fans had seen so many times before. Hank Gathers received the alley-oop pass from teammate Terrell Lowery and delivered his signature tomahawk dunk.

The best player on the nation's highest scoring team then did exactly what he always did. He gave a high five to a teammate and then started playing defense.

There was 13:34 left in the first half when Gathers fell to the court. Moments later, officials canceled the game. Hours later, Hank Gathers passed away.

Gathers was not a college basketball superstar in the traditional sense. His close friend and high school and college teammate Bo Kimble recalled that Gathers rarely played on their junior varsity or freshman teams. "He worked twice as hard as most players," Kimble said. "Nothing came easy to him."[1]

After one year of college basketball at the University of Southern California, the six-foot-seven forward from North Philadelphia transferred with Kimble to the much smaller Loyola Marymount.

Under head coach Paul Westhead's fast-paced style of play, Gathers flourished. As a junior, Gathers led all of college basketball in scoring and rebounding. He became only one of two players in history who have accomplished that feat. Many scouts believed he would be selected as an NBA lottery pick after his senior season.

Despite the sudden nature of his death a few months later, signs of a problem began to appear early in that senior season.

On December 9, 1989, Loyola Marymount played a regular-season game against UC Santa Barbara. After a routine drive down the lane and foul by a defender, Gathers stepped to the free-throw line. Seconds later, he collapsed.

Gathers's mother later recalled how she was woken from sleep and told of her son's collapse. "I thought they were kidding," she said, "because he always had trouble at the foul line."[2]

It turns out Gathers had a much more serious problem than free throws. His heart was racing before he fell. With medical assistance, he rose to his feet and walked off the floor.

Dr. Michael F. Mellman, an internal medicine physician at Centinela Hospital Medical Center, treated him after that December collapse and referred him to cardiologists for treatment of an arrhythmia, or abnormal heart rhythm. Dr. Vernon Hattori and Dr. Charles Swedlow reportedly cleared Gathers to return to basketball and monitored his condition. According to a statement from the Daniel Freeman Marina Hospital, Gathers had been diagnosed with the arrhythmia and placed on an anti-arrhythmic medication to treat it. The statement added that Gathers was regularly monitored following the incident.[3]

As his coach, Westhead worried about Gathers returning to play. "I had fears and concerns about him coming back. But we were on top of the situation." He noted that electrocardiograms were performed several times per week. In the opinion of team athletic trainer Robert Schaefer, "He was given the best workups that could be had. No stone was left unturned."[4]

The doctors treated Gathers's arrhythmia with propranolol. This beta-blocker is a common heart medication that blocks stimulation of the sympathetic nervous system that increases heart rate.

Gathers returned to the court after only missing two games, but his medication's side effects proved to be a formidable opponent. He complained frequently of feeling tired. He could not run or play at his desired level.

He asked doctors and his coaches about the medication. He pleaded to be allowed to stop taking the medication or cut back on the dose. The autopsy performed shortly after the fateful event of March 4 showed no signs of propranolol in Gathers's system. Presumably he had not taken his medication for at least eight hours before his death.[5]

March 4 should have been just like any other night. Loyola Marymount was playing in a semifinal game of the West Coast Conference tournament, where they were heavy favorites over upstart Portland. Gathers warmed up for that game as for every game before it, jogging and then sprinting around the court three times. The team opened the game as it often did, amassing a quick 12-point lead in the game's first eight minutes.

At 5:14 p.m., everything changed. Gathers's crumpling body hit the court so hard that fans throughout Gersten Pavilion could hear the impact.

Portland's Josh Lowery offered his hand to help Gathers to his feet. Loyola Marymount's medical staff, including Schaefer, orthopaedic surgeon Dr. Benjamin Schaeffer, and team physician Dr. Dan Hyslop, rushed to the star's side. Gathers initially sat up but fell back to the floor before his body began convulsing. Portland athletic trainer Tom Fregoso began chest compressions. The player's aunt, Carol Livingston, and soon his mother and brother, ran onto the court.

"Somebody please do something! Somebody please do something!"[6]

Carol Livingston's pleas accompanied quick action from the medical staff. They took the player off the court and outside the gym, placing him on a stretcher. After three shocks with a defibrillator, Gathers briefly lifted his hand and took a few breaths before collapsing again. Paramedics arrived and continued CPR and shocks with the defibrillator as they took the player to nearby Daniel Freeman Marina Hospital.

Emergency physicians and staff tried to resuscitate the fallen player for over an hour, to no avail. Just 23 years old and one of the best players in college basketball, Hank Gathers's life ended suddenly.[7]

Loyola Marymount teammates and players on the opposing team were understandably stunned. Coach Westhead tried to comfort players and family. "Words are hard right now. This is the hardest thing I've experienced—to be so close to a player and to see him fall and for it to be over. I feel a deep hurt for his family."[8]

Hours later, West Coast Conference officials canceled the game and the tournament.

Gathers's death rocked the sports world. How can a seemingly healthy athlete performing at such a high level simply drop dead on the basketball court? And playing in a system based on running up and down the court for 40 minutes, Loyola Marymount players should have been some of the fittest athletes in basketball.

In fact, Hank Gathers frequently described himself as the strongest man in America.

How could this happen?

Days later, the cause of Gathers's death was declared to be idiopathic cardiomyopathy with interstitial myocarditis. Doctors found patches of scarring in both ventricles and enlargement of some muscle cells that had likely occurred over time. These changes could have created an arrhythmia.[9]

Arrhythmias can decrease the volume of blood the heart can pump, resulting in inadequate oxygen delivery to the brain and other body organs. These events can surprisingly manifest in outwardly healthy athletes as fainting spells. Collapse and even sudden death represent the most tragic results.

Hypertrophic cardiomyopathy is a primary disease of the heart muscle. The muscle cells of the involved heart are larger and often cause the walls of the left ventricle of the heart to thicken. With thicker walls, the ventricle holds less blood than normal. The heart might also struggle to pump blood out of that thickened ventricle.

Some patients with hypertrophic cardiomyopathy have symptoms like shortness of breath and arrhythmias, while others have no symptoms at all. Sometimes an athlete has no knowledge of his condition, but strenuous physical activity causes an arrhythmia that causes sudden cardiac arrest.

Sudden cardiac death (SCD) is more common than sports fans might think. The CDC estimates that approximately 2,000 patients younger than age 25 die of sudden cardiac arrest in the United States each year.[10]

The incidence rate of SCD in sports is difficult to estimate. There are few national registries for collection of information on these deaths across the country. Much of the information comes from media reports rather than standard scientific surveillance systems. Also, accurate numbers of athletes playing sports in this country are imprecise, so the estimates vary in different scientific studies. Estimates for the incidence rates of SCD during sports in the United States range from 1 in 25,000 athletes to 1 in 200,000.

Young athletes bear much more risk for SCD than their nonathletic peers. In a study performed in the Veneto region of Italy, adolescent and young adult athletes were 2.5 times more likely to experience these events than age-matched controls who did not participate in sports.[11]

In terms of demographics, male athletes seem to have a much higher chance of SCD in sports than females. African American athletes have a dramatically higher rate of sudden death caused by hypertrophic cardiomyopathy, the most common cause of SCD in athletes. Finally, certain sports, especially basketball and football, seem to have much higher numbers of SCD death than other sports.[12]

A 2011 study published in the journal *Circulation* aimed to determine the incidence of SCD in NCAA student-athletes. Between January 2004 and December 2008, 45 athletes suffered a cardiac death. The incidence of SCD in NCAA student-athletes, based on these data, was 1:43,770 per year.

Kimberly G. Harmon, MD, and the other authors of that study found that the rate of SCD was 2.3 times higher in male than female athletes. Likewise, black athletes had a much higher rate of SCD.

Cardiac deaths were most common in basketball, with 14 during the period studied. Among Division I male basketball players, the incidence of SCD was 1 in 3,126 athletes.[13]

Sudden death can be the first manifestation of an athlete's underlying heart condition. While symptoms such as shortness of breath with exertion, chest pain, feelings of a racing heart, dizziness, or fainting spells, or family history of premature SCD would potentially arouse suspicion for underlying cardiac risk in athletes, studies show that these findings are only present in 25% to 61% of SCD cases.[14] Studies estimate that 30% to 50% of these SCDs are "first clinical events" among all age groups, and that first event is even more likely for younger athletes.[15]

March 3, 2011

On the eve of the 21st anniversary of Hank Gathers's fatal collapse on a basketball court, another tragedy would strike a basketball game.

Wes Leonard was the star of his varsity basketball team in Fennville, Michigan. He had already scored 1,000 points in his high school career despite only being a junior.

This was not just any game. Fennville was facing its rival, Bridgman. The Fennville players entered the game undefeated. A victory tonight would complete a perfect regular season.

The outcome was just as magical as the season had been. Leonard hit the game-winning shot—in overtime no less—with less than 30 seconds remaining.

"And then 10 seconds later . . . everything's pulled out from under you, from out of nowhere," coach Ryan Klingler later described.[16]

Seconds after the teams shook hands, Leonard collapsed in front of approximately 1,400 stunned fans. He was taken immediately to Holland Hospital, but soon Wes Leonard was pronounced dead.

An autopsy later determined that Leonard died of cardiac arrest due to dilated cardiomyopathy.[17] Like Gathers, Leonard's condition created a heart that was enlarged and too weak to pump blood to his brain and body efficiently.

Due to the possibility of heart failure or sudden collapse, the American Heart Association (AHA) advises that children with dilated cardiomyopathy should not be allowed to play competitive sports.[18]

By all accounts, Wes Leonard never experienced symptoms. Unlike Gathers, no precipitating event signaled an underlying medical condition. In fact, Leonard was felt to be in terrific shape. Before the fatal game, his coach even remarked that the junior took "care of his body better than probably anybody I've ever coached."[19]

The fallen star's mother, Jocelyn Leonard, has courageously tried to use her son's death to help other athletes. The Wes Leonard Heart Team honors athletes who die of SCD. It raises money for schools to purchase automated external defibrillators (AEDS) and lobbies lawmakers to provide AEDS and education on SCD to schools.

"If you have an AED, you can give someone a chance. That's just what we want."[20]

While Jocelyn Lenard's push to get AEDS in schools is an admirable goal, it is difficult to know if an AED would have saved her son.

Data on the survival of episodes of sudden cardiac arrest in children and adolescents is frightening. Most studies report statistics for these episodes among pediatric patients for all causes and not only sports. Nevertheless, early studies reported the proportion of young patients who survive the arrest and are later discharged from the hospital to be approximately 10% or less. Many of the kids who do survive experience serious and lasting neurological damage.

A recent review of nine studies looking at out-of-hospital cardiac arrests among children and adolescents that occurred at schools showed somewhat more encouraging results. Survival through discharge from the hospital or one month after the event ranged from 31.9% to 71.2%.[21]

Most evidence for the benefits of AEDS has been demonstrated with their use for cardiac arrest in adults. For arrest with ventricular fibrillation, a disturbance of the cardiac rhythm in which the heart cannot beat normally, survival due to AED use has been shown to be greater than 70%.[22] An AED should be used within the first three minutes of arrest. Brain damage, which can become irreversible, develops in as little as three to five minutes without a pulse. In fact, among adults with out-of-hospital ventricular fibrillation arrest, the chance of survival drops by 7% to 10% for each minute these devices are not used.[23]

Little data on the use of AEDS on younger athletes currently exist. A study looking at nine cases of sudden cardiac arrest among college athletes provides discouraging results. In five of the nine cases, athletic trainers applied the AED at an average of 1.6 minutes after the event started. In the other four cases, emergency medical services utilized AEDS at an average of 5.2 minutes after the event. Eight of the nine athletes died.

Researchers at the University of Washington identified 486 cases of exercise-related sudden death events. These occurred in young patients ranging from elementary school to college age, from January 1, 2000, through December 31, 2006. The overall survival rate in these arrests was a dismal 11%, although the survival rates improved in the more recent years of the study.

The authors obtained details of defibrillation used in 40 of the 55 patients who survived: 93% of them (37 out of 40) received defibrillation, 35% received AED by a bystander, and 58% underwent defibrillation by emergency medical services personnel.[24]

Health-care organizations do recommend the availability of AEDs and advocate their use in children. The National Athletic Trainers' Association (NATA) recommends public access to AEDs, development of emergency action plans, and the use of CPR and AED when these events occur.[25] More studies on the use of AEDs with young athletes are needed to demonstrate the effect of AEDs for improving survival of sudden cardiac arrest.

The bigger question from Leonard's death is not treatment, but prevention. If any doctors involved—the team's physician or other physicians who performed the preparticipation physical exam, or even his primary care physician—had detected that Leonard had dilated cardiomyopathy, he likely would have been restricted from playing sports. He never would have played on that Fennville High School team, but he might be alive today.

The fundamental questions that Gathers's and Leonard's deaths create seem straightforward at first.

Can physicians screen for and effectively detect the underlying conditions that cause sudden cardiac death?

If we can effectively identify athletes at risk for sudden cardiac death, is it feasible to screen every young athlete preparing to play sports?

Parents, coaches, and sports fans likely assume that the answers to these questions are easy. It seems reasonable that if we can prevent an athlete from dropping dead on the field or court, physicians should do whatever it takes to do so.

Unfortunately, the answers to those two questions are among the most debated topics in all of sports medicine.

In 1971 Italy instituted a law that required every athlete aged 12 to 35 to undergo an annual evaluation in order for athletes to participate in competitive sports. In 1982 the law was revised to specifically stipulate that preparticipation screening be conducted annually and include a general physical examination and 12-lead electrocardiogram (ECG).

The law did not only mandate the necessary components of cardiovascular screening. It held physicians criminally negligent for improperly clearing an athlete to participate in sports if that athlete later was determined to have died as the result of an undetected cardiovascular abnormality.

Researchers argued that under this law, the incidence of SCD dropped significantly with the addition of routine ECG. Studies by Domenico Corrado showed that the incidence dropped from 3.6 deaths per 100,000 person-years between 1979 and 1981 to 0.4 death per 100,000 person-years in 2003–2004. These data suggested an 89% reduction in deaths among screened athletes. In the early years of this program, 1.8% of the athletes in the Veneto region of Italy were excluded from competition due to cardiovascular conditions.[26]

Using data largely from the Italian model, the European Society of Cardiology recommended a policy that included ECGs for all athletes as part of a screening process.[27] The International Olympic Committee followed suit with its recommendations for screening of Olympic athletes.[28]

Approximately 4,000 athletes play in the four major professional sports in the United States. Each sport utilizes its own standard for cardiac evaluation of its athletes, but clearance of these athletes largely involves some combination of ECG, echocardiogram, or exercise stress test. In fact, a 2006 study found that 92% of major North American professional sports teams use ECGs in routine preparticipation screening.[29]

With the top athletes in the United States undergoing ECG, and countries in Europe forcing doctors to utilize them for screening athletes, why are ECGs not required screening tests for athletes in this country?

To better explain the arguments for and against mandatory ECGs, it's important to understand the current standards.

The AHA and its Sudden Death Committee (Clinical Cardiology) and Congenital Cardiac Defects Committee (Cardiovascular Disease in the Young) issued guidelines for the evaluation of cardiac risk in the athletic population in 1996. These guidelines were largely retained in the 2007 and 2014 AHA updates.

As part of a preparticipation physical exam, health-care providers perform a 14-point screening. These points include questions asked while taking an athlete's history and findings on physical examination.

The information specifically asked as part of the medical history includes a personal history of chest pain or discomfort with physical exertion, unexplained syncope or near-syncope, unexplained or excessive fatigue or shortness of breath with exercise, a heart murmur, or high blood pressure.

The questions regarding family history include death due to heart disease in one or more relatives, heart-related disability in relatives under the age of 50, and the presence of a number of cardiac conditions among family members.

The physical examination looks for abnormalities with respect to pulses in the legs, blood pressure, heart murmur, and signs of the presence of connective tissue diseases.

These questions alert the examiner to current symptoms possibly signifying an underlying cardiac condition or to a family history of a condition that might increase the risk that the athlete being screened also has that heart condition. Given the likelihood that a young athlete might not know about heart conditions in other family members, parents are strongly encouraged to fill out the questionnaires with their children.

An affirmative answer to any of the heart questions or a positive finding on the physical exam alerts the examiner that the athlete could have an underlying heart problem. That examiner then would refer the athlete for further diagnostic testing (such as an ECG or echocardiogram), for evaluation by a cardiologist, or both.

Does the current system in the United States work?

Proponents of the current system point to the incidence of SCD among young athletes. A study of 1.9 million high school student-athletes in Minnesota in 24 sports over 26 years reported 13 deaths, which correlated with an incidence rate of 1:150,000 per year.[30] Some studies even show that the SCD rates are even lower than the postscreening rates after the Italian mandate.

On the other hand, the current system has flaws, including discrepancies in how preparticipation physical exams are administered.

Mass screenings are commonly employed at American middle schools and high schools. These sessions, with hundreds of athletes spread across gymnasiums or examined after standing in lines, are certainly efficient. Health-care providers can perform huge numbers of preparticipation physical exams with the fewest resources in a short period of time.

These mass screenings are complicated by noise, which could hinder physicians hearing subtle heart murmurs. After waiting for hours, young kids might not mention symptoms, in order to finish as quickly as possible. While it's efficient in completing the largest number of exams, mass screening is likely far from being the most thorough and effective process.

A one-on-one preparticipation physical exam (PPE) between an athlete and a physician is ideal. While many athletes see their primary care physician for the exam, it is believed that a large percentage of these examinations are performed in urgent care facilities. These physicians (or midlevel providers such as physician's assistants or nurse practitioners) are often unfamiliar with the athlete and likely have no sports medicine training.

In terms of level of training, there is wide variation in the training and education of the examiners. Even among physicians, there is no specific requirement that a pediatrician or family medicine physician perform the exam. Certainly there is no guideline mandating experience with athletes. Physician's assistants and nurse practitioners often perform PPEs as well. The AHA update in 2007 noted that over one-third of PPEs of US high school athletes are performed by nonphysicians. At the time of the update, 18 states allowed chiropractors to clear athletes to play.[31]

The history and physical examinations of 134 athletes who fell victim to SCD were reviewed retrospectively. Only 3% of the athletes were considered to have a cardiovascular condition based on this preparticipation 12-point screening. None of those athletes were excluded from athletic competition.

With the flaws in our current PPE system, the data from Italy, and the use of ECG among Olympic athletes and most American professional athletes, it is no wonder that many experts advocate ECG screening for young American athletes.

Within the modern version of the Hippocratic oath lies a pledge applicable to this debate. "I will prevent disease whenever I can, for prevention is preferable to cure."

If technology to identify someone at risk for illness or injury exists, it is only natural to assume that as physicians we should do whatever it takes to prevent that injury, or in this case, potentially save that life.

Critics of the AHA guidelines argue that the value of a life saved could be greater in this population. Because a young athlete potentially has many more years to live, screening to prevent these deaths could be more beneficial than programs to screen for illnesses in older people. Also, these screening programs could identify cardiac conditions with a familial predisposition. If one identifies a heart condition in an athlete, one could find it in his brothers, sisters, parents, or extended family.

Lawmakers could enact legislation requiring every athlete to undergo an ECG prior to being allowed to play. The development of the system or organization to oversee such a plan would be challenging and expensive. The actual tests, though, are relatively simple to perform. Even nonphysicians, such as athletic trainers, could be instructed to place the leads and start the ECG recording.

The first challenge, though, lies in determining who could, and would, interpret the tests. Primary care physicians, such as family medicine doctors and pediatricians, are certainly qualified to interpret ECGs. Possibly more debate might arise concerning physician's assistants, nurse practitioners, or even physicians covering urgent care facilities. Would they consistently recognize the subtle changes that might signify a cardiac abnormality?

There is wide variability in what is considered to be abnormal findings on an ECG. What is normal for an adult might be abnormal for a young athlete. Also, high-level athletes have been shown to develop adaptive changes in their hearts, and thus heart tracings might appear slightly different than in the nonathletic adolescents.

With increased attention on cardiac events in athletes and larger numbers of athletes undergoing cardiac testing, findings that represent a normal "athlete's heart" and not signs of structural problems are being recognized. Approximately 40% of athletes have abnormal ECGs, and most of those are felt to be physiological adaptations from training.[32]

It is reasonable to ask whether family medicine physicians or pediatricians would recognize ECG findings of hypertrophic cardiomyopathy and other causes of SCD in the first place. These conditions are somewhat rare in the young population, so it is unlikely that many primary care physicians who do not have a sports medicine background have seen many such patients in their careers.

The purpose of a screening test is presumably to alert a physician to a possible condition and initiate a workup to determine if that condition truly exists. In this model, an abnormal ECG would lead to a formal cardiac evaluation. This workup could include testing—most likely an echocardiogram—or referral to a pediatric cardiologist.

What percentage of these workups would be unnecessary? In other words, how many false positive ECGs would occur? How many ECGs would show heart tracings that suggest cardiac abnormalities, when in fact no such problem exists?

Data regarding the false positive rate of ECG in this population vary. When ECG was used as part of the screening of 510 college athletes, the tests proved to have a false positive rate of 16.9%. Applying newer criteria for ECG findings that are considered normal for changes in the hearts of athletes dropped the false positive rate to 9.6%.[33]

The AHA estimated that 15% of young athletes would have positive findings on the history, physical examination, or ECG. That 15% includes both truly positive findings and false positive findings. Assuming that roughly 10 million middle school and high school athletes would be screened, approximately 1.5 million athletes would require further cardiac workup.[34]

In its 2014 statement, the AHA suggested that even if the false positive rate of ECGs could be brought down to 5%, screening 10 million athletes would still identify roughly 500,000 who would then need further testing to rule out underlying heart disease. The authors suggest that very few of those athletes would ultimately prove to have heart disease placing them at risk for SCD that would require disqualification from sports.[35]

An American College of Cardiology Workforce Task Force noted that 2,039 board-certified pediatric cardiologists practiced in the United States. At the time of its 2009 report, 30%, or nearly 800 pediatric cardiologists, were expected to retire within the next 10 years.[36]

Many feel that these specialists are already saturated with patients known to have cardiac conditions. Can this small number of pediatric cardiologists add a large number of patients to their clinics, especially in a timely manner? And what would young athletes in small towns do? Access to a pediatric cardiologist could be particularly challenging in smaller, more rural areas.

Interestingly, at the time of this writing, Fennville, Michigan, the hometown of Wes Leonard, does not have a practicing pediatric cardiologist. The nearest one practices in Holland, Michigan, about 14 miles away.

The cardiac evaluation based on positive ECG findings introduces an even bigger question. How much would such a program cost? One can't stop with the cost of each test. Further studies, referrals to specialists, and even program administration must be considered.

In its 2007 guidelines, the AHA calculated an enormous potential cost. It assumed a cost of $50 per ECG plus $25 for the preparticipation physical itself.

With a population of 10 million athletes needing screening, that would be $750 million for the screening process alone.

With the earlier calculated 1.5 million athletes who would require an echocardiogram (estimated at $400 per test) and/or referral to a specialist (estimated at $100 per visit), the estimated cost would skyrocket to $1.5 billion. Factoring in an estimated $500 million for administration of the nationwide program, the AHA concluded that mandatory ECG screenings would cost $2 billion per year.[37]

Critics of the AHA recommendations argue that this estimate is too high. They point to cost efficiencies that could come with performing large numbers of ECGs rather than individual tests in an office setting. In addition, creation of a health-care or government infrastructure to administer and oversee the program would create mostly one-time costs rather than the $500 million per year the AHA suggests. Finally, many point out that an athlete might not need to undergo an ECG each year.

Whatever the true amount would be, who would pay that cost? Schools? Athletes and their families? Taxpayers?

While disease prevention is certainly a noble and desirable goal in modern health care, the issue of finite resources, especially money, must be considered. Would the $2 billion per year, or even the lower estimates, be better spent screening for more common killers? Would screening and prevention measures for childhood obesity, which affects far more children and adolescents, be more effective from both fiscal and overall population health standpoints?

There is another way to look at whether spending that amount of money should be a priority in American health care. What would it cost with a mandatory ECG program to save the life of a single young athlete?

Again the estimates vary widely. The AHA estimated the cost of preventing a single death using its calculation of $2 billion per year. Factoring in both the incidence of the common underlying causes of SCD among children and adolescents and the risk of sudden death of those athletes, it believed that it would cost $3.4 million to prevent one theoretical death.[38]

Since these are young athletes with many years to live, it might be better to look at the cost of the tests in terms of life-years saved. Most public policy debates use $50,000 per life-year saved to consider a health-care intervention to be cost effective. The ECG screenings in both the Italian system and a similar program in Japan have reportedly cost well below this $50,000 per life-year saved threshold.[39] Even a study looking at ECGs among Nevada high school athletes estimated that the tests cost $44,000 per year of life saved.[40]

The last category of arguments against ECG comes from the legal angle, and there are many potential legal issues.

First, would this policy drive physicians away from performing clearance physicals? Some worry that fear of litigation over missing a fatal cardiac condition would lead to fewer physicians being willing to perform them. The AHA even articulated this possibility. Pediatric cardiologists and primary care sports medicine physicians might feel comfortable interpreting ECGs in young athletes. Would general pediatricians, family medicine physicians, or even physician's assistants or nurse practitioners, who do not regularly treat athletes, feel as confident?

Would public and community-based preparticipation screening programs using volunteer efforts and/or fee-for-service vendors effectively identify at-risk athletes at individual high schools, even if not used on a widespread basis?

Also, what are the legal ramifications if an athlete is felt to have a condition such as hypertrophic cardiomyopathy? Could an athlete and his family choose to play against medical advice? Or could the athlete refuse an ECG in the first place? These legal questions could arise in our current system, but one wonders if legal battles would increase with mandatory testing.

Dr. Jordan Metzl, a primary care sports medicine physician at the Hospital for Special Surgery in New York City, believes ECG screening will eventually become a mandatory component of preparticipation physical exams.

"I think it's probably coming," Dr. Metzl predicted. "I'm not, personally, a huge fan. I don't think it makes a lot of sense just from a dollars and cents point of view. I just think we could spend our resources better somewhere else. But, I think we're probably headed in that direction is my guess."[41]

Exactly 25 years after the Loyola Marymount star's SCD, the NCAA's chief medical officer, Dr. Brian Hainline, announced that he would recommend electrocardiogram screening for college athletes at higher risk of cardiac defects.

According to Sharon Terlep of the *Wall Street Journal*, Hainline based his recommendation to screen male college basketball players on the 2011 study that found the rate of sudden cardiac death among Division I male college basketball players to be roughly 1 in 3,100 per year.[42] Medical experts disagree on the rates for all college athletes, with some placing that figure around 1 in 43,000 athletes and others feeling it is closer to 1 in 100,000.[43]

A study published in *Circulation*, a journal of the AHA, in May 2015 found an incidence rate of SCD in Division I male basketball athletes of 1 in 5,200 athlete-years.[44] While opponents criticized the study and how it calculated the incidence rate, Dr. Hainline stressed that the study proved the issue deserves attention.

His announcement renewed the debate among medical professionals about cardiac screening for athletes. While Dr. Hainline alone cannot create a rule that would require NCAA schools to implement ECG testing for their athletes, it is conceivable that his recommendation could have placed an NCAA school refusing to use the tests in legal jeopardy if one of its athletes died suddenly.

Barry J. Maron, MD, the cardiologist who served as the lead author of the AHA's position statements on cardiac screening for athletes, told the *Wall Street Journal* that Hainline's recommendation could create more problems than it solves. "This idea of screening selectively with [ECGs] is an unfortunate decision and initiative that will undoubtedly lead to unnecessary targeting (including by race), confusion, misdiagnosis, overdiagnosis and ultimately many unnecessary college-athlete disqualifications."[45]

One hundred university team physicians signed a petition opposing Hainline's plan. Dr. Hainline did ultimately change his mind about pushing for ECG testing, but he aims to keep urging that more attention be paid to the issue, with the hope of preventing another death like Hank Gathers's.

The issue now is no longer whether we could identify silent but potentially deadly cardiac abnormalities. Parents, physicians, and lawmakers will have to decide whether we should universally screen athletes for these conditions.

11 / *KOREY STRINGER*

Exertional Heat Stroke

July 31, 2001

The northern latitude of Mankato, Minnesota, offered little relief from the brutal summer heat as the Minnesota Vikings began the second day of training camp.

With temperatures in the 90s and the heat index hitting 110, the Vikings practiced for two and one-half hours. The players wore full pads as they engaged in one-on-one drills with intense hitting.

The team's medical staff, including head athletic trainer Chuck Barta, treated several Vikings players for heat-related problems that day. "You recognize you have the heat, you recognize you have to force fluids down them and you also have ice towels to keep them cool," Barta said in an article days later in the *New York Times*.[1] Most of those Vikings players recovered uneventfully. Korey Stringer did not.

According to a press release issued by the team the following day, the offensive lineman walked off the field to an air-conditioned shelter. He reported feeling dizzy and weak before starting to breathe rapidly. Athletic trainers attended to him and called emergency medical services.

Documents submitted to the court in a suit filed by Korey's wife Kelci and his family against the Vikings and its coaches and medical staff paint a much scarier picture of the events of July 31.[2] While attorneys for the team likely contested specific details of this account, it is at least worthwhile to present the family's version of the key events on and off the field that morning.

Stringer reported for practice Tuesday morning as he had promised after his struggles with the heat the day before. During the formal practice, Vikings center Matt Birk saw Stringer vomit clear fluid.

After the formal practice ended, Stringer reportedly dropped to his knees, then lay on his back. Stringer collapsed at approximately 11:15 a.m.

Athletic trainers took Stringer to a nearby trailer. Attorneys for Stringer's family claimed that the athletic trainers involved offered insufficient attention to Stringer once he arrived in the trailer. They argued there was little to no assessment of Stringer's medical condition, including measurements of his temperature or his vital signs. They claimed that the athletic trainers showed little concern for Stringer's lack of verbal responses to comments and questions or his inexplicably lying on the floor and humming and bobbing his head to "music."

According to court documents, athletic trainer Paul Osterman noticed that Stringer was "unresponsive" and did not move when asked to get onto a cart about 30 minutes after arriving in the trailer.

When Osterman took Stringer's pulse, he described it as "weak" but "steady." Another athletic trainer, Fred Zamberletti, arrived and observed Stringer's rapid, shallow breathing. Assuming Stringer was hyperventilating, they put a plastic bag over his nose and mouth.

Osterman called Dr. David Knowles, a family practitioner in Mankato and physician for the training camp. Dr. Knowles reportedly told him to call an ambulance. Osterman called for an ambulance at 12:00 p.m. and noted a "glazed stare" in the player's eyes.

On the way to the hospital, emergency medical providers measured Stringer's pulse at 140 beats per minute. He was comatose.

The ambulance took Stringer to Immanuel St. Joseph's-Mayo Health System, arriving at 12:24 p.m. When his body temperature was checked at 12:35 p.m., it measured 108.8°F.

Korey Stringer passed away at 1:50 a.m. on August 1, 2001.[3]

Wide receiver Cris Carter remained at the hospital until Stringer's death, along with head coach Dennis Green, fellow wide receiver Randy Moss, and the rest of the offensive line. Carter spoke at the news conference after Stringer's death.

"We thought everything was going to change (at the hospital). There's nothing that can prepare you for something like this. It's far graver than any football (game). The amount of hurt this has on our team. . . . [W]e are devastated."[4]

Korey Stringer was born in Warren, Ohio, on May 8, 1974. After playing for Ohio State, he was the first-round draft pick of the Minnesota Vikings in 1995. Ultimately Stringer was named to the Pro Bowl in the 2000–2001 NFL season, his last before his death.

Stringer lived all year in the Minneapolis area. He volunteered in community service programs in schools and at the St. Paul Library, which made him a local fan favorite.

The Minnesota Vikings would take the field for a preseason game only 10 days later, but Green recognized the immediate needs of his players. He woke his team at 6:00 on the morning of August 1 to deliver the news of Stringer's passing.

"We think we have the type of young men who can go on and play football," Green told reporters. "But right now, we are concerned about the Stringer family. We have lost a 27-year-old man and we are going to miss him. He had a great ability to give, and he was one of our gifts from heaven."[5]

Korey Stringer left behind his wife, Kelci, who was also 27 years old at the time, and his three-year-old son, Kodie.

Korey Stringer was the first NFL player to die from heat stroke.

Exertional heat stroke is arguably one of the most serious medical conditions that can affect athletes. Up to 15% of patients die. Others suffer permanent organ and neurological damage.

If we are going to successfully protect football players and other athletes from the youth recreational levels to high school, college, and the pros, we must focus both on the treatment of heat stroke and on recognizing the risk factors and taking steps to correct them.

In terms of treatment of this potentially fatal condition, medical providers actually can successfully prevent an athlete from dying by quickly recognizing the problem and taking immediate efforts to cool his body.

By definition, exertional heat stroke encompasses a core body temperature greater than 40°C (104°F) and altered mental status. It is believed to be the culmination of overheating from either dangerous environmental conditions or increases in body temperature from exertion, or both.

Heat stroke is thought to be the most serious condition in a spectrum of heat-related illnesses. Milder forms of heat illness, like heat rash, heat edema, heat cramps, and even heat syncope, can usually be treated with rest, fluids, and cooling the athlete's body. Heat exhaustion often causes nausea, vomiting, and dizziness, but the athlete demonstrates normal cognitive function.

Evidence of altered mental status suggests an athlete could be facing life-threatening heat stroke. That abnormal mental state might manifest as confusion, disorientation, impaired judgment, abnormal motor coordination, seizures, or loss of consciousness.

The excessive core body temperature in heat stroke can quickly cause multi-system organ failure. Seizures, cardiac arrhythmias, and liver failure can develop. The patient's blood pressure can drop to dangerously low levels. Muscle tissue can break down, dumping waste products into the bloodstream and potentially shutting down the kidneys—a condition called rhabdomyolysis. Acute respiratory distress syndrome, a lung condition in which little oxygen gets into the blood, and disseminated intravascular coagulation, a condition in which blood clots develop in the small vessels, causing organ failure and widespread bleeding as clotting factors are consumed, can occur rapidly.

It is critical that athletic trainers and other medical providers present recognize an athlete struggling before he reaches the point of heat stroke. Often they aren't aware of an athlete developing heat illness. The athlete might be reluctant to report feeling sick, so other players and coaches should watch for nausea, vomiting, dizziness, and fatigue and bring any ill player to the attention of the medical staff.

Moving the athlete to a cooler location, preferably an air-conditioned environment, and encouraging him to drink fluids is important. A baseline measurement of the athlete's core body temperature is critical. The athletic trainer should take a rectal temperature, as it is better at determining core body temperature than other methods of taking a person's temperature.

If an athlete does suffer heat stroke, athletic trainers and doctors can still prevent the athlete from dying if they recognize it and start treatment immediately, according to Douglas J. Casa, PhD, a professor in the Department of Kinesiology at the University of Connecticut, as well as chief operating officer of the Korey Stringer Institute and a leading expert on heat stroke.[6]

It's critical that doctors and athletic trainers recognize any alterations in mental status or other central nervous system dysfunction and obtain a rectal temperature to properly assess core body temperature. Then the medical staff must treat the athlete on site first. They should use cold water immersion—putting him in a cold bath—to get his temperature down below 104°F. Then the athlete can be transported to a hospital.

Medical providers have a roughly 30-minute window to decrease the athlete's core body temperature. If they skip cold-water immersion and instead wait for an ambulance, they lose 5 to 7 minutes or more before it arrives. Then the paramedics might need 8 to 10 minutes to assess the athlete and load him into the ambulance. The transport to the hospital could take 10 to 15 minutes. It will then take several minutes for the emergency room doctors to assess him before initiating treatment. Now far more than the critical 30 minutes have passed.

That 30-minute window is vitally important. Approximately 105.5°F appears to be a critical threshold for cell damage. If an athlete's core body temperature falls below that level within 30 minutes, the athlete survives and has no long-term complications. If his temperature remains above 105.5°F for 30 to 60 minutes, he might survive but suffer long-term complications. If he remains above 105.5° past 60 minutes, he will either die or survive but suffer permanent damage.

Let's say an athlete's core body temperature is 108° when an athletic trainer first takes a rectal temperature. That temperature is a reasonable estimate given that the vast majority of athletes are between 106° and 110° in these cases. It takes about three minutes to lower an athlete's temperature 1°F. To get him down to a safe 104° level, it would take at least 12 minutes.

That's 12 minutes once the medical staff starts cooling the player. Getting the athlete off the field, taking his helmet and pads off, assessing him, taking his rectal temperature, and preparing the cold tub add several minutes before the cooling starts. Finally, the athletic trainers and doctors must realize that the athlete's temperature probably exceeded the critical threshold for several minutes before anyone recognized his illness.

With quick and appropriate action, doctors and athletic trainers can prevent deaths in controlled sports environments like football fields or road races. "Deaths from EHS within controlled environments are always preventable," Dr. Casa stressed. "Meaning, exertional heat stroke is 100% survivable if you get their core body temperature under 104° within 30 minutes of collapse. Over 2,000 cases of heat stroke—all have survived when this is accomplished."[7]

"All Korey wanted to do was get better. Everybody wants to talk about the heat, but it's hot everywhere. This is really difficult. We really don't understand. It's a shock. There is nothing in life to prepare you for something like this," Cris Carter remarked at a press conference held shortly after Stringer's death.[8]

Commissioner Paul Tagliabue of the NFL praised the league's medical treatments and preparedness while also urging teams to review their assessment and treatment procedures. "N.F.L. medical staffs are extremely knowledgeable regarding hydration of players, fluid replacement and other methods used to prevent heatstroke," he noted in a statement released shortly after Stringer's death.[9]

Even with rapid medical assessment, conditions in Mankato that day could have created a perfect storm of sorts for any athlete trying to play football. Reviewing the conditions and circumstances on that hot July day can help us better understand the extrinsic risk factors for exertional heat stroke. These factors include the temperature, humidity, physical activity, and clothing.

The weather conditions on the first day of training camp, July 30, 2001, were the most difficult that the Minnesota Vikings had experienced in a decade, with extreme temperatures and heat index levels. To understand the risk that Vikings players faced that day, we must recognize the different ways an athlete's body eliminates heat.

Essentially, heat travels from a hotter surface to a cooler one in one of four ways. Conduction of heat involves the direct transfer of heat through contact with a cooler object, such as an ice pack. Convection allows heat to transfer from the player's warm skin into cooler air passing around the body, such as a breeze or wind. Radiation involves direct release of heat into the environment. Evaporation allows heat to be released through perspiration.

All of these mechanisms of heat dissipation could have been altered that day. High outside temperatures decrease an athlete's ability to dissipate heat as he gains radiant heat from the environment. Excessive humidity impairs his body's ability to dissipate body heat through evaporation of sweat. Helmets and layers of clothing and pads add weight and interfere with his ability to cool.

In Monday's first practice, players wore only shorts and "shells," or essentially pads and helmets. As Stringer took the field Tuesday morning, players wore the full uniform, helmet, and shoulder pads. Stringer wore a dark-colored jersey and a knee sleeve under his football pants.

During that first day of practice, offensive line coach Mike Tice reportedly noticed that Stringer appeared sluggish. Stringer told Tice that his stomach was "killing him." Stringer vomited multiple times before athletic trainers took him into a trailer.

According to court documents in the lawsuit filed by Kelci Stringer against the team and its coaches and medical staff, Dr. Knowles recorded that Korey Stringer had experienced an episode of heat exhaustion on that first day of camp.

In the same court documents, attorneys for the Stringer family asserted that this was not the lineman's first experience with heat issues. They claimed that Stringer had been treated for heat-related illnesses prior to the 2001 training camp.[10]

When he returned to practice on what would prove to be that fateful Tuesday, the heat was still scorching. The National Weather Service issued two heat advisories for Mankato, projecting that the heat index could reach 105° to 110°F. According to court documents, the weather advisories cautioned, "extremely humid conditions will team up with hot weather to produce potentially life-threatening conditions."[11]

Approximately 400 people die from heat-related illness in the United States each year. While only a fraction of these deaths results from athletics, exertional heat stroke is the third leading cause of death among athletes, after cardiac arrests and brain injuries. According to the National Center for Catastrophic Sports Injury Research, football is associated with the greatest number of heat stroke deaths.[12]

Football players can't control how hard they work or when to quit, putting them at risk for heat illness.

"The reason you see it in the football environment is that the person often doesn't get to control his own intensity," Dr. Casa explained. "It's controlled for him. If you had football players just out doing their own conditioning sessions, football players are not going to ever drive themselves to heat stroke. They're only driven to heat stroke because they're trying to keep up with teammates or the coach is telling them they have to do a certain amount in a certain amount of time. Thankfully, people don't, on their own usually, or almost ever, drive themselves to have a heat stroke. Meaning, if you and I went out for a 10-mile run in brutally hot conditions, we would back off when we started feeling like crap. We wouldn't go to the point of killing ourselves if we were just out on a recreational run together on a trail."[13]

In terms of intrinsic risk factors for heat illness, an athlete's fitness level, his hydration, his heat acclimatization status, and other personal factors influence his risk.

The size of most football players is one of the most important intrinsic risk factors. People with more body weight produce more heat metabolically. Unfortunately, that increased body mass does not cause a proportional increase in body surface area. With a relatively lower surface area, overweight athletes would be less capable of dissipating heat through evaporative means.

Dr. Casa estimated that about 80% of all heat strokes in football involve linemen. Dr. Barry Boden agreed that football linemen are especially at risk. Boden published a study on fatalities in high school and college football, many of which were related to heat.

"Exertional heat stroke deaths are more common in overweight patients such as the 300-plus linemen. The problem with these obese patients is that they have increased heat production, but a relatively low surface area necessary to dissipate the heat for evaporation. These overweight athletes are the ones that really need to be monitored carefully."[14]

This combination of increased physical exertion and body mass could predispose athletes to heat illness. A study of military recruits in the Israeli army found that half of the cases of heat stroke occurred in the recruits' first six months of service. During this period, a recruit's desire to push himself to new limits physically might have been more important than the outside temperature, as many of the events occurred in the spring. Of the soldiers who suffered exertional heat stroke, 60% were overweight.[15]

Korey Stringer stood six-foot-four and weighed 335 pounds. Weight was an issue throughout his playing career. In fact, he frequently tipped the scales at over 350 pounds. Heading into what would have been his seventh season, Stringer claimed that he had arrived at training camp in the best shape of his life.

In an interview with Clifton Brown of *Sporting News* 10 years after Stringer's death, Kelci said that she believed many people think Stringer's size, health, or supplement or substance use might have led to his heat stroke. In fact, during the legal battle between Kelci Stringer and the Minnesota Vikings, lawyers for the team claimed Stringer was taking a supplement containing ephedra.[16]

Certain medications and supplements can increase the risk of heat illness. Stimulants like amphetamines, thyroid medications, and ephedra can increase the body's heat production. Ephedra, a supplement used for weight loss and increased energy and athletic performance, can be dangerous when used while training or competing in hot temperatures. In 2001 the NFL banned ephedra.

In addition to obesity and stimulants, there are many other risk factors for heat illness. Different classes of medications increase the risk in different ways: decreasing sweat production, increasing heat production, or altering the cardiovascular response to dehydration.

Coexisting medical conditions, recent illnesses in which the athlete has had a fever, sickle cell trait, sunburn, skin conditions like psoriasis, and alcohol abuse are all believed to be risk factors for heat illness. And kids under the age of 15 are thought to have a higher risk as well.

In sports, dehydration likely plays an enormous role in the development of exertional heat stroke. Both excessive loss of body fluids through sweating and inadequate fluid intake can increase the risk for heat illness.

While watching athletes drink bottles of sports drinks and swallow gulps of water during games seems commonplace now, proper hydration was not recognized as important decades earlier.

In a 1984 article in the *American Journal of Sports Medicine*, the team physician at The Ohio State University, ironically where Korey Stringer later played college football, described the evolution in prevention of heat issues in the 25 years up to that point.

Robert J. Murphy, MD, recounted the story of five Ohio State football players who had collapsed on a hot and humid day decades earlier. Four of the five players had recovered with intravenous fluids in the training room, but the fifth player had lost consciousness and was taken to the hospital. He was found to have a rectal temperature of 106.2°F. He suffered kidney and liver damage but ultimately recovered.

Murphy also recalled another Buckeye player who battled multiple episodes of heat exhaustion. The medical staff began weighing the athletes before and after practices and observed up to a 22-pound weight loss within a given practice.

Dr. Murphy then described reviewing the procedures at Ohio State in order to prevent these episodes of heat illness. Water, which was not even on the field 25 years earlier, was now given to players throughout those practices and games. Likewise, weighing each player before and after practices became the norm.[17]

Today sports medicine organizations have created guidelines for fluid management. For example, the NATA recommends that athletes drink 16 to 20 ounces of fluid in the two to three hours before physical activity. Just before training, they should consume 6 to 10 more ounces of water or sports drink. They should drink 6 to 10 ounces every 15 to 20 minutes during training. If an athlete weighs himself after practice and finds that he has lost weight, he should replace every pound lost by drinking 16 ounces of fluid.[18]

While we must teach athletes about proper hydration and other risk factors for heat illness, it is critical that parents, coaches, and medical providers who work with athletes learn to prevent and recognize heat illness and treat athletes at risk.

To that end, Korey Stringer's tragedy ultimately might have a positive outcome. Since the time of his death, Kelci has been an advocate for the prevention of sudden death in sports, especially exertional heat stroke.

Kelci Stringer partnered with Dr. Casa and the University of Connecticut Neag School of Education to create the Korey Stringer Institute. In conjunction with its corporate partners—the NFL, Gatorade, and others—the institute opened in 2010.

The organization focuses on four areas. First, it conducts research into sudden death in sports, including heat stroke. It provides education to physicians, athletic trainers, coaches, paramedics, athletic directors, schools, and athletes. The institute works with leagues and at the state level to promote policy changes.

Finally, it works with athletes to perform heat tolerance testing and help athletes who have suffered heat stroke recover.

Outside of sports, the Korey Stringer Institute works to change policies in the military and industrial settings as well.

Dr. Casa especially recognizes the importance of treatment and prevention of heat stroke, as he suffered an episode of heat stroke himself:

> When I was 16 years old, I grew up in New York, so we have something called the Empire State Games, which was like a summer Olympic-style festival for the best athletes in the state that came and represented their region. I qualified out of Long Island for the 10-K, and the 10-K on the track is 25 laps on the track. They decided to run that in Buffalo during a heat wave in the middle of the day.
>
> On the 25th lap, I was vying for a medal. I collapsed at 200 meters to go, got back up, and then collapsed again with about 50 meters to go and was in a coma for most of the afternoon. Very luckily I had amazing care on-site and at Millard Fillmore Hospital in Buffalo and had a physician there who knew about aggressively bringing someone's temperature down.
>
> From that day in August of '85, now 31 years later, the concept of prevention, recognition, and treatment of exertional heat stroke has consumed me.[19]

Since Korey Stringer's death in 2001, no NFL player has died due to heat stroke. Unfortunately, heat stroke does still occur in college and high school football.

Dr. Boden and other researchers analyzed data regarding fatalities in high school and college football reported to the National Center for Catastrophic Sports Injury Research between July 1990 and June 2010. Among the 243 fatalities in that 20-year period, 38 deaths were related to heat—almost 2 per year.

When the authors looked at specific factors in these heat-related fatalities, many common factors emerged that existed in Stringer's death as well.

On the days of the high school and college heat stroke deaths, the average temperature was 79.8° F. The average high temperature was 89.6°. The average maximum humidity on the days of these events was 87.7%.

The exact temperature and humidity were not known at the specific time each athlete became ill. If the practices had been held during times of maximum temperatures (89.6°F) and maximum humidity (87.7%), the Wet Bulb Globe Index, which is thought to be the best measurement of environmental conditions related to heat illness, would have measured 104°F. This level would far exceed the levels representing a hazardous risk, in which case sporting events should be canceled.

The average weight of the players who died of heat stroke was 265 pounds. The average body mass index was 33.9. A person with a BMI of 30 is generally considered obese.

All 38 deaths occurred in July, August, or September, and 97% of the heat stroke events occurred during practices. In cases where the circumstances were known, 83% of the events occurred during two-a-day practice sessions, and 44% occurred on the first day of practice.

The athletes were wearing helmets in 60% of the heat stroke deaths, and 25% occurred in players wearing full equipment.[20]

Even if heat and humidity do not exceed critical levels, athletes and coaches must exercise caution when practicing in summer months. Players' bodies must grow accustomed to these conditions. This process, called acclimatization, involves the body "learning" to increase its sweat rate and decrease its electrolyte loss.

Generally, athletes require about 7 to 10 days to acclimatize to hot and humid conditions. This period of time gives the athlete time to safely adjust by increasing physical activity and exposure to the conditions, as well as adding clothing and equipment.

In 2009 the NATA developed heat-acclimatization guidelines for secondary schools. The NCAA has similar guidelines for its schools.

The NATA designated the heat-acclimatization period as the first 14 consecutive days of preseason practice. Its practice, clothing, and equipment recommendations aim to gradually enhance exercise heat tolerance of the athletes and their ability to exercise safely and effectively in hot weather.

In the first five days, athletes may not participate in more than one practice per day. The total practice time should not exceed three hours in any one day. A one-hour walk-through is permitted during these first five days, but teams must place a three-hour recovery period between the practice and walk-through.

On the first two days, players can only wear helmets. On days three through five, players may wear helmets and shoulder pads. Only starting on the sixth day of practice may players wear full uniforms and equipment. Teams may start full contact on day six.

Teams can start two-a-day practices on day six, but they must follow them with a single-practice day. On a single-practice day, the team can also add a walk-through that is separated from formal practice by at least three hours. A double-practice day can be followed by a rest day and then another double-practice day.

On days when teams have two practices, neither of the practice sessions should exceed three hours. Players should participate for no more than five total hours, including warm-up, stretching, cool-down, walk-through, conditioning, and lifting weights. The two practice sessions must be separated by at least three hours in a cool environment.

Finally, due to the high risk of heat illness during this period of acclimatization, athletic trainers should be present before, during, and after each practice.[21]

Approximately 14 states currently have guidelines that meet the minimum NATA standards. Fortunately, these are largely states in the southeast United States, where the risk of heat illness is highest. Getting all 50 states to adopt these guidelines will take tremendous effort.

"It's such an uphill battle getting policies changed," Dr. Casa noted. "Just take ten important policies for high school sports. Let's say AEDs, coaching education, immersion tubs being available, wet bulb globe temperature policies. Just take our ten most important ones, and you have to get all ten of them changed for each of the 50 states. One of them might take an entire winter to get a state to approve. So that's one state, one policy, and then you've got to go back again and hit the next policy. It's just incredibly daunting sometimes. It just takes time."[22]

The reason for states to adopt these guidelines is clear. There has not been a single heat stroke death in high school football in August at a school in any state that followed guidelines passed in that state or the 2009 NATA guidelines.[23]

These acclimatization guidelines are the best—but not the only—evidence that heat stroke events are fundamentally different from almost every injury described in this book. We could largely—maybe even completely—prevent every athlete from dying from exertional heat stroke in sports. In that sense, our efforts to decrease noncontact ACL injuries through neuromuscular training programs—discussed in the next chapter—might represent a similar attempt to prevent an injury from happening in the first place.

A parent of a high school football player might worry about her son suffering a head or cervical spine injury, but those events might never be completely avoidable. She can, however, encourage her son to take steps that would dramatically decrease his risk of heat illness.

All of the risk factors described in this chapter should be addressed through prevention efforts and education programs, not just for professional athletes, but also for youth athletes. In fact, given the fact that adolescents appear to be more susceptible to heat illness than adults, it could be even more important for them.

Proper hydration is crucial. Athletes can consume sports drinks if the practice sessions are long. Teams must allow frequent rest breaks, during which every athlete goes to a shady area and removes his helmet and pads. Finally, an acclimatization period is critical.

Many young athletes try to get in shape and adjust to the heat at the same time, which can create an extra burden on their bodies. Instead, athletes should work to get in shape in the early part of the summer, especially June and early July. Then they can add in heat exposure, starting with relatively easy exercise in heat and then training harder as they get used to it.

Physicians performing preparticipation physical examinations for high school and college athletes should screen for sickle cell trait and other medical conditions that could predispose an athlete to heat illness. They should educate kids about the dangers of ephedra and other stimulants in nutritional supplements. Withholding an athlete from practice or competition while he recovers from a gastrointestinal, respiratory, or other illness is also important.

Teaching athletes proper hydration strategies is paramount. Coaches and athletic trainers must not only provide adequate water and sports drinks, but also learn to recognize the signs of dehydration. Daily weigh-ins before and after practice are a good start, but everyone involved with a sports team must understand and individually watch for any athlete demonstrating early signs and symptoms of heat illness.

Without a doubt, proper evaluation and initial field management of heat illness are vital. A survey of athletic trainers who treated athletes with exertional heat stroke in high school football during the 2011 preseason found that only 0.9% of them used rectal thermometers to measure core body temperature.[24] Oral, axillary, and forehead temperatures do not provide accurate measures of core body temperature, so this finding is discouraging. While ingestible heat sensors that can provide core body temperature data are currently available, all athletes participating in a practice or game must swallow them before heat stroke occurs. The cost might also prohibit their use in high school programs.

It is evident that adopting and following heat acclimatization guidelines is critical. We might eliminate most heat stroke events with these basic prevention measures. We can prevent deaths due to heat stroke if we recognize and treat affected athletes immediately.

Kodie Stringer was a three-year-old at the time of his father's death. By the time he turned 13, Kodie was big like his dad—six-foot-one and 280 pounds. He even played offensive line, as his father did for the Minnesota Vikings.

With the help of his mother's Korey Stringer Institute; athletic trainers and team doctors adopting treatment and prevention guidelines; and comprehensive education about heat illness for all parents, coaches, and athletes, maybe we can rid sports of heat stroke for Kodie and all young athletes.

12 / BRANDI CHASTAIN
Prevention of ACL Injuries

July 10, 1999

A 30-year-old native of San Jose, California, stood outside the penalty box in the Rose Bowl. A record crowd of 90,185 and an estimated 40 million American fans watching on TV held their breath.

After 90 minutes in the 1999 Women's World Cup final, the United States and China were scoreless. Two 15-minute sessions in extra time did not produce a victory. After four out of five successful penalty kicks by the Chinese and four kicks netted by the Americans, Brandi Chastain stepped up to take the final penalty kick. A ball past China's Gao Hong meant victory—and the Women's World Cup title—for the United States.

Less than four months earlier, Chastain had faced an almost identical situation. In the Algarve Cup in Portugal, she had lined up for a penalty against China. Years later, in a speech to the graduating class of her alma mater, Santa Clara University, she recalled that moment: "I put the ball down. I looked up, and the goalkeeper was standing there, and she unnerved me. She got me out of my zone, and I missed, and we ended up losing that tournament."[1]

After China's Sun Wen kicked to even up the penalties at 4–4, Chastain calmly stepped up.

Chastain now had the opportunity to avenge that miss and bring home the World Cup for her country. Using her left foot to take a penalty kick for the first time, she sailed the ball past Hong into the top right corner of the net.

It became "The Kick Heard 'Round the World."

That kick and Chastain's ensuing celebration—taking off her jersey and swinging it wildly in the air—became an iconic moment in the history of women's soccer.

One injury has also become synonymous with women's soccer. It has sidelined many of Chastain's US Women's National Team (USWNT) teammates—past and present. That injury is an ACL injury.

Chastain has suffered that injury—twice.

Chastain loved playing soccer from the first time she played in a girls' league in San Jose. She told Joann Weiner of the *Washington Post*, "as soon as that ball hit the ground and I kicked it the first time, I fell in love, and it has been my passion ever since."[2]

That passion helped her excel. She led her high school team to three California state titles. As a freshman at the University of California at Berkeley, Chastain earned the Soccer America Freshmen Player of the Year award.

Then injury struck.

Chastain tore her ACL in the spring of 1987. It took her about a year to get back to 100% with no issues on the field.

"This is not something you get over very quickly," Chastain explained. "I would say that there was a lot of sadness about not being on the field. I absolutely love playing soccer and have never needed to be on the sideline before."[3]

She later transferred to Santa Clara University. In the same month that she accepted the scholarship to go there, she tore the ACL in her opposite knee. Since the season would start months later, she pushed to return. "I was back on the field in six months, but not fully 100%, but I probably could play through the season," she recalled.[4]

Brandi Chastain missed two entire years of college soccer recovering from those ACL tears.

Those injuries were not the only setbacks in a career capped by triumph in Pasadena.

Chastain made that USWNT in 1988 and played on the 1991 team that won the World Cup. Only two years later, coach Anson Dorrance cut her from the team.

She claims that getting cut from the US team was critical to her later success. "Getting cut was the most important thing in my career," Chastain told the *Monterey County Weekly*. "Not being on first World Cup team [in 1991], not scoring the [1999 World Cup] goal, but coming back."[5]

That dismissal sparked a change. Chastain trained at a relentless level until she finally made it back into the pool of eligible players for the national team.

The US coach, Tony DiCicco, told her that to make it back to the team, she would have to transition to defense, despite a career as a goal-scoring striker.

Even that 1999 dream moment almost failed to happen. Early in the quarterfinal game against Germany, she attempted to pass the ball back to the goalkeeper, Brianna Scurry. Amid the noise of 75,000 fans in Jack Kent Cooke Stadium in Landover, Maryland, Chastain and Scurry got their signals crossed. Scurry came out of goal just as Chastain passed the ball. It trickled into the Americans' net.

Carla Overbeck, the us team captain, consoled her. "Don't worry. It will be all right. There's a lot of game left, and you will be part of the reason why we win," Chastain recalled in the Santa Clara graduation address.[6]

She did, in fact, overcome her mistake that put the Germans up 1–0. She scored in the 49th minute and helped her team advance.

Each time Brandi Chastain faced adversity, she responded and succeeded, ultimately helping return the USWNT to glory. Few challenges, though, have caused as much physical and emotional adversity for her and so many other female athletes as ACL injuries.

President Richard Nixon signed Title IX of the us Education Amendments of 1972 into law on June 23, 1972. According to the us Department of Education, Title IX aims to protect individuals from sex-based discrimination in education programs or activities that receive federal funding. Specifically, the legislation mandates:

> No person in the United States shall, on the basis of sex, be excluded from
> participation in, be denied the benefits of, or be subjected to discrimination
> under any education program or activity receiving federal financial assistance.[7]

Senator Birch Bayh authored and introduced the Title IX legislation. Speaking on the floor of the Senate, Bayh argued, "While the impact of this amendment would be far-reaching, it is not a panacea. It is, however, an important first step in the effort to provide for the women of America something that is rightfully theirs—an equal chance to attend the schools of their choice, to develop the skills they want, and to apply those skills with the knowledge that they will have a fair chance to secure the jobs of their choice with equal pay for equal work."[8]

Title IX applies to all sorts of educational opportunities, such as school admissions, financial aid, and treatment of students who are pregnant or parents. Perhaps the most widely discussed—and debated—aspect of Title IX legislation is its effect on athletics.

Prior to the enactment of Title IX, roughly 1 in every 27 females played high school sports. Fewer than 32,000 women participated in college athletics. Few college athletic scholarship opportunities existed, and only 2% of college athletic department budgets supported female sports.

In the four decades since Title IX was signed into law, participation in sports by females has exploded. In the 1971–1972 school year, just before Title IX was passed, girls comprised only 7% of all high school athletes. By the 2010–2011 season, females made up 41% of all high school athletes.[9] In the 2013–2014 school year, 3,267,664 females played high school sports—the highest number ever. In fact, the number of females who play high school sports has increased over 25 consecutive years.[10]

At the college level, female participation has also grown significantly. In 2010–2011, 191,131 female athletes played collegiate sports in Division I, Division II, and Division III. There were 9,746 women's teams in all sports—an increase of 2,703 teams from 1988–1989.[11]

This increased participation in sports could at least partially explain the rising rates of injuries in those sports. The more opportunities to practice and compete female athletes have, the greater are their chances of suffering an injury in those practices or games.

Anterior cruciate ligament injuries might be the best example of an injury for which females are at higher risk. When we look specifically at sports that both men and women play with essentially the same equipment and rules, females face a much higher risk of tearing their ACLs.

According to Timothy Hewett, PhD, the sports medicine director of research and biomechanics at the Mayo Clinic, soccer is the number one cause of ACL injuries in female athletes.[12]

In a five-year study of college soccer and basketball players, Elizabeth Arendt, MD, and Randall Dick found that female soccer players had an incidence rate of ACL injuries 2.4 times greater than male college soccer players. Female basketball players had an incidence rate 4.1 times greater than male college basketball players.[13]

Over a 13-year period between 1990 and 2002, Julie Agel and others found a similar discrepancy between male and female athletes—essentially that female soccer and basketball players had a much greater risk of suffering ACL injuries than did their male counterparts. This fact appears to be especially true when ACL injuries resulting from noncontact mechanisms are considered.[14]

A study looking at musculoskeletal injuries suffered by midshipmen at the US Naval Academy also found the risk discrepancy between males and females. Among candidates accepted to the Naval Academy, 2.41 times as many females as males had previously undergone ACL reconstruction. Women's varsity soccer athletes there had a nine times greater relative risk than the male varsity soccer players.

Overall, female midshipmen had a relative injury risk for ACL tears that was 2.44 times greater than that of the male midshipmen, which was even more noteworthy given the fact that the females did not participate in football, wrestling, or lacrosse at the Naval Academy during the study period.[15]

The difference in ACL injury risk for females exists at the high school level as well. A study looking at high school basketball in Texas found that girls had a 3.79 times greater injury risk for exposure than boys.[16]

A recent study showed that female collegiate athletes suffer between 2.8 and 3.2 ACL injuries per 10,000 athlete-exposures.[17] We define an athlete-exposure as one practice or one game. Using these data, if we followed two female soccer teams of 20 players who practiced four times per week and played one match per week for 50 weeks, we could expect roughly three of the players to suffer an ACL injury.

Regardless of the sport, most studies show that female athletes at the high school level or older have a 2 to 10 times higher rate of ACL injuries than male athletes in those same sports.

September 2, 2002

Rachel Buehler, a senior at Torrey Pines High School in San Diego, lunged for a ball 10 minutes into the final for the US Women's U-19 team in the FIFA U-19 World Championship.

Buehler, who had already accepted a scholarship to play at Stanford University, had an injury-free soccer career leading up to the World Championships. "I never had been seriously injured before," she told Mark Zeigler of the *San Diego Union-Tribune*. "I thought I was really lucky. I have pretty muscular legs, too, and you look at other people and you say, 'Oh, they're not strong enough.' I never thought it would happen to me."[18]

Buehler had torn her ACL.

The defender worked hard in rehabilitation and successfully returned to play soccer in only five and one-half months. Two weeks later, exactly six months out from her ACL injury with the U-19 team, she ran in a scrimmage, stepped awkwardly, and felt a pop in her opposite knee.

Rachel Buehler had injured her opposite ACL.

A host of risk factors have been proposed to explain the higher rate of ACL injuries in female athletes. Setting aside some of the external factors that could be involved—shoe types, field or court surfaces, weather, and playing conditions—there are some factors that could explain the risks for female athletes.

First, female athletes simply have different anatomical features than males. They have a wider pelvis, which could increase the valgus alignment of the knee. In essence, a more valgus knee is what we commonly refer to as a "knock kneed" appearance, in which the angle between the hip and knee and the knee and ankle is greater. The knee is closer to the midline relative to the ankle. Some experts feel that this increased angle could increase the risk of ACL injuries.

Within the knee, females are thought to have smaller ACLs than males as well as narrower intercondylar notches—the space in the femur where the ACL sits.

Generalized joint laxity, hamstring laxity, and a higher body mass index might increase the risk of ACL injury in some female athletes.

Genetics could play a role. In a study published in the *American Journal of Sports Medicine*, Kevin Flynn and others showed that patients with an ACL injury were twice as likely to have a first-, second-, or third-degree relative who has had one than people without an ACL tear.[19]

One of the more controversial risk factors proposed to explain the higher risk in female athletes is hormones. Receptors for the hormones estrogen and progesterone have been discovered within the ACL. It is possible that these hormones could affect the composition of the ligament and its biomechanical properties.

Multiple studies have examined the incidence of ACL injuries in different phases of the menstrual cycle and found conflicting results. Likewise, different researchers have observed more laxity in different phases of the menstrual cycle.

The challenge for definitively proving a hormonal component or even that females are at increased risk in certain phases of the menstrual cycle comes down to testing. Studies have rarely obtained blood samples to accurately determine an injured athlete's current menstrual phase, but instead have relied on surveys and guesses as to which phase of the menstrual cycle she is in.

To accurately conclude that the risk of ACL injury increases in certain menstrual phases, a researcher would have to enroll an enormous number of female athletes in the study and follow them for years until a certain number suffered ACL injuries. In addition, he would have to collect blood samples every day on every subject—injured and uninjured. Such a study would be challenging—if not impossible—to perform.

There have been studies, though, that suggest oral contraceptives might lower the rate of knee injuries. It's unclear what the exact mechanism is that the contraceptives could influence, however. It is possible that they might prevent large swings in hormone levels or alter hormonal effects on neuromuscular control.

Anterior cruciate ligament injuries peak in girls around age 16. These injuries begin to increase when girls start adolescence, which for the average American girl is around age 11.

Dr. Hewett explained that a neuromuscular imbalance develops in adolescent girls that contributes to the risk of ACL injury:

> If you used a car analogy, you say both boys and girls start out as small Toyotas, a Toyota Prius with a Toyota Prius engine. Then what happens is they get a much bigger chassis, a bigger machine. They both get a Cadillac. Then what happens is, boys very soon after that get a Porsche engine. They have an over-match. They're more powerful relative to the size of their machine. But girls stay about the same, or even have more of a mismatch, so even though they get a Cadillac chassis, all they'd get is somewhere between say a Chevy and a Cadillac engine. They don't get an overpowered engine.[20]

Neuromuscular imbalance leads girls to become "ligament dominant." Instead of using the large muscles of their legs to control the forces from landing and cutting, the forces go to the joint, specifically the ACL. The ligament can't withstand high forces, and it can tear when it faces a high force.

Girls and women tend to be more quadriceps dominant than boys and men. This term implies that females use their quadriceps muscles to absorb force instead of the hamstrings like males do. Quadriceps contraction pulls the tibia forward and puts more strain on the ACL when girls land and cut.

Along the same lines, the gluteal muscles are crucial in controlling and dissipating forces at the knee and hip. Females don't activate the gluteal muscles nearly as well as males do.

Several body positions and movement patterns have consistently been shown to be associated with ACL injury: decreased flexion of the knee, decreased flexion of the hip, increased knee valgus, and increased tibial rotation.

Females are also trunk dominant. They often cannot control their core, the center of mass, when they land and cut. The trunk moves around more, allowing the forces to go outside the center of the knee, pushing the hip and knee inward.

Hewett explained that these imbalances can be measured. Using these measurements, he can predict, with about 80% sensitivity and specificity, the young female athletes at high risk for ACL injury.[21]

Another Santa Clara University alumna, midfielder Leslie Osborne, tore her ACL in a practice shortly after starting her professional career.

While guarded by Heather Mitts, who had only recently returned from her own ACL injury, Osborne pivoted her body in response to Mitts's position. Osborne's body rotated, but her leg did not.

"It was the loudest noise I've ever heard," Osborne recalled to Women's Professional Soccer contributor Karyn Lush. "It didn't even hurt. . . . [W]e were the only ones who heard it but we knew right away that something was wrong because of that noise, that pop."[22]

That pop has afflicted an unbelievable number of players from the USWNT. In addition to Chastain, Osborne, Buehler, and Mitts, Alex Morgan, Megan Rapinoe, Christie Rampone, Amy LePeilbet, and Ali Krieger have suffered ACL injuries.

Dr. Bert Mandelbaum, an orthopaedic surgeon in Santa Monica, California, has worked with the US national teams. His group performed the physicals on the 2015 USWNT, which won the Women's World Cup. Nine of the twenty-five players had undergone ACL reconstructions.[23]

Maybe because an ACL tear usually requires surgery and up to 12 months or more for an athlete to return to sports, many people assume that a direct force causes the ACL to rupture. For instance, Kansas City Chiefs safety Bernard Pollard rolling into Tom Brady in the first game of the 2008 season caused Brady's ACL injury, and the Patriots quarterback missed the entire season. Or a direct blow to a planted leg, like what caused USWNT defender Ali Krieger's ACL and medial collateral ligament injury, should be responsible.

Surprisingly, those direct forces—direct contact injuries—are much less often the reason than what usually happens.

Roughly 70% of ACL injuries result from noncontact mechanisms. A women's soccer player might jump to head a ball and land on her feet with her knee extended. As she lands, her knee buckles. She might feel or hear a pop as the ligament ruptures, and she crumples to the ground as her knee gives way.

She could also simply run and change directions. She plants her foot to turn. The foot stays planted while her knee rotates. She feels a pop, and her knee buckles. Again, what seems to be a trivial event leads to a major injury.

Female athletes who have seen so many of their teammates go down with these injuries increasingly understand their significance. Surgery. Time in a brace and on crutches. Months of work with a physical therapist. And, of course, no soccer for a long time.

Jo Hannafin, MD, the orthopaedic director of The Women's Sports Medicine Center at the Hospital for Special Surgery in New York City and past president of the American Orthopaedic Society for Sports Medicine, uses the term "grief reaction" to describe some of the emotional effects on the injured athletes. She observed that unlike high school boys, who often accept the injury knowing that they will return to play, high school girls often struggle more emotionally. "They've lost their sport, and they've lost the kinship of their friends, which is almost as bad as not being able to play," Hannafin noted.[24]

Not being able to play is bad enough. Add the distance created by not being around your teammates and experiencing the camaraderie of team travel and celebration of victories, and these injuries can take an emotional toll on the athlete on top of the physical damage.

A huge percentage of Dr. Hannafin's young female patients with ACL injuries are devastated when they hear the news, often bursting into tears. They have a hard time dealing with the injury. She stressed the importance of creating a plan to help get the athlete through the recovery process.

Dr. Hannafin outlines a detailed timeline for her female patients, describing the surgery and the length of rehabilitation, and she helps them find a physical therapist they really like. She even gives them a choice to watch the surgery.

Hannafin recounted her own experience with an ACL injury. She planned to become a pediatrician but decided to become an orthopaedic surgeon after she tore her ACL in medical school.

She said that her experience changed her perspective. Now she draws pictures of the surgery for her patients and shows them exactly what she's going to do.

"Honestly, if I can turn like one out of every 20 of those girls into orthopaedic surgeons 15 years from now, that would make me really happy."[25]

Given that many elite US soccer players have suffered these injuries, and tens of thousands of young females in a variety of sports do so each year, it's worth asking if it is possible to prevent them. Clearly surgery can be performed, and the athlete has a reasonably good chance of returning to play.

If there was a way that we could keep even a portion of these injuries from ever occurring, it could benefit the athletes and the teams on which they play.

In June 1999 a group of concerned surgeons, physical therapists, athletic trainers, and others in sports medicine met in Hunt Valley, Maryland, to devise an intervention that might decrease the risk of ACL injuries. According to Dr.

Mandelbaum, they watched 15 videotapes trying to determine how this injury was occurring. They reviewed available scientific research on injury risk factors as well as prevention programs already in use.[26]

In 1990 Henning and Griffis found that a program aimed at emphasizing knee flexion on landing, accelerated rounded turns, and using a multistep stop after deceleration reduced ACL injuries 89% in two Division I basketball programs.[27]

Ettlinger and others implemented a training program to teach skiers to avoid high-risk behaviors and positions and better respond quickly to difficult conditions. Approximately 4,700 ski instructors and patrollers at 20 ski areas in the United States completed the program during the 1993–1994 ski season. They found that the people who participated in the program had a 62% lower rate of serious knee injuries than those who did not do the training.[28]

Myklebust and other researchers began a training program for elite female handball players in Norway between 1999 and 2001. Throughout the preseason, as well as once a week during the season, the handball players practiced floor exercises as well as activities on a wobble board and balance mat. In the season before the program began, 29 ACL injuries occurred among 942 athletes. In the first season using the program, 23 injuries occurred. Only 17 ACL injuries occurred in the second season using the program.[29]

Dr. Hewett studied the use of a neuromuscular training program among 15 high school female soccer, basketball, and volleyball teams. Fifteen female teams in the same sports did not participate in the training and served as controls. Thirteen male teams also served as controls. The athletes in the training group performed exercises for 60 to 90 minutes three times a week for six weeks prior to their seasons.

The athletes who underwent the neuromuscular training had a 72% lower incidence of noncontact ACL injuries than the athletes who did not do the program. Five untrained female athletes in basketball or soccer suffered noncontact ACL injuries, while none of the trained female athletes suffered any.[30]

This study and others suggest that a neuromuscular training program could decrease the risk for ACL injury among female athletes. Dr. Mandelbaum, physical therapist Holly Silvers, and others at the Santa Monica Orthopedic and Sports Medicine Group developed the Prevent Injury and Enhance Performance (PEP) program to try to decrease the incidence of ACL injuries among female athletes, especially young female soccer players.

Dr. Mandelbaum explained what happened after the Hunt Valley meeting:

I felt that we needed to do something more. We need to do it now rather than wait for more science. We came back from the Hunt Valley meeting. Holly and myself brought together a team of people. Coach Steve Sampson at the time had just finished up being the National Team coach. We put together a program that was simply named Prevent Injury, Enhance Performance. My design motif was I didn't want it to smell like alcohol or have a white coat on it. I wanted it to be a warm up that would be something that anybody in the world could do. All you need is a grass field, a ball, and some cones and kids. You can do it. The goal was to develop this program and then test it to see its efficiency. We did that. Amazingly when Holly and I went for our first meeting in Orange County, because there were so many ACL injuries, everybody was saying, "Can I participate? Can I participate?"[31]

Holly Silvers, a physical therapist and the director of research at the Santa Monica Sports Medicine Foundation, described why she felt it was important to work with Dr. Mandelbaum on this injury: "Bert and I have been working together since late 1999, and we just had such an influx of young women coming in with acute ACL injuries and recurrent ACL injuries. When we looked at our Under-20 team at the time, over one-quarter of them had been reconstructed. I just thought we had to do something about this. It just seemed—I hate using the word epidemic—but sort of epidemic in proportion."[32]

The PEP program is a series of exercises aimed to correct strength deficits and lack of coordination of the stabilizing muscles around the knee. After learning the program and the proper ways to do each exercise, athletes use these programs as their warm-up before practices and games, requiring about 15 to 20 minutes to perform. Athletes perform the program three times per week.

The program is also inexpensive, requiring no special equipment other than some cones. Hopefully the simplicity helps with compliance by removing a lack of fancy equipment as an excuse for athletes and their coaches to not use the exercises. In addition, the efficiency of the program is especially important in youth club sports, in which the teams might only have two practices and a game each week.

The PEP program, like many other neuromuscular programs, addresses proper deceleration and landing techniques. It emphasizes hip and knee flexion upon landing and lateral, side-to-side maneuvers. It tries to correct valgus alignment of the knee upon landing, in which the knee is situated closer to the midline of the body in relation to the hip and ankle—a knock-kneed position, so to speak. And it develops hamstring, hip, and gluteal muscle strength.

The PEP program consists of five sections: warm-up, strengthening, plyometrics, agilities, and stretching. In the warm-up, the athlete starts with jogging line-to-line or cone-to-cone. She focuses on good running technique, especially maintaining good alignment of the lower extremities. Next she performs side-to-side shuttle runs, again concentrating on bending at the knee and keeping proper alignment of the knee. She last performs backward running, making sure to land on her toes and keeping her knees bent.

In section 2, the athlete performs walking lunges, Russian hamstring exercises, and single toe raises to increase strength in the quadriceps, hamstrings, and calf muscles, respectively. Proper technique, again, is critical.

The plyometrics phase builds strength, power, and speed. Exercises here include lateral hops over a cone, forward and backward hops over a cone, single leg hops over a cone, vertical jumps with headers, and scissor jumps. Not only is proper technique when doing the exercises important, but the athlete must also focus on landing softly on the balls of her feet with her hips and knees flexed.

To start the agility section, the athlete performs forward runs with three-step deceleration. She does lateral diagonal runs, keeping good alignment of the lower extremities without the knees caving in, and ensuring her knees are bent. Finally, she does close to 50 yards of a bounding run, bringing her knees up to her chest, landing properly with each step.

Either after the warm-up or after completion of the strengthening, plyometrics, and agility exercises, each athlete performs stretching exercises, including calf stretch, quadriceps stretch, figure-4 hamstring stretch, inner thigh stretch, and hip flexor stretch.

Mandelbaum and his team at the Santa Monica Orthopaedic and Sports Medicine Research Foundation tested this program among female soccer teams in the Coast Soccer League of Southern California, from which 1,041 female athletes between the ages of 14 and 18 who played on 52 soccer teams participated in the first year, and 1,905 soccer players on 95 teams did not. In the following season, 844 female soccer players did the PEP program, and 1,913 did not.

After completion of the first season, the researchers found that only two athletes involved in the PEP program had suffered ACL injuries, compared to 32 control athletes.

In simpler terms, the study showed an 88% overall reduction in ACL injury among athletes who performed the program. Year 2 of the program showed a similar drop—74%—among female athletes who used the PEP program.[33]

Dr. Mandelbaum believed this initial study validated the PEP program. A pediatrician at the CDC approached him about performing a randomized controlled trial.

The CDC partnered with the organization to study the PEP program among 61 Division I NCAA women's soccer teams. In 2008 Julie Gilchrist, MD, and others published the results of the study—supported not only by the Santa Monica Orthopaedic and Sports Medicine Research Foundation, but also by the American Academy of Orthopaedic Surgeons, the American Orthopaedic Society for Sports Medicine, Fédération Internationale de Football Association (FIFA), and the NCAA—in the *American Journal of Sports Medicine*.

The researchers randomized 26 soccer teams to use the PEP program, while 35 teams did not use it. The rates of noncontact ACL injuries among athletes on the teams that used the PEP program were 3.3 times lower than among control athletes. The rate of all ACL injuries was 1.7 times lower among the trained athletes than among the control athletes.

The authors made other important findings as well. Athletes using the PEP program suffered no ACL injuries in practice, while six of the control athletes suffered tears. No athlete in the PEP program suffered an ACL injury in the second half of the season, compared to five in the non-PEP soccer players, suggesting a possible cumulative benefit to the neuromuscular training.

The study also looked at athletes who had previously suffered an ACL injury. Five athletes with a history of ACL injury who did not perform the training program suffered a second ACL injury. Among the PEP participants, no athlete with a history of ACL tear suffered another one.[34]

"This study shows tremendous promise for female collegiate soccer players, especially those with a history of ACL injuries," Gilchrist, the lead author of the paper, concluded in a press release for the study. "Enjoying sports is a great way to stay fit. And to stay healthy, we encourage coaches, athletic trainers, and athletes to consider adapting this program into their routine."[35]

Soccer's governing body, FIFA, wanted to go further and prevent more than ACL injuries. Mandelbaum's team tweaked the PEP program into the FIFA 11 and then the FIFA 11+ programs to minimize ankle and hip injuries as well.

Despite the attention given to female athletes, Mandelbaum argues that the program can benefit male athletes as well. His team studied the use of the FIFA 11+ in Division I and II male athletes and found a 42% reduction in ACL injuries.[36]

Lindsay DiStefano, an assistant professor in the Department of Kinesiology at the University of Connecticut, has researched ACL injuries for the past 10 years. When she implements an ACL prevention program, she often hears boys complain that they shouldn't do them because "it's a girls' injury." Yet she feels strongly that these programs offer protective benefits for males, too.[37]

Finally, Mandelbaum pointed to a study his group did with Dr. Christopher Ahmad and his group at Columbia University. They looked at the cost efficiency of using these programs to train all athletes, versus screening them and training only the high-risk athletes, versus training none of them. They found that the fewest injuries occurred when they trained everyone, and it was the most cost-effective method as well.

"We found that we can make a significant difference. Not only is it significant, but it's also cost effective," Mandelbaum concluded.[38]

If performing the PEP program or another neuromuscular training program can prevent one female athlete from suffering an ACL injury and make surgery, rehab, and the possible grief reaction less likely, that would be a significant advance. An ACL injury can have long-term consequences as well.

First of all, we know that ACL injuries have good, but not necessarily great, success rates for athletes returning to sports.

Robert H. Brophy, MD, and other orthopaedic surgeons collected data on ACL reconstructions performed at centers across the United States. They specifically analyzed the data from soccer players in their database. Overall, 72% of the soccer players who underwent ACL reconstruction returned to the sport an average of 12.2 months after surgery. Of those who did return, 85% made it back to the same or a higher level of play. While 76% of male athletes returned to soccer, only 67% of females did.

Viewed over the long term, the numbers are not quite as encouraging. At follow-up after 7.2 years, only 35% were still playing soccer, and only 46% of those athletes were playing at the same or a higher level. Those statistics cast doubt on the success of reaching elite level soccer—like the USWNT—if a player tears her ACL early in her soccer career.

In addition, it is certainly possible to suffer a second ACL injury. In Brophy's study, 12% of the soccer players underwent a second ACL surgery at some point after the first one; 9% injured the contralateral knee, or the side opposite the initial injury; and 3% injured the graft and required a revision ACL reconstruction of the initially injured knee. Female athletes were much more likely than male athletes to require a second ACL surgery.[39]

Other studies have found a similar risk for second ACL injury among athletes who have suffered one compared to athletes who have never suffered an ACL injury. For example, John Orchard and other researchers observed that a prior ACL reconstruction is a risk factor for a second noncontact ACL injury in Australian football players. An athlete who had an ACL injury more than 12 months before is 4.4 times more likely to tear the graft in the surgical knee or injure the opposite ACL than an uninjured athlete. If an athlete suffered an ACL injury within the previous 12 months, the risk of a second injury was 11.3 times greater than for an athlete without a prior ACL injury.[40]

Essentially the same neuromuscular imbalances and deficits that lead to the first ACL injuries in female athletes put them at risk for a second tear.

Dr. Hewett estimated that between 20% and 30% of patients who undergo ACL reconstruction eventually suffer a second injury. He is starting a randomized controlled trial to determine if adding neuromuscular training on top of the standard rehab protocol reduces the risk of reinjury.[41]

Not only does a second ACL surgery mean another 6 to 12 months out of sports, but those injuries and surgeries also might have worse outcomes in terms of return to play and patient satisfaction, especially for young athletes.

Even if an athlete does return to play and does manage to avoid a second injury, she's not necessarily out of the woods. Anterior cruciate ligament reconstruction can restore stability to the knee to allow her to successfully land from jumps and cut and change directions quickly in sports and exercise. That surgery and recovery don't preclude her from developing degenerative changes in that knee later in life.

Regardless of the treatment for an ACL tear—whether the athlete undergoes ACL reconstruction or treats it by wearing a brace and going through physical therapy without surgery—osteoarthritis develops much more often than in a patient who has not suffered an ACL injury.

Osteoarthritis develops in 41% to 51% of ACL-injured knees. The opposite, uninjured knee develops these degenerative changes only 4% to 8% of the time.[42]

So many possible outcomes can make ACL injuries devastating, including time away from the team, loss of scholarship, not returning to play sports or at least not returning to the same level of play, a second ACL injury, and development of osteoarthritis in the future.

On top of all of those factors, these injuries are expensive. A 2013 study of all lifetime costs involved with ACL reconstruction—the surgeon's fee, anesthesia fee, physical therapy, work status, disability, and so forth—found the total cost to society of a single ACL reconstruction to be $38,121. On the other hand, the lifetime cost for nonoperative treatment was $88,538. The cost of an ACL tear over the lifetime of a patient is tremendous, suggesting that efforts to prevent these injuries could be beneficial for financial reasons as well.[43]

Everyone involved in the field of sports medicine should be concerned by these statistics.

Still, not everyone is convinced that these neuromuscular programs work.

Dr. Donald Shelbourne, an orthopaedic surgeon in Indianapolis, says the mechanism of noncontact ACL injuries implies that these programs wouldn't work. The athlete's quadriceps contract as she anticipates the foot hitting the ground. If the foot doesn't hit the ground exactly when it is supposed to, the quad still fires, pulling the tibia forward. Then the tibia is out of place when the foot hits the ground. Essentially, noncontact ACL tears result from violent muscle contractions and mistimed landings. Dr. Shelbourne doesn't believe that an exercise program can prevent those events:

> You can't tear your ACL playing basketball by yourself. You can't tear your ACL playing soccer by yourself. You have to have the element of unknown and surprise in there to make you have a mistimed foot plant. That's how you tear your ACL.
>
> People don't tear their ACLs because they can't jump and land. Everybody can jump and land and not tear their ACL. You can't jump and land by yourself and tear your ACL. You have to jump and land with somebody bumping you, pushing you, and having a landing that is mistimed so your muscle firing doesn't coincide with foot plant.[44]

There are studies that question the effectiveness of these injury prevention programs.

In 2014, J. Herbert Stevenson and other researchers at the University of Massachusetts Medical Center performed a systematic review of 10 studies of neuromuscular programs and their efficacy in preventing ACL injuries. They found that only 2 of the 10—Mandelbaum's first study of the PEP program at the Coast Soccer League and Hewett's program with female soccer, basketball, and volleyball players—produced statistically significant drops in the incidence of ACL injuries. Two others—Gilchrist's CDC study and Myklebust's study of Norwegian handball players—showed statistically significant decreases within certain subgroups.

In their systematic review, Stevenson and his colleagues did find that the programs that involved different aspects of training, such as strength, agility, and balance, provided a decrease in ACL injury incidence. Incorporation of plyometrics seemed particularly important.[45]

Dr. Stevenson started the study expecting to find that these programs were effective. He believes many variables in the studies could affect the results. How are the programs implemented? Who supervises the athletes? How compliant are the athletes with the programs?[46]

DiStefano agreed that fidelity and compliance play a role in these studies. When we look specifically at the training programs that have been implemented with high fidelity and high compliance, we see the greatest reduction and injuries.

"Despite public perception, ACL injuries are a relatively rare injury compared to an ankle sprain," DiStefano pointed out. "We finished a multi-year prospective study for ACL injury risk factors. We had to collect close to 12,000 man-years to illicit 150 primary ACL injuries. So in the spectrum of proving an injury reduction, you have to get so much data on so many athletes to prove it from a research standpoint, it's a really challenging thing to do."[47]

Dr. Hewett says that these collective studies do show a benefit to the programs. He points to a meta-analysis of 14 studies published by his group. "If you look at it, the P value is less than one in 1,000 that this effect is by chance. It's clear that the effect is there. They do reduce risk, and they reduce risk by somewhere between a half and two thirds. The data clearly shows that."[48]

But where do these data leave us? These programs seem beneficial, but we cannot definitively promise a young athlete or her parents that we can prevent her from tearing her ACL. These are complex injuries that involve athletes and active people in different sports and exercise. A myriad of risk factors exists—not just neuromuscular but genetic, anatomical, hormonal, and so forth—and we likely can't eliminate all ACL tears by focusing on only one of those risk factors.

This doesn't mean that we shouldn't try. Convincing athletes and coaches to use these programs can be challenging, however.

Silvers noted that getting coaches and teams to use these programs is the biggest obstacle. When she and Dr. Mandelbaum did their 2012 study on NCAA teams, they personally called the coaches at every Division I and Division II college in the country. Of over 400 teams, only 61 participated—about 14%.[49]

Coaches often don't want to use any time available on the field for anything other than practice. In fact, DiStefano noted that she has better luck convincing coaches to have the players perform the exercises regularly when the program will only take 5 or 10 minutes each day rather than 15 or 20. And while these programs can replace the traditional series of warm-up exercises and thus not add any time, coaches must still monitor the athletes for correct landing and cutting techniques.

Many coaches worry that if the players do these exercises before practices, they won't be able to train as well. DiStefano argued that research has shown that the programs don't impair performance during practices and may actually improve it through movement efficiency.

DiStefano also pointed out that no research has ever shown any harm from an injury standpoint with these programs.[50]

Silvers has a simple message for hesitant coaches. "I always tell coaches if you can look down in the last week of the season, and you have a full bench available to you of healthy athletes willing and able to play for you, that's fantastic."[51]

Even athletes with good neuromuscular control and balance can improve by performing these programs. In a team environment, there is no reason to isolate these high-risk athletes. Instead, sports medicine programs can help teams implement them with every athlete participating. It just becomes a normal routine for everyone on the team.

The earlier an athlete begins the neuromuscular training program, the more it might help. A meta-analysis of 14 studies looking at the outcomes of this program showed a noticeable difference based on whether the athlete was older or younger than 18. These programs proved to have a 72% reduction in risk for female athletes younger than 18, while females older than 18 only had a 16% decrease.[52]

Silvers, Hewett, and DiStefano all acknowledged these programs work best the earlier girls start them. If we can start these programs with 8- or 9-year-old girls, such as U-10 recreational or travel teams, we could fix pathologic movement patterns before they start in the first place. If we wait until 16, 17, or 18 years old, it's almost too late.

In addition to club sports, getting these programs into the school systems might be the best way to reach and impact the largest number of young female athletes.

"I think if we get them young and teach them quality movement and how to move well and biomechanically sound, we have a really great opportunity to prevent the faulty movement patterns from being entrenched down the line," said Silvers.[53]

Retraining a young athlete on how to land and how to cut properly takes time, though. Darin A. Padua and others at the University of North Carolina compared teams who performed the programs for three and nine months. Only athletes who completed the extended duration training exhibited the improved movement patterns three months after the programs ended.[54]

Not only would young high-risk athletes need to start learning and using these programs early, but they would need to stick with them week after week for a long time to keep the risk of ACL injury low.

Young athletes should really do them year after year. Doing them on a continued basis would reinforce proper movement patterns and also improve compliance as these programs become a normal part of their training.

"What I usually tell athletes is, like a basketball player, you don't stop practicing foul shots the minute you make the foul shot. Even professional basketball players continue to shoot foul shot after foul shot after foul shot. Movement, neuromuscular control is the exact same thing," DiStefano explained.[55]

While there is still much we need to know about using neuromuscular training programs to try to prevent ACL injuries, they still offer hope. Most of the injuries in this book have focused on efforts to treat them: surgeries, rehabilitation, PRP, and so forth. This is one of those few occasions that sports medicine has sought to prevent injuries in the first place. Maybe these programs won't stop every athlete from tearing her ACL. Maybe they will only prevent a few injuries.

"I honestly can't think of a downside," Silvers concluded. "Other than maybe it's a little bit boring because you are doing a similar program over and over throughout the course of the season, but I think if you tell any athlete, 'Hey, we can effectively reduce your risk of injury' say on the low side, 40 percent, I think any athlete would sign up for that.

"We cannot prevent every one of them, we can't. But I think we can do a heck of a lot better than we are now," Silvers argued.[56]

For an athlete who could tear her ACL, these programs could have a dramatic impact. Simply changing warm-up exercises every day could possibly prevent an

ACL injury that could cause her to miss the playoffs, sit out a season while her friends play, require her to undergo surgery and a year of rehab, and increase her risk for future injuries and arthritis. I bet most athletes would gladly do the exercises if they considered that kind of impact.

The USWNT captain, Carla Overbeck, consoled Brandi Chastain after she accidentally kicked the ball into her own goal in that 1999 World Cup. Chastain described Overbeck as her "impact player."

Now Chastain serves on the advisory council of the Bay Area Women's Sports Initiative. The program's mission is to impact the lives of young girls by improving their health and self-esteem. The organization uses sports as a vehicle to promote wellness. They came up with the name BAWSI because they want young girls to be bossy about who they are and who they want to be.

Chastain described her experience with one young Bay Area female while working with a group of girls on a playground:

> I said, "One time I scored a goal, and I celebrated and tore off my shirt and I whipped it around my head. Does anyone here have a celebration for when they do something really good?" One girl that was standing around raised her hand. I was so happy because I didn't want to pull anyone to the middle that didn't want to be there. She came to the middle, and I said, "Are you ready to show everybody your celebration dance?" And she froze. I thought, "Oh my gosh. I can't force her to do it." So I said, "Okay, would you like me to do mine first?" She nodded her head. So I jump up, and I pumped my fists, and I let out a "woo hoo." And the girls clapped.
>
> I said, "Okay, are you ready to do yours?" She said yes. She pulled off this Mary Lou Retton double back handspring with a twist and a perfect landing. The girls went bananas. "That is the kind of excitement and joy that I want you to go back to the playground with, and you be bossy." So they all run back to their stations, and it's more energy, a lot of excitement, a lot of smiles and laughter.
>
> We concluded about a half hour later. As I was talking to someone, I felt a tug on my sleeve. I turned around, and it was the little girl from the middle. She looked up at me with these big brown eyes and said, "Thank you for not giving up on me."
>
> It literally makes me emotional today as it did that day. I thought how simple was it to stand next to her and to let her know that I believed that she could

do it and that I was there to support her. And together we can make nervous situations or uncomfortable situations or maybe what we think might be unrealistic situations for us actually happen.

So I walked away from that afternoon with the BAWSI girls with this new enlightenment about how impactful every person can be to somebody else if we're just willing to take the moment and to make a difference.[57]

Brandi Chastain returned from two ACL injuries and years of rehab and struggles to impact women's soccer forever. Maybe sports medicine, with these injury prevention programs, can impact the health and success of young female soccer players who dream of achieving that same success one day.

13 / TOMMY JOHN

Tommy John Surgery and Youth Baseball Injuries

July 17, 1974

Chavez Ravine has been the site of many legendary baseball moments. Sandy Koufax pitched a complete game in game 4 of the 1963 World Series to clinch a championship for the team in only its second season playing in Dodger Stadium. Koufax threw a perfect game in 1965. Kirk Gibson hit a walk-off home run in the 1988 World Series. But it was a single pitch in a regular-season game against the Montréal Expos that ultimately would affect the careers of baseball pitchers for decades to come.

Thirty-one-year-old Tommy John entered the game against the Expos with a 13–3 record and 2.59 ERA. With a 4–0 lead entering the fourth inning and runners on first and second base, John threw what he thought was just one pitch to get one batter out. It turned out to be much more.

"As I came forward and released the ball, I felt a kind of nothingness, as if my arm weren't there, then I heard a 'pop' from inside my arm, and the ball just blooped up to the plate. I didn't feel soreness or pain at this point, but just the strange sensation that my arm wasn't there. It was the oddest thing I'd ever felt while pitching. I shook my left arm, more baffled than concerned," he later wrote in his book *T.J.: My 26 Years in Baseball.*[1]

John tried to throw one more pitch—another sinker—before he took himself out of the game. "My next pitch would be the last one I threw in a big league game for the next twenty-one months. I released the ball, and this time I heard a slamming sound, like a collision coming from inside my elbow. It felt as if my arm had come off."[2]

"I got to the bench, I got my jacket and I told our trainer, I said 'Billy, let's get Dr. Jobe—something's wrong, get Dr. Jobe,' and the rest is history," John said in an interview years later.[3]

Tommy John was born and raised in Terry Haute, Indiana. Living two blocks from school, Tommy and his friends would race home, change clothes, and play sports every day. He recalls that they would play whatever sport was appropriate for that season. "If it was fall, we'd play football. In the winter, the sport was basketball," he explained.[4]

Not surprising for a young athlete living in Indiana, Tommy had a successful high school career in basketball. In fact, by his senior year he had received scholarship offers from 35 colleges to play basketball. Although he enjoyed basketball, he really loved baseball. The choice between sports would become his first major career decision.

Tommy worried that his six-foot-two size would only let him be an average college basketball player. He probably would never become a pro. He also believed that he was better at baseball than basketball. "If I were to make it as a professional athlete, it would be on the diamond and not on the hardwood."[5]

John recalled in his book how his father realized early on that his son was serious about becoming a baseball pitcher. While drinking a cup of coffee in the kitchen, Thomas E. John Sr. looked out the window to see his eight-year-old son struggling to move a wheelbarrow full of dirt. "'What's Tommy doing?' Mom asked. 'I'm not sure, but I think he's trying to build himself a pitcher's mound,' Dad answered."[6]

Perhaps it was this love of baseball that led Tommy John to make the difficult decision he did.

Dr. Frank Jobe, the Los Angeles Dodgers team doctor and orthopaedic surgeon, examined John's elbow in the training room after that painful pitch. Jobe knew immediately the injury was bad. John had torn a ligament in his elbow.

Like pitchers with these injuries before him, John tried to rest his elbow to get the ligament to heal. After three weeks of rest, he tried to throw batting practice. Not only could he not throw a strike, he struggled to even get the ball to the plate.

At that point, Tommy John faced the possibility that his injury might mean the end of his MLB career. Dr. Jobe, whom John considered a close friend, discussed possible surgical options for his UCL injury. If Jobe found that the ligament had pulled off of its bony attachment, he could simply reattach it to the bone. That recovery would be fairly straightforward. On the other hand, if he found that the UCL had ruptured in the middle of the ligament, he proposed a never-before-attempted surgery to fix the problem. He would take a tendon from the right forearm and use it to create a new ligament in John's left elbow.

Tommy's wife Sally asked the surgeon about his chances for a successful outcome. Dr. Jobe admitted that the chances would be slim. Exactly how slim?

He estimated that there would be about a 1 in 100 chance of returning to the mound. When she asked how likely it was that her husband would return to pitch without undergoing the surgery, Jobe responded frankly, "Zero chances in a hundred."[7]

"Well, I was valedictorian of my high school class and 1% or 2% in 100 is far better than zero percent in 100," John later remarked.[8]

Dr. Jobe recalled to FOX Sports the moment that Tommy John made the daunting decision. "He looked around my office very seriously. He looked me in the eye and said, 'Let's do it.' And those are three words that changed baseball."[9]

Although this surgery was first performed on Tommy John, the injury itself was first reported decades earlier among elite javelin throwers.

The anterior bundle of the UCL is the elbow's primary restraint against valgus force during overhead motions such as throwing. During the late cocking and early acceleration phases of the throwing motion, there are large tensile forces across the medial aspect of the elbow. With each throw, the ligament works to resist these forces and stabilize the joint.

While occasionally injuries to the UCL occur acutely—are torn in a traumatic event with no underlying history of ligament damage—far more often they gradually fail over time. The pitcher often remembers the one throw during which the UCL finally gave way. But the ligament—and the pitcher's performance—usually has been slowly worsening for months or even years.

While occasionally the UCL pulls off the bone on one side, and therefore can be simply reattached, most are intrasubstance tears.

Like fixing ACL tears in the knee, repairing a torn UCL has had poor results. Imagine a rope that gradually frays in one spot until it breaks. Trying to sew the frayed ends of the rope—or ligament—would not yield sufficient strength for it to perform its stabilizing duties.

Surgery for UCL injuries almost always involves reconstruction. A ligament from another part of the body—usually the palmaris longus tendon in the opposite wrist—is placed in the elbow to make a new ligament. The graft is passed through drill holes in both the humerus and the ulna. It is held in place by tying it to itself in figure-eight fashion or anchoring it in other ways.

There have been some technical modifications in the last few decades, but the surgery still closely resembles the one Dr. Jobe tried for the first time on Tommy John.

Ulnar collateral ligament reconstruction has largely proven effective to help baseball pitchers and other overhead athletes return to sports. A 2008 review of all published reports of these surgeries by Vitale and Ahmad showed that 83% of patients had an excellent result. They found an overall complication rate of 10%. Ulnar neuropathy—a temporary or permanent dysfunction of the ulnar nerve that provides motor function and sensation to parts of the hand—was the most common complication. It occurred in 6% of patients.[10]

In 2010 E. Lyle Cain, MD, reviewed the data on 1,281 athletes, 95% of them baseball players, who had undergone UCL reconstruction by Dr. James Andrews between 1988 and 2006. . Of the 743 athletes available for follow-up at a minimum of two years after surgery, 617 (83%) had returned to their previous level of competition.[11]

"Those patients prior to 1974 probably would not be pitching anymore," Dr. Cain explained. "They probably would be out of the sport. Having 83% return is, in my mind, a very good number."[12]

Brett W. Gibson, MD, and his colleagues reviewed the outcomes of UCL reconstructions specifically among MLB pitchers. They reviewed data on 68 pitchers who underwent UCL reconstruction between 1998 and 2003. Even in this high-demand group, the success of the operation was evident. Of those pitchers, 82% returned to play at an average of 18.5 months after surgery. By the second season back from surgery, those pitchers threw similar numbers of innings as control pitchers. The researchers found no significant change in ERA, walks, or hits after pitchers returned to play from surgery.[13]

Some studies place the success rate for return to pitching even higher. In 2006 George A. Paletta Jr., MD, and Rick W. Wright, MD, reported a 92% success rate for return to the same or higher level of pitching among 25 elite professional or scholarship college pitchers after reconstruction.[14]

It is difficult to determine the exact number of major league pitchers who have undergone UCL reconstruction since Dr. Jobe first performed the surgery to try to save Tommy John's career. It is believed that 25% of current MLB pitchers have had Tommy John surgery.[15]

Tommy John was one of those pitchers who did successfully return to the mound. After missing the entire 1975 MLB season, he returned in 1976 and pitched 13 more seasons. He finished his pitching career with 288 wins, 2,245 strikeouts, and a 3.34 career ERA. Never missing another start due to elbow pain, he pitched until age 46.

"It's unreal, isn't it?," he said in an interview with FOX Sports. "It's like when you go to Vegas, you've won $1,000 and you put the original money back in your pocket. Now you're playing with their money. That's what I was doing in baseball. I was playing with the house's money. I was doing what I had done my entire life, only this time I knew that it was the house's money, and not my money."[16]

Today MLB pitchers don't face UCL reconstruction with the pessimistic prognosis that Dr. Jobe gave the Dodgers southpaw in 1974. They now expect to return to their previous performance after surgery and rehab. But to this day, no pitcher has had more wins after the surgery—164 of them—than did Tommy John. Now the surgery he decided to undergo, facing 1 in 100 odds of ever pitching again, is commonly referred to as Tommy John surgery.

September 8, 2012

The most noteworthy date in the history of Stephen Strasburg's UCL injury wasn't the day on which he tore the ligament. It wasn't when he had surgery, or when he returned to pitch. It was the day when the Washington Nationals shut him down.

Of course, baseball fans across the country had known this day was coming for months. It was one of the most debated topics in all of sports in 2012. Teammates, pitching coaches, former players, and orthopaedic surgeons argued for and against the Nationals' decision. Even Washington, D.C., mayor Vincent Gray weighed in on the Stephen Strasburg issue.

Perhaps the most hyped pitcher in years, Stephen Strasburg was the overall number one pick in the 2009 MLB draft. Almost immediately, the phenom seemed to live up to the hype. In his debut against the Pittsburgh Pirates, Strasburg struck out 14 (including every batter in the Pirates' lineup at least once). In 12 appearances during that 2010 season, he amassed a 5–3 record, with a 2.91 ERA and 92 strikeouts. Fans packed the stadiums to watch him pitch.

Even before Strasburg made his remarkable MLB debut, Washington Nationals general manager Mike Rizzo had planned to shut him down as he approached 105 innings. Unfortunately, his season ended after only 68.

In the fifth inning of a start against the Philadelphia Phillies on August 21, Strasburg threw a 1–1 changeup to Domonic Brown. Clearly in pain and grabbing his wrist, he left the game. After an initial MRI suggested a flexor tendon strain in his forearm, a follow-up MR arthrogram revealed a torn UCL.

"Bottom line, this is a game. I'm very blessed to play this game for a living. It's a minor setback, but in the grand scheme of things it's just a blip on the radar screen," Strasburg told reporters after learning the diagnosis.[17]

Days later, Strasburg underwent Tommy John surgery.

Although almost four decades have passed since Tommy John's experimental surgery, rehab from UCL reconstruction has remained largely unchanged.

Surgeons must protect the graft as the body incorporates it. Surgeons and physical therapists can slowly work to increase a pitcher's elbow motion and strength, but must protect the healing graft. When the graft is believed to be strong enough to withstand the forces on it from throwing—usually at least four months after surgery—the pitcher starts a progressive long-toss program.

Modern long-toss programs vary, but the principles are fairly consistent. The pitcher gradually increases the distance he throws each week—45 feet, 60 feet, 90 feet, 120 feet, 150 feet, and 180 feet, for example. Throwing every other day, he might increase the number of throws or the intensity of the throws. If he completes those sessions without any pain, he increases to the next level and distance. If he feels any pain or has any other symptoms, he drops back a level and resumes as his arm will tolerate it.

Compare that modern program with the one Tommy John followed.

He threw a baseball to his wife because he knew he wouldn't throw too hard to her. Then he threw to a neighbor who played softball. At spring training in Vero Beach, he threw against a wall. Over and over, he threw the ball, fielded it, picked it up, and threw it again.

John threw every day but Sunday. When his arm felt bad, he didn't throw much. He used how his arm felt to guide his personal rehab.[18]

One day after the one-year anniversary of his landmark surgery, Tommy John pitched in an Instructional League game in Mesa, Arizona. John threw 39 pitches in three perfect innings, with four strikeouts. He wanted to keep pitching, but the coaches stuck to their pregame decision. They would limit him to 50 pitches or three innings, whichever came first.

"When I left the mound after the third, I felt as if I had won the seventh game of the World Series," Tommy John wrote years later.[19]

Like Tommy John, Stephen Strasburg returned to pitch around the one-year mark after his surgery. Pitching for the Hagerstown Suns in the South Atlantic League, he threw 31 pitches in one and two-thirds innings on August 7, 2011.

After five rehab appearances in the minors, Strasburg returned to pitch for the Washington Nationals. He pitched 24 innings over 5 games for the Nationals and compiled a 1.50 ERA with 24 strikeouts.

Entering the 2012 season, Washington Nationals general manager Mike Rizzo decided to shut down Stephen Strasburg at a certain point. It was arguably one of the most controversial decisions in baseball in many years.

Initially the idea that a team would end a pitcher's season after a certain number of innings didn't get much attention. While it was widely reported in the media that the Nationals placed his ceiling at 160 innings, Rizzo denied that a magic number of innings existed. Instead he would use the eye test. Basically Rizzo, and not manager Davey Johnson or the Nationals' owners, would watch Strasburg and determine when he would be shut down based on how he was performing on the mound.[20]

Not much was expected of the Nationals before the 2012 season. After all, they had finished 21.5 games back of the division-winning Philadelphia Phillies the previous year. Baseball experts picked the team anywhere from second to fourth in the National League East before the 2012 season. In addition to questions about the center fielder and closing pitcher as well as the team's propensity to strike out, no one knew exactly what to expect from the Nationals' ace pitcher returning from Tommy John surgery.

Strasburg turned out to be sensational. By the All-Star break, he had a 9–4 record, with a 2.82 ERA. And his remarkable efforts helped to propel his team to first place in the National League East division. By August it was clear that the Nationals were a legitimate World Series contender.

The city of Washington, D.C., hadn't seen its team make the playoffs since the Washington Senators did it in 1933. The years of futility that had followed the 1933 season often led cynics to remark that Washington was "first in war, first in peace, and last in the American League." In fact, the Nationals franchise, which began when the Montréal Expos relocated to DC, is the only National League team to have never appeared in the World Series. Why would the team consider shutting down its ace now?

Knowing that it could ruin his reputation, Rizzo repeatedly told the media he would stick to the decision he made months earlier because he believed it was best for the long-term health of the pitcher and long-term success of the team. Nothing would change his mind, including the opinions of critics.

Those critics included legendary pitching coach Leo Mazzone, who coached Hall of Fame pitchers Greg Maddux, John Smoltz, and Tom Glavine, among others, in his time with the Atlanta Braves. In an interview with a radio station in San Francisco, Mazzone argued that it was totally ridiculous to shut down Strasburg when the team had one of baseball's best pitching rotations and a good chance of making the World Series.[21]

As the regular season end neared, stories surfaced quoting Nationals players—Strasburg's teammates—as being unhappy with the decision to shut down their best pitcher.

According to Thomas Boswell of the *Washington Post*, even Strasburg's father questioned Rizzo when they met at an August game.

Rizzo responded, "Mr. Strasburg, don't ask the question if you don't want to hear the full answer."[22]

As mentioned previously, many studies have shown good outcomes after UCL reconstruction. However, data on the results of recurrent UCL injury and risk factors for re-tearing the ligament are lacking. In the 2015 study performed by former Los Angeles Dodgers athletic trainer Stan Conte that found that 25% of current MLB pitchers had undergone Tommy John surgery, only 3 of 96 had undergone two reconstructions.[23]

As for many ligament reconstructive surgeries, orthopaedic surgeons assume that the outcomes are worse for repeat operations. The tunnels drilled in the bones of the elbow during the first operation could compromise the bone quality in the humerus and ulna. A second operation could require use of a backup tendon—maybe from the knee or from a cadaver—since the preferred option might already have been used.

Despite roughly 83% of pitchers returning to the same or a higher level of pitching, the outcome has proven to be worse after a second operation. A 2015 study by Nathan E. Marshall and other researchers found that only 65.5% of MLB pitchers returned to that level after revision UCL reconstruction.[24] Even worse, researchers at Dr. Jobe's Kerlan-Jobe Orthopaedic Clinic in Los Angeles found that only 5 out of 15 baseball players on whom they had performed revision surgery returned to their previous level of play for at least one season.[25]

Likewise, while we assume that the risk factors for a recurrent injury would be the same as those for a primary one—namely too much pitching and poor throwing mechanics—we don't have evidence to prove it. Specifically, no study has shown a threshold number of innings above which a pitcher is more likely to tear the graft during his first season back.

Some MLB team physicians use soft limits, aiming to keep the recovering pitcher between roughly 100 and 200 innings in the first full season back. If the team is contending for a playoff spot, then the doctor can work with the team to adjust the innings the pitcher pitches during the regular season to allow him to pitch in the postseason. The pitcher might get extra days of rest or even miss a start occasionally. Others might not use a specific innings limit but could monitor the pitcher's performance and technique by video, looking for signs of a problem.

Ultimately Strasburg presented a short-term versus long-term risk and reward dilemma. He was the best pitcher on a team that wasn't just a World Series hopeful in 2012. The Nationals might be a playoff contender for years to come. There was no absolute right or wrong answer.

In explaining his decision to Jim Strasburg, Rizzo included the perspective of Dr. Yocum, Strasburg's orthopaedic surgeon. Based on his experience with hundreds of UCL reconstructions, Yocum believed that the second season back often wrecked the pitcher. Both shoulder and elbow injuries could destroy the pitcher's arm, as well as his career, if he rushed back too fast.[26]

Rizzo and Dr. Yocum seemingly decided before that 2012 season—Strasburg's first full season back—they would carefully watch his starts and how well he was pitching. They would limit his innings for the season as well. Strasburg, only 22 years old when he suffered the Tommy John injury, had never pitched a full MLB season.

Strasburg struggled through what turned out to be his final 2012 start. The looming possibility of being shut down for the rest of the season when he was pitching well and the team was leading the division took a toll on him. Manager Davey Johnson believed it was affecting him mentally and affecting his sleep. Strasburg didn't want to let his teammates down.[27]

Strasburg finished that first full season after Tommy John surgery with a 15–6 record, 3.16 ERA, and 197 strikeouts in 159⅓ innings.

The Washington Nationals did make the playoffs for the first time since the Washington Senators had done so in 1933. In fact, they entered with the best record in all of baseball. Without Strasburg, they lost their opening round series against the St. Louis Cardinals.

Two of the main risk factors for UCL injuries are thought to be poor mechanics and overuse. Having both problems presents a real risk for any pitcher.

The Washington Nationals chose to modify Stephen Strasburg's risk for another UCL injury by preventing overuse. They did not alter his pitching technique.

Multiple flaws might exist in Strasburg's delivery. Rotating too far toward second base in the wind up, stepping too far toward a right-handed batter's box, and keeping his elbow above his wrists and shoulder could lead to trouble over time. His timing and positioning could force him to use the smaller muscles around his shoulder, arm, and elbow to generate force rather than the powerful core muscles and lower body.

Strasburg heard the criticisms of his mechanics but brushed off suggestions that he should try to fix them. He had been pitching that way since he started playing baseball, after all. He wouldn't try to change at this point.

Late in Strasburg's brief return toward the end of the 2011 season, Washington Nationals television commentators F. P. Santangelo and Bob Carpenter had an enlightening exchange during an outing when the right-hander appeared to be struggling.

"He's getting out front, and his arm was dragging," Santangelo noted, pointing out Strasburg's known arm lag. Carpenter later responded that Nationals pitching coach Steve McCatty was "scared to death every time Strasburg goes to pitch."

"I don't want to be the one that screws the kid up," McCatty reportedly remarked.[28]

Major League Baseball teams might have little incentive to correct a pitcher's mechanics. After all, the job of the team's manager and general manager is to win games and World Series titles. To do that, the pitcher and his pitching coach have to do their jobs—namely get the batters out. If athletic ability can overcome technical flaws and help get batters out, why fix a problem that may or may not lead to injury?

Despite the availability of video analysis that can break down into millisecond snapshots every aspect of the pitcher's mechanics—shoulder and elbow position, spine rotation and alignment, head tilt, grip and position of the ball, and much more—many big league pitching coaches seem unwilling to use them. The pitching coaches might resist the use of video analysis, instead relying on watching the pitchers themselves and making any necessary tweaks to the technique. Or they might believe that the pitchers' mechanics are fairly ingrained by the time they reach the majors.

Glenn S. Fleisig, PhD, is the research director of the American Sports Medicine Institute (ASMI). He and his team have worked with many hundreds of major and minor league pitchers. He does believe it is possible to change a minor leaguer's mechanics.

When he evaluates a minor league pitcher, he gives the feedback on ways to improve his mechanics to the coaches and team management, not the pitcher. Then the coaches can work with him to make those changes. The pitcher will take the advice because he wants to make it to the majors. He believes that those changes are what he needs to make it to the next level.[29]

Still, fixing flaws in technique is not easy.

"It's very difficult to change their mechanics," Dr. Cain remarked. "It's like changing a golf swing. You have a lot of coaches and a lot of people telling you what to do, but actually changing that is a difficult process."[30]

Ulnar collateral ligament injuries are essentially preventable injuries. Recall the analogy comparing the UCL to a rope. If stress is abnormally concentrated on one section of the rope, over time that rope will gradually fray, until it snaps.

As previously mentioned, the two critical risks for UCL injuries appear to be poor mechanics and overuse. Poor pitching mechanics place increased stress on the ligament. Overuse—manifested as too many pitches, innings, starts, and seasons over a career—frays the ligament until it finally ruptures.

If major league clubs can't—or won't—change a pitcher's mechanics, that's one issue. But both overuse and poor mechanics of a pitcher can be—and should be—corrected in youth baseball.

If this is done, rates of UCL injuries should gradually decline. Unfortunately, they aren't decreasing. We are headed in the opposite direction.

Ulnar collateral ligament reconstructions used to be performed almost exclusively on professional athletes. Now we are witnessing what appears to be an epidemic of these injuries and surgeries among younger kids.

Among the 1,607 UCL reconstructions performed by Dr. James Andrews between 1994 and 2010, the percentage performed on youth and high school pitchers rose significantly. In 2010, 31% of the surgeries were on youth pitchers, compared to only 18% a decade earlier.[31]

"I used to see just a handful of those kids each year," Dr. Andrews told *Orthopedics Today* in 2010. "Now I am seeing 50, 60, 70 a year. I will bet this year I will see 100 of them."[32]

Dr. Cain said that his group at ASMI recently presented a study of their Tommy

John surgeries over the last 15 years, looking at the prevalence in different age groups. They have seen a dramatic shift in the age population from older, more mature professional pitchers to high school and youth pitchers.[33]

A study done by Damon H. Petty, MD, looked at UCL reconstructions specifically in high school baseball players. Unlike the 80% and higher rates of return to baseball at the same or higher level in older players, they found a success rate of only 74%.

More striking were the risk factors these injured high school players exhibited. Of the injured pitchers, 85% were overused in at least some way; 69% were found to have been throwing year-round or had less than two months of rest during the year. In addition, 62% had been overused during the season, meaning that they had pitched more than the recommended limits per game or week or did not get the minimum rest after pitching, while 42% were overused in some fashion during a particular game, series of games, or event. Two-thirds of the injured pitchers had been throwing curveballs before age 14.[34]

Overuse is the primary culprit for these injuries. To understand the rise in youth pitchers who suffer shoulder and elbow injuries, look for the young kids who pitch for multiple teams and pitch year-round without rest.

Kids who pitch more are more likely to suffer shoulder or elbow problems regardless of mechanics or whether they threw curveballs. Dr. Fleisig has seen kids with seasonal and career pitch count numbers that are dramatically higher than younger pitchers had in previous generations.[35]

Youth pitchers dramatically increase the risk of suffering throwing injuries with these habits. Those who throw more than 80 pitches per game have a 360% increased risk. Pitching for more than eight months per year leads to a 500% increased risk. And pitching while fatigued increases the injury risk 3600%.[36]

All of these risks can be stopped, or at least modified, but it doesn't appear to be happening. At some point, parents, coaches and yes, the young athletes themselves, will have to recognize the problem that currently exists and change it.

To understand why UCL injuries and surgeries are increasing among younger kids, and why the risks are largely being ignored, it is important to understand the perspective of the kids and their parents and coaches.

Pitcher Hayden Hurst underwent Tommy John surgery in eighth grade. He remarked to ESPN.com, "I can definitely feel the difference. Before the surgery it felt like I had a bum arm. Now it feels alive."[37]

Jeff Fish, father of a 16-year-old pitcher who had the surgery in order to pitch in college, heard a teammate claim to gain 3 to 5 mph on his fastball after surgery. "I'm not saying that's the reason to do it," Fish explained to the *New York Times*. "It's encouraging to think he might get more velocity."[38]

A 2012 study by Christopher S. Ahmad and others surveyed youth, high school, and college baseball players, as well as parents and coaches, regarding the injury and its risk factors, the benefits of surgery, indications for doing the surgery, the rehab, and return to baseball.

The authors found that 30% of coaches, 37% of parents, 51% of high school athletes, and 26% of college athletes believe that Tommy John surgery should be performed on players with no injury in order to improve performance. All groups also thought the surgery improved a pitcher's control, speed, and performance to levels above what they were before injury.[39]

"That's just not true," Dr. Gary Green, the medical director of MLB, argued. "It leads to a lot of parents feeling, 'I'll just have my kid throw as hard as he can for as long as he can. When his elbow blows out, we'll just pop a new ligament in and then he's good to go.'"[40]

There is no scientific evidence to support the beliefs of these parents, coaches, and young athletes.

Kids might feel like they pitch better after surgery, but the surgery alone probably isn't what makes them feel stronger.

First, they often compare their velocity after surgery to what it was when that ligament was slowly failing, not when it was healthy.

Second, over the 12 to 18 months between the surgery and return to baseball, their bodies are maturing. They grow taller and develop stronger muscles.

During the rehab and throwing program, they might correct their technical flaws. Finally, they don't have chronic shoulder and elbow pain and have time to rest instead of throwing all the time.

Kids and the parents and coaches pushing them must do everything they can to avoid this injury. While the overall success rate is 83%, that statistic means that 17% never make it back to play. Those players have the same dreams as the 83%. On top of that, it is a long road back, and complications do occur. Having Tommy John surgery at a young age is not good for your future.

"Having a Tommy John surgery when you're a young athlete begins the wear and tear process much earlier than the typical professional athletes," Dr. Cain observed. "Even then you may make it to the college level. You may even sign a professional contract. I think most of us believe now that it probably shortens your overall career length because you're potentially laying a foundation of injury earlier in life."[41]

Dr. Fleisig claimed that it will take a three-pronged approach to fix this problem. First, the baseball leagues and the medical community must inform parents and young athletes about the realities of and misperceptions about these injuries and surgeries. Second, the baseball leagues have to buy into these limits and this approach to safe pitching.

The third prong is perhaps most interesting. The pro teams, Fleisig argued, need to remove the reward for kids abusing their arms. If MLB teams started drafting kids who didn't pitch year-round or for multiple teams, that behavior might start to correct itself.[42]

ESPN *the Magazine* pointed out that the salaries paid by MLB teams to players on the disabled list rehabbing from Tommy John surgery alone over a recent five-year period exceeded $193 million.[43]

"It's not a Major League Baseball problem, and it's not a Little League baseball problem. It's a baseball problem," Fleisig admitted.[44]

Recently, former MLB commissioner Bud Selig and Major League Baseball formed an elbow task force. Dr. Fleisig, Dr. Green, and others serve on this committee, PitchSmart.org. The website offers tips to young athletes and their parents and coaches for players to avoid injury and have long baseball careers.

Dr. Green pointed to PitchSmart.org as a positive step toward correcting the epidemic of youth pitching injuries. "As with most things in medicine, prevention is a whole lot better than treatment in most cases."[45]

One of the key challenges we must overcome to correct these overuse injuries is the trend toward earlier single-sport specialization. Tommy John, like most kids in the 1970s and 1980s, played different sports growing up. Instead of kids playing different sports every season—baseball in the spring, football in the fall, and basketball in the winter, for example—now more and more kids are pressured to play one sport only, starting as early as seven or eight years old.

Playing the same sport every season, especially if a kid does it all year with no rest, places stress on the same parts of the body over and over. Essentially that wear and tear can cause injuries, like these UCL injuries. Playing different sports shifts those stresses to other parts of the body and gives the stressed areas needed time to rest.

Even if a young athlete really likes baseball, he doesn't have to pitch all the time. Many current major league pitchers played other positions growing up.

As evidence of the problem of early single-sport specialization and year-round pitching, Dr. Green said that a disproportionate number of pitchers in MLB grew up in northern states, where playing baseball all year long is not possible.[46]

In fact, two studies published in the *Orthopaedic Journal of Sports Medicine* observed that trend. One study found that more MLB pitchers who pitched in high schools in warm-weather states had undergone UCL reconstruction than those who pitched in cold-weather states.[47] Another study found that college pitchers who pitched in southern states in high school had an increased risk of UCL surgery. Pitching in the Southeastern Conference also led to a greater likelihood of undergoing Tommy John surgery than did pitching in the Big Ten Conference.[48]

Dr. John DiFiori, the current director of sports medicine of the NBA, surveyed 296 NCAA Division I male and female athletes, finding that 88% participated in two or three sports as kids, and 70% did not specialize in one sport until after the age of 12.[49]

This is not just a problem in youth baseball. Brandi Chastain also sees this problem in soccer:

> I didn't choose to play only soccer until my senior year in high school. That was because someone said, "Hey maybe you should play soccer only because you have a chance to play on these other teams." Honestly, it never really dawned on me that I would only play soccer because I played sports just for fun. There was no other reason to be playing sports. I loved all sports. I participated in baseball, basketball, volleyball, soccer, track and field, and I loved them all. Soccer just happened to be the one that I excelled at a younger age. Ultimately as a senior, that's when it was clear. At that time, you start talking to colleges. Whereas now you're going into your freshman and sophomore year, and you start thinking about where you're going to college.[50]

Chastain claimed that almost all of her 1999 USWNT teammates—if not all of them—played other sports growing up.

It isn't just the physical wear and tear that accumulates for kids as they play only one sport. Chastain learned many skills while playing basketball and baseball that ultimately made her a more well-rounded soccer player as she got older. In the long run, playing different sports helped her soccer career.

"It's like going to school and only studying math or only studying English. There's a lot to each person, and you can't develop a full, well-rounded person with ultra-specialization at an early, early age."[51]

Dr. Green stated it quite simply. "Playing multiple sports is a really good way to avoid injury."[52]

Efforts by orthopaedic surgeons to promote youth pitching injury prevention have increased in recent years. But the message often falls on deaf ears.

North Reading High School baseball coach Frank Carey, one of the most victorious baseball coaches in Massachusetts history, once let one of his pitchers throw 16 innings and 223 pitches in a game. He stated that coaches focus too much on pitch counts. "You hear a story about a kid pitching a 12- or 14-inning game," Carey told Christopher Smith of the *Eagle-Tribune*. "People today think that's heresy. I don't think there's anything wrong with it."[53]

Parents are often quick to point to major league pitchers from Latin America. They argue that "these Dominican kids" throw year-round and throw breaking pitches when they're young and have no problems.

To argue that young pitchers from other countries, or even from the United States, can ignore risks and avoid injury is misleading. Stories like those are anecdotal experiences of one or a small number of kids who might have defied the odds. But we ignore—or never hear about—the kids who get hurt and never pitch again. Why would we? Shows like *SportsCenter* feature highlights of stars, not injuries of kids who never make it.

Parents often ignore the risks of injury because the lure of pro contracts, college scholarships, and media exposure is just too great. To chase the money in pro baseball, parents often believe they have to force their young athletes to play year-round, often on more than one team during a single season. If their son takes the season off to play a different sport and rest his arm, he will get behind his eight-year-old neighbor who is playing nonstop.

Parents and coaches alike push kids to play in showcase events so that college and professional scouts might "find" their kids. Frequently these kids participate while tired from a grueling season. Then they throw harder than normal in an attempt to impress the scouts. They might even pitch through pain.

Parents must begin to recognize that more is not better when it comes to pitching at a young age.

And while it would be easy to blame "those parents," many coaches are equally to blame. They often ignore opportunities to correct poor pitching mechanics and limit overuse of growing arms.

Why? Coaches, even at the youth level, need to win. If their teams don't win, parents will pull their kids out and take them to play for another coach whose teams do win.

And how does a youth baseball coach whose team might only have one or two gifted pitchers on his team win? By pitching those one or two pitchers all the time. They use these pitchers for too many innings, in too many games, and for too many consecutive seasons.

It doesn't matter to the coach if that amount of pitching leads to shoulder and elbow injuries in those kids two or three years later. They will be in high school then, pitching for a different coach. That's not this coach's problem. He needs to win now.

Without a doubt, there are parents and coaches who do it the right way, who work with the kids to teach mechanics, and who try to prevent overuse. But there is far too much emphasis placed on winning, statistics, and pursuit of scholarships and money—and too much reliance on the notion that Tommy John surgery can serve as a cure-all to reverse the damage those activities caused.

We must take action if we are going to stop this epidemic of Tommy John injuries or even simply stem the tide. Dr. Fleisig argued that should be our first goal. "That's my first humble vision, which is not that the number of pro pitchers, pro being major or minor league pitchers, having Tommy John injury is going to go down right away. My hope just for the next few years is it stops going up."[54]

For all the good—and possibly the bad—that his injury and surgery have caused, Tommy John seems to understand his place in baseball history. "I thank God that Dr. Jobe did what he had to do and I did what I had to do. And it will be forever known as Tommy John surgery. I'll be dust in the ground and Tommy John surgery will probably be living on."[55]

CONCLUSION

I met Bill Walton in the late spring of 2015 during a meet-and-greet session for a conference in Chicago. He told me about his 37 orthopaedic surgeries, so naturally I asked to interview him for this book. I didn't even have to explain its premise to him.

"Hopefully this book is about, 'This is the way it used to be. This is the way it is now. How can we be better for the future so that our athletes, our young people, our guys who want to test themselves and are willing to go for everything out there, that they have the best chance of success, but they also have a future?'"[1]

I couldn't have expressed the purpose of *That's Gotta Hurt* any better.

The injuries described in this book span roughly four decades of sports. Chronologically the first landmark surgery presented was Tommy John's surgery, and it exemplifies the fundamental shift that has occurred over those 40 years.

Tommy John suffered an injury that up to that point had ended pitchers' careers. Orthopaedic surgeons had diagnosed the injury previously; after all, it was first reported back in 1946. Prior to the advent of the MRI and a thorough understanding of the elbow injuries, we did not recognize these injuries in elite pitchers. Dr. Frank Jobe reportedly once remarked that he thought Dodgers great Sandy Koufax might have had a UCL injury.[2]

Jobe devised a surgical technique that probably sounded ridiculous at the time: taking a tendon from the wrist and implanting it through drill holes in the bones of the elbow. Tommy John himself took an enormous chance by undergoing that surgery; he had a 1 in 100 chance of ever pitching again, Dr. Jobe believed. But what choice did John really have? If he didn't undergo the untested surgery, he would never pitch again. Today approximately one of every four MLB pitchers has extended his career by undergoing a surgery very similar to the one performed in 1974.[3]

Sports medicine hasn't just developed solutions that simply keep people playing sports and exercising; these solutions help athletes and active people return to their activities faster than ever. Instead of a complex knee surgery involving a long incision and months of rehab, Joan Benoit underwent arthroscopic knee surgery to compete in—and win—the US Olympic marathon trials 17 days later.

Bernard King suffered a horrific knee injury and yet overcame surgery and a grueling rehab to return to play and excel in the NBA. Now over 100,000 people undergo ACL reconstructions every year in the United States alone.

Professionals in the field of sports medicine continually aim to better treat injuries, but we also want to prevent the injuries from occurring in the first place. With the help of an institute that bears his name, Korey Stringer's death from exertional heat stroke, along with deaths of athletes at the youth, high school, and college levels, has brought attention to heat illness in sports and led to changes in sports training and on-site management to make it one of the most preventable injuries or illnesses in sports.

Orthopaedic surgeons, athletic trainers, and physical therapists continue to develop and promote neuromuscular training programs to try to prevent ACL injuries—the injury Bernard King and countless numbers of football, basketball, and soccer players and athletes of all sports have suffered. If doing an exercise program for 10 or 15 minutes a day can lower the chances of suffering one of these injuries, it seems reasonable to try. In the process, we just might impact sports for an entire generation of female athletes.

Dr. Norman Scott, the former New York Knicks team physician who performed the landmark ACL surgery on Bernard King discussed earlier in this book, summarized just how far sports medicine has come; "I just think when you put it into perspective, sports medicine in the '70s was somewhat of a joke, and it was nothing more than general orthopaedics in most people's minds. The sports world has done a spectacular job in making it much more of a science, and that had so much to do with the successes we're seeing today."[4]

As sports medicine moves forward, surgeons, physicians, and other medical professionals have an amazing opportunity. We can improve the careers and performance of elite athletes. We can have an even greater impact, though, on the future stars who dream of one day joining the ranks of pro athletes. And we can improve the health and happiness of the millions of regular people who just want to play sports recreationally and exercise to stay in shape.

As I have tried to show with these injuries and the effects they have had, those opportunities also present questions and challenges. Everyone involved—the doctors, athletic trainers, parents, coaches, and teams—must address these issues in the coming years.

The Role of Sports Medicine Surgeons and Doctors

With the growth and increasing importance of sports in modern society, it should be no surprise that sports medicine has exploded in popularity.

After orthopaedic surgery residents complete their training, they can go on to practice as general orthopaedic surgeons. They can also choose to perform fellowships and specialize in one of orthopaedic surgery's many subspecialties: joint replacement, trauma, pediatrics, oncology, spine, shoulder and elbow, foot and ankle, hand, and sports medicine. With all of the practice options, today more orthopaedic surgery residents go on to orthopaedic sports medicine fellowships than any other subspecialty.

Likewise, physicians who want to work in sports medicine are more abundant than ever. Many primary care fields, including family medicine, pediatrics, physical medicine and rehabilitation, and emergency medicine, offer fellowship training in sports medicine. These primary care sports medicine physicians often work in large hospital-based sports medicine programs or in orthopaedic surgery practices. They provide diagnosis and nonoperative treatment for musculoskeletal injuries. They also serve as the medical providers for sports teams at the professional or college levels while the orthopaedic surgeons treat the bone and joint injuries.

Even medical fields not typically associated with sports have joined in to treat athletes and active individuals. Entire fields have developed—sports psychology, sports neurology and neuroscience, sports nutrition, and many more.

All of this growth has undoubtedly led to more thorough care of athletes. Today, health-care providers with more experience with these injuries than ever treat athletes at all levels. With the growth of specialists, many problems that largely fell outside the training of orthopaedic surgeons serving as team doctors in the past—concussions, sudden cardiac arrest, depression, eating disorders, and much more—are better recognized, treated, or prevented.

Perhaps it is this growth in the numbers of sports medicine professionals—and the money involved in professional sports—that has led to a shift in how professional teams select team doctors. In the past, a franchise would select a doctor, group, or hospital that it deemed to be the most capable of providing top care to its athletes. Over the last 20 years or so, financial arrangements have entered the picture.

In a 1995 editorial entitled "Job Auction," the editor of the *American Journal of Sports Medicine*, Robert E. Leach, MD, commented on a *Sports Illustrated* article claiming that the new NFL franchises in Charlotte and Jacksonville were both accepting bids for the rights to be medical providers for the teams. Leach recognized the criticism sports medicine had already received throughout medicine due to the high-profile treatment of famous athletes. He worried that this "team physician job for sale" set a much worse precedent.[5]

Now such financial arrangements are common. Some groups might not pay for the right to serve as team physicians specifically, but they might agree to pay a certain amount—sometimes in the hundreds of thousands or millions of dollars—for the marketing rights.

After all, the right to announce that a hospital or group of doctors is the exclusive medical provider for the New York Yankees or Dallas Cowboys on television, radio, or billboards would seem to be extremely valuable.

In a position statement, the American Orthopaedic Society for Sports Medicine (AOSSM) admits that the selection process for team physicians can be a complicated one. The organization asserts that the selection of team physicians should be based fundamentally on the ability of the physicians and medical group. They should have the appropriate credentials, including sports medicine fellowships after completing residency training programs. They should have experience caring for teams at the level of the team with whom they are negotiating. And they should have a network of appropriate specialists, ancillary personnel, and facilities to serve the team's required level of care.

Selection should not be based solely on financial incentives offered by a hospital or medical practice. Bidding for these contracts exposes both the team and physicians to conflicts of interest, AOSSM believes. Yet some marketing may be involved between a hospital or physician and a professional team, so some latitude for these negotiations can be entertained.[6]

Since these are some of the best athletes in the world, we might assume that these teams want the best doctors. And while most orthopaedic surgery groups are qualified, adding a financial relationship into the equation might cause the athletes to question whether their team doctors are capable.

Professional athletes can easily travel to get second opinions. We hear about athletes undergoing surgery by a surgeon other than the team doctor all the time. College athletes, though, might be limited to having surgery done by the physician selected by the school, given a college athlete's limited personal resources and distance from home. The athlete and his parents might feel that the school's surgeon is the best in the area, but a pay-to-serve contract might cast doubt on that assumption.

The appeal of these relationships for a practice lies in the potential gain of new patients, not from the players on the team as much as from fans and other people who live in the area. The mother of a high school football player might pick the Chicago Bears' doctor to do her son's ACL reconstruction because she assumes he must be the best in Chicago if the Bears trust their players to him. She might be surprised to learn that a hospital could have persuaded the team to pick it as its health-care provider with an expensive marketing arrangement.

This discussion is not meant to cast doubt on any team doctors—quite the opposite. Most sports medicine–trained orthopaedic surgeons and their groups provide excellent care to teams and patients. The selection process, though, can generate confusion and controversy.

Doctor-Patient-Team Relationship?

If you go to the doctor and discuss an injury or illness, you have a fairly straight-forward relationship. He or she asks you about your condition, examines you, orders and then reviews any necessary tests, makes a diagnosis, and suggests treatment options. You and the physician are the only participants in the treatment decision.

In professional sports, coaches or general managers who want to be involved complicate the doctor-patient relationship. The athlete is a patient, but the coach wants to know if the player can return to the field or court. The general manager wants to know how long the player might be out in case he needs to bring in another player.

One could argue that the professional team is an employer and thus has the right to be involved in treatment decisions. Regardless, this doctor-athlete-team triad creates some challenging scenarios.

Let's say the point guard of a leading NBA team strains his hamstring one week before the playoffs begin. The coach pressures the doctor and the team's athletic trainer to do whatever it takes to get the player back on the court as soon as possible. The athlete has concerns that he is much more likely to suffer a repeat hamstring strain if he returns to play before he is completely healed. The doctor could be caught between siding with the player and the team.

On the other hand, it is also common, as we have seen with concussions and musculoskeletal injuries in the NBA, that athletes often want to return quickly.

They want to play to help their teams. They might fear losing their starting spots on the team. Or they might fear getting cut from the team entirely. College athletes might worry about losing their scholarships.

Regardless of the treatment decision, when working with pro teams today, a team doctor opens himself or herself up for scrutiny in the media. If a surgery goes well and the athlete returns in the expected timeframe, little mention of it will be made. If the athlete takes longer to return to play than expected—even if the surgery went well—expect fans to criticize the doctor or the athlete on the Internet or sports talk radio.

With the explosion of money generated by professional and college sports and their ever-growing prominence and popularity in society, we can expect even more attention from fans who have 24/7 access to information. Expect far more scrutiny of sports injuries—and the players who suffer them and the doctors who treat them.

Working with Top Athletes—and the Rest of Us

The dilemma of what treatment is most appropriate can affect all athletes and active people, not just pros. Often the decision is one of short-term versus long-term choices.

Say, for example, a varsity soccer player tears a meniscus in her knee four weeks before the state playoffs begin. The orthopaedic surgeon finds a bucket-handle meniscus tear that he feels is reparable. Surgery would involve repairing the meniscus, or sewing it together. It would require four to six months to heal and for the patient to recover. The athlete's hopes for playing in the state playoffs would be dashed.

Instead she insists on having a partial meniscectomy. The surgeon would trim out the torn portion of meniscus instead of repairing it. She might return to play in as little as three to six weeks, possibly in time to play for the title. But the orthopaedic surgeon worries that trimming out the meniscus tear could lead to the development of arthritic changes years later. How does the surgeon balance what the athlete wants now versus problems that could arise in the future?

In an alternative scenario, continuing to play the sport could jeopardize the health of the athlete. It might be a football player with a history of multiple concussions. It might be a hockey player determined to play a few more years despite a bad knee, on which he has had three or four surgeries. Or it could be a basketball player with chronic foot pain. Even though the athlete can earn a paycheck for a few more years, when does the doctor stop him before his condition causes disability and pain later in life?

Perhaps more important, we must decide our role in optimizing the long-term health of the regular athlete. Whether it's a 45-year-old recreational tennis player or a 32-year-old woman who just wants to run occasional 10K road races, we must find a way to allow people to pursue their sports and exercise passions, but we must also do it in a way that allows them to stay active in them for decades. There are so many benefits to sports and exercise—improved physical health, emotional well-being, camaraderie with friends, just to name a few—that we want people to participate. We must find ways that they can do so safely.

Screening of Athletes

With so much money involved in professional sports, teams will increasingly scrutinize every draft pick and player they sign. In the coming years, a thorough review of an athlete's medical history and in-depth physical examination could become just as important as the scrutiny of his or her physical abilities and play.

Expect statistical analyses to better predict which players might develop certain injuries. For example, seven-foot-tall basketball players with certain types of foot anatomy might be more likely to suffer stress fractures of the bones in the feet. Statistics will soon be able to determine which injuries an athlete has had will have little effect on his future injury risk—an MCL injury of the knee, maybe—and which ones could shorten his career—like a meniscus tear in that same knee.

Teams might scrutinize more than the health of the player. In the Tommy John chapter, I discussed some recent data on the part of the country where kids grow up and their importance in predicting elbow injuries. Several recent studies have shown that major league pitchers who played youth baseball in warm-weather climates are more likely to suffer UCL injuries of the elbow and require Tommy John surgery. They also undergo the surgeries at younger ages and earlier in their careers than do those who pitched in cold-weather climates as kids. Expect teams to study whether they should lean toward drafting an above-average pitcher from New Hampshire over a top-level prospect from Florida, out of fear that the star from the Sunshine State has already jeopardized the health of his arm by pitching year-round in the South.

How do athletes respond to this intense medical scrutiny? In the coming years, teams could push for more sophisticated tests. They might want screening for certain genes that increase the risk of prolonged recoveries from concussions and later CTE. Teams might want to use more advanced cardiac tests, like echo-cardiograms or even genetic screenings, to identify basketball players at risk for SCD. Will some athletes understand the risks and still refuse to undergo the tests?

At the youth and high school sports levels, we must decide whether we will institute mandatory screenings to identify a small percentage of athletes at risk for a very serious medical condition. Will the United States invest tremendous financial resources—hundreds of millions or even billions of dollars—as well as physician specialists and an administrative infrastructure, to perform screening electrocardiograms on every young athlete?

Testing does present some questions that teams and medical staffs will have to answer. For example, teams might want to start genetic testing for the APOE ε4 allele if a definitive link to CTE is established one day. What would happen if the results of genetic tests became publicly available or available to insurance companies? Could an athlete conceivably lose his or her health insurance? Could professional teams choose not to honor a player's contract?

Along the same lines, we will certainly see more advanced psychological testing of athletes in the next few years. Up until now, we have basically used simple interviews of prospective players. The medical evaluation process will grow to include not only musculoskeletal and medical screening, but also complex batteries of tests of athletes' emotional health and neurocognitive function, and even brain imaging. Dr. Erin Shannon, doctor of clinical psychology and energy medicine practitioner who works with top athletes and the NFL's St. Louis Rams, said some of this neurocognitive screening has already quietly begun, given how many millions of dollars are on the line when pro teams draft players.[7]

Mental and Emotional Aspects of Sports

On the topic of psychological health and mental performance, we will likely also see a much greater role of sports psychologists and mental health professionals in sports. Soon sports psychologists will be embedded in every professional sports team, traveling with them just like the coaches and team physicians do. Dr. Shannon expects teams to have multiple specialists, such as one who focuses on the mental and neurological side and another who addresses the psychological issues.[8]

Her husband, Gregg Williams, who is the defensive coordinator for the Rams, noted that the ability of players to talk about what is wrong and what they feel is light-years ahead of where we were just a few years ago. By combining the mental and physical aspects of recovery, Williams has seen his players recover from injuries in half the time with less atrophy and fewer injury setbacks.[9]

In addition, sports psychology will become a more critical tool to improve the performance and production of athletes, optimizing their attention and mental focus. After all, there is little physical difference between elite athletes. Obviously nutrition, genes, training methods, and even luck provide some advantages to certain athletes who become superstars over others. But what's "above the neck" plays an enormous role, no matter what sport an athlete plays. Training an athlete to maximize his or her psychological and neurological potential has just begun.

Right now, there are only a handful of professionals like Dr. Shannon in pro sports, and teams largely keep quiet about them to maintain an advantage. Soon, she said, they won't be a secret because each team will have 1, 2, or 10 of them.[10]

Rules Changes in Sports

It is critical that the sports medicine community continue to research risks for injuries in different sports and look for ways to make sports safer. While concerns about brain injuries in football are prevalent, there is much more we need to know before physicians can advocate that young athletes stop playing the sport. We need more information in order to properly educate the public.

What happens if we as a profession decide that the health and injury risks of certain sports are just too great? If CTE ultimately does prove to be a significant risk for football players, should we try to ban the sport, much as medical organizations have consistently tried with boxing? What should doctors advocate about extreme sports, like freestyle snowmobiling or motocross?

Medical organizations will need to work with sports leagues to implement changes to decrease injuries. This could involve making small adjustments, like moving kickoffs up five yards in football, mandating helmets in hockey, and eliminating home-plate collisions in baseball. Or we might consider more radical steps, like banning hits to quarterbacks in football or eliminating heading in soccer.

These are just philosophical questions, but each sport will likely face questions like these in the coming years.

We cannot forget that fans are critical to the success of the sports. Without fans attending the games, watching on television, and buying the merchandise, these sports will cease to exist. If we make fundamental changes to the nature of the sports themselves, will fans continue to watch? Or will fans grow even more concerned about serious injuries and stop watching altogether?

The Role of Coaches and Athletic Trainers in Sports

Let's be fair. Coaches are usually very good at what they do: teaching their sports and coaching athletes and teams to play them as well as they can. What they generally don't do well is evaluate and treat injuries. Unfortunately, many parents believe that they can send their kids off to play football or other sports and everything is going to be fine.

It is critical for coaches to have some sort of first aid background. Even basic medical training isn't enough, though. Coaches focus their attention on the players and actions on the field or court. It is difficult for them to also watch an athlete's tackling technique, his symptoms of heat illness, or his dizziness after a tackle. That is a fundamental reason we need athletic trainers involved at every level of sports.

Make no mistake. Athletic trainers are not "personal" trainers or "strength and conditioning" trainers. While many athletic trainers do hold additional strength and conditioning credentials, these are highly trained health-care professionals focused on evaluation, treatment, rehabilitation, and prevention of injuries and illnesses.

Athletic trainers unquestionably play critical roles in athletic programs. In addition to serving as first responders to injured athletes, they can develop emergency action plans; monitor field, environment, and weather conditions; develop and coordinate injury prevention programs; prepare athletes for practice and games; communicate with physicians about injuries; treat and rehabilitate injured players; and help determine return to play for injured athletes.

A 2015 study published in the *Journal of Athletic Training* by the National Athletic Trainers' Association surveyed secondary schools in all 50 states and Washington, D.C., and found that 70% of the 8,509 responding schools had access to athletic training services at games or practices, but only 37% had full-time athletic training services.[11] It isn't enough. All schools that field teams in contact and collision sports need athletic trainers. Ideally they would be present at youth sports games and tournaments as well, especially since physicians rarely cover those competitions.

Coaches have a role to play in the safety of young athletes. They can invite parents at the start of the season and demonstrate the equipment that the kids will wear and what their plan is for medical illnesses and injuries. Coaches, however, shouldn't be responsible for the life or death decisions about the children. Athletic trainers are skilled medical professionals who should be present.

Parents of Young Athletes

How will the parents whose kids want to play the sports react to the growing concerns about athletes' long-term health? We've started to see evidence that some parents might be growing increasingly concerned about the long-term effects of concussions. Participation rates in youth football have dropped slightly in recent years, and media attention to brain injuries could have played a part.

At some point, it is at least conceivable that parents on a large scale will start holding their kids out of sports out of fear of injury. Football is the most visible sport that presents that dilemma, but what about extreme sports? Will parents discourage kids from sports like freestyle snowmobiling? What about allowing their kids to snowboard for fun in terrain parks?

Will parents push their children to take more and better precautions than the pros do? For example, major league pitchers and batters have resisted the idea of wearing helmets. The helmets would feel unnatural or alter their performance in some way. Younger players, though, wouldn't know the difference if they started using them early in their playing days. Will concerned parents ask their children to wear less comfortable and more protective equipment?

On the other hand, with the explosion of sports at the professional and college levels, more opportunities for fame and financial success exist for athletes now than ever before. How aggressively should parents push their children in pursuit of these opportunities? Should kids start playing in elite leagues before they hit their growth spurts? Should kids only play one sport year-round as early as seven or eight years old? Or are the parents who pressure kids in that way risking their children's health, burning them out, and actually hurting their future athletic success?

Few parents truly realize just how unlikely playing college sports or even making the pros one day really is. In 2014, *Elite Daily* published statistics on sports participation in the most popular American sports that illustrate how few kids progress from high school to college or the professional ranks. For example, 1,121,744 boys play high school football. One in forty of them will play in college. Only 1 in 1,010 of those high school players will be drafted into the NFL. In men's basketball, of the 535,569 boys who play high school basketball,

1 in 17 will play in college, but only 1 in 8,926 of the high school players will be drafted into the NBA. Some 373,391 girls play high school soccer in the United States. One out of every ten of them will play soccer in college, but only 1 in 10,316 will be drafted into the National Women's Soccer League.[12]

If parents push their kids too hard, they risk creating a situation in which the young athletes burn out and quit. The STOP Sports Injuries campaign estimates that 70% of kids stop playing sports by age 13, and pressure from parents and coaches is thought to be one of the key reasons.[13]

We need to stop focusing on winning, statistics, and hiring individual coaches for seven- and eight-year-olds. We need to stop pressuring kids to play one sport only before they enter middle school. We need to make sports fun for kids again.

Brandi Chastain made a passionate plea to parents:

> The most important thing for parents out there to do is be supportive. The majority or our children, mine included, who will play sports as their occupation or their career is very minimal. The most important thing we can do is support our kids in a loving, open, thoughtful and supportive way. Allow our kids to make mistakes, and to not make the team, and to sit on the bench, and to score a goal, and to save a goal, and to hit a home run, and to have a ball go between their legs. It will allow them to experience all that sports have to offer because the lessons they are going to learn from their teammates, from their coaches, from the game itself are so rich. If we get in the way with "We have to win," "We have to win," "We have to be better every time," we are going to lose that. Ultimately we lose them sports and all the lessons that go with it. So enjoy sports for what it has to offer your children. Be supportive, educate yourself, but don't make it about you, and let the kids enjoy it.[14]

There are so many benefits to sports for children and adolescents. On top of the support for their physical health, there are social, emotional, and even mental benefits. Test scores and academic performance are thought to be better among athletes.[15] In addition, playing sports likely helps achieve career success later in life. A study commissioned by Ernst & Young surveyed senior managers and executives who work at companies with annual revenues in excess of $250 million; 96% of the females in senior executive leadership positions played sports either in primary and secondary school or during college or other tertiary education.[16]

We want our kids to play sports. We must keep them healthy enough to do it.

The Rest of Us

How do all of these injuries and improvements in injury treatments affect every-one else: the adult recreation league soccer player, the older woman who does Zumba every day, the investment banker who loves lifting weights and doing CrossFit? If we suffer injuries, will we rush back to play as soon as possible, or will we work back slowly to protect our bodies long term? Will we try unproven treatments—such as PRP and stem cells—in the hopes of extending our days of playing sports or exercising?

And do we continue to play sports or perform an exercise if we learn that we risk making an old injury worse and potentially harming our health down the road?

Spreading the Message of Safety and Prevention

Orthopaedic surgeons and sports medicine physicians really haven't had a platform for spreading messages about safety and prevention. We see patients in our clinics and treat them surgically in our operating rooms. We publish studies in academic journals that only our peers read, and we speak at medical conferences only attended by our colleagues.

We have traditionally done a poor job of getting our message out to the general public—the athletes, parents, coaches, athletic directors, and fans—who often have little medical knowledge. We have failed to educate, to motivate, and to inspire people to discover what they really need to do.

Dr. Mandelbaum, who works to decrease ACL and other lower extremity injuries, is working with members of the USWNT, most of whom have extensive social media platforms, to spread information about the importance of injury prevention programs.[17] The collaboration among orthopaedic surgeons, youth pitching experts like Dr. Fleisig, and MLB to use the league's platform to poten-tially reach millions of young baseball players and educate them about injuries is another step in the right direction.[18]

Since 2010 I have tried to provide commentary and education on injuries, injury treatments, and prevention in sports and exercise so that athletes and active individuals can stay healthy and perform their best. I have worked to build a platform through my website, podcast, newspaper column, social media, and so forth. That is the main reason I wrote this book, so that everyone can understand where sports medicine started, where we are now, and where we need to be in the future. But we need more team doctors, orthopaedic surgeons, primary care sports medicine physicians, athletic trainers, and other health-care professionals to speak up and share their messages as well.

Hopefully *That's Gotta Hurt* has demonstrated just how far sports and sports medicine have come in the last 40 to 50 years. Yet with all of our advancements, we still have a long way to go.

ACKNOWLEDGMENTS

My father actually came up with the idea for this book. He sent me a text message one night saying that I should write a book and call it *That's Gotta Hurt: The Injuries That Changed Sports Forever*. He offered Joan Benoit, Bernard King, and Dave Duerson as examples of athletes whose injuries and injury treatments have changed their sports and the treatment of athletes of all ages. After a few more hours of texting, we had almost the entire list of athletes I discuss in this book.

In fact, he insisted I use the *Wide World of Sports* opening montage, with Vinko Bogataj crashing at the base of a ski jump, as my introduction. While I remembered watching the show almost every Saturday afternoon as a kid, I couldn't figure out how "the agony of defeat" would apply to what I wanted to write. After researching the crash and learning the effects that footage had on the sport of ski jumping, I had my introduction. As always, my dad's instincts were right.

He has been more helpful through this process than I can ever describe. He has read multiple drafts of every chapter. He convinced me to stick with my message when agents and publishers wanted a more prescriptive medical book. I could not have written this book without his time, wisdom, support, and love.

Much of the information on the injuries I describe came from hundreds of hours of research in newspapers, magazines, and online publications. I could not have told these stories and explained their significance, though, without the insight and experiences of people close to the events. So many people selflessly gave their valuable time to talk to me, and I could not be more grateful to them.

Among the athletes and their coaches, teams, and family, I am deeply appreciative of Sam Bowie, Rory Bushfield, Brandi Chastain, Michael Duerson, Max Eisenbud, Bob Sevene, Bill Walton, and Gregg Williams. I am also thankful for the time and insight shared by many journalists and experts in their fields, including Ken Anderson, Timothy Epstein, Andrea Kremer, Mike Oliver, Alan Schwarz, and Doug Wilson.

In writing this book, I relied on the knowledge and research of a huge number of physicians, health-care professionals, and medical experts who graciously offered their time and perspectives. Many thanks to Barry Boden, James Bradley, Peter Brukner, Lyle Cain, Robert Cantu, Douglas Casa, Lindsay DiStefano, Julie Eibensteiner, Gary Green, Glenn Fleisig, Tom Hackett, Jo Hannafin, Tim Hewett, Barry Jordan, Steve Lombardo, Bert Mandelbaum, Matt Matava, Chris Mazoué, Ann McKee, Jordan Metzl, Fred Mueller, Norman Scott, Erin Shannon, Donald Shelbourne, Holly Silvers, Robert Stern, Herb Stevenson, Jeff Stotts, Dania Sweitzer, and Vehniah Tjong.

I cannot say enough about Dana Newman, my amazing literary agent. Many publishers wanted me to write a prescriptive book, suggesting what readers could do for a rotator cuff tear or meniscus tear. This is the book that I wanted to write. She understood it immediately and supported it completely.

Thank you to Stephen Hull and the team at ForeEdge and University Press of New England. You are all great at what you do, and you were a pleasure to work with.

Thank you to Erik Calonius for reading and helping me craft my book proposal, reading my initial chapters, and offering much-needed encouragement.

I am indebted to my longtime assistant, Jen Streckfuss. She tracked down contact information for people I wanted to interview and helped assemble the citations for the hundreds of sources I used. In addition, she helped with many of the daily functions of my website, podcast, videos, and Sports Medicine University so that I could devote much of my limited free time to this book.

Along the same lines, thank you to Stephanie Coffin for her help with both this book and my website and social media. And thank you to Prateek Prasanna for letting me bounce ideas about injuries and injury trends off him.

Malcolm Dewitt, the sports editor at *The Post and Courier*, offered me my first real opportunity to write for an audience outside of my website. I started by writing what he and I thought readers in Charleston would want to read from an orthopedic surgeon: explanations of injuries among local athletes. Honestly, my first few columns were not good at all. Malcolm stuck with me as I worked to improve. Gradually he allowed me to expand my column to discuss my passions: arguments for rule changes in sports and ways to make sports safer. Those passions largely shaped the theme of this book.

Thank you to Heather Woolwine and Tony Ciuffo for encouraging me to write that newspaper column and promote those messages online and in the media.

Special thanks go out to Joy Groblebe and Brian Scheer, who have helped me build my platform and encouraged me to share my message with audiences across the world, and to Roger Love, who has helped me improve the delivery of that message.

I am deeply grateful to Jenny Blake, who has coached me through this process from beginning to end. She guided me through the roller coaster of emotions of trying to get an agent and publisher and writing chapters on weekends after long weeks of clinics and surgeries. Her encouragement and wisdom even helped me restart my writing after I gave up after only three chapters. I could not have completed this book without her.

I have made a number of difficult career decisions in order to share my message with people around the world. To my family who have supported me the entire way, I want to say thank you. I love you so much.

Finally, and perhaps most important, thank you to all of my readers, listeners, and viewers. I had no idea when I started my website in 2010 that I would actually get excited to open my laptop and spend hours writing after a long day at work. I am eternally grateful that my information and commentary on sports and exercise injuries, injury treatments, and prevention have resonated with so many people. I cannot express how much the hundreds of questions and comments I receive every week mean to me. I hope that in some way this book and all of my work inspire you to stay healthy and perform your best.

Introduction

1. Rich Hoffmann, "These Moments of Defeat Pale in Comparison with Bogataj's," *Philadelphia Daily News*, February 14, 2014.

2. Dave Seminara, "Vinko Bogataj and the Ecstasy of Defeat," *Real Clear Sports*, March 20, 2010, accessed September 14, 2014, http://www1.realclearsports.com /articles/2010/03/20/vinko_bogataj_and_the_ecstasy_of_defeat_96904.html.

3. Ibid.

4. Patrick Hruby, "'Wide World of Sports' Crash Hits Home," ESPN.com, April 29, 2011, accessed September 14, 2014, http://espn.go.com/espn/page2/story?page=hruby /110429_vinko_bogataj_wide_world_of_sports.

5. Dave Seminara, "Vinko Bogataj and the Ecstasy of Defeat."

6. Hoffmann, "These Moments of Defeat Pale in Comparison with Bogataj's."

7. *The Agony of Defeat—Vinko Bogataj (Yugoslavia)*, uploaded September 8, 2007, accessed June 9, 2016, https://www.youtube.com/watch?v=M-RumbnQZTE&feature =related.

8. Dave Seminara, "Vinko Bogataj and the Ecstasy of Defeat."

9. Doug Wilson, in discussion with the author, June 2015.

10. Ken Anderson, in discussion with the author, July 2015.

11. Ibid.

12. Oslo Sports Trauma Research Center, "FIS Injury Surveillance System," International Ski Federation, n.d., accessed March 8, 2016, http://www.fis-ski.com/mm /Document/documentlibrary/Medical/03/31/94/fis-iss-brochure-081_Neutral.pdf.

13. Ken Anderson, in discussion with the author, July 2015.

14. Doug Wilson, in discussion with the author, June 2015.

15. Dave Seminara, "Vinko Bogataj and the Ecstasy of Defeat."

16. George A. Snook, "The History of Sports Medicine: Part I," *American Journal of Sports Medicine* 12, no. 4 (July–August 1984): 252–54.

17. George A. Snook, "The Father of Sports Medicine (Galen)." *American Journal of Sports Medicine* 6, no. 3 (May–June 1978): 128–31.

18. George A. Snook, "The History of Sports Medicine: Part I."

19. Ibid.

20. Ibid.

21. Ibid.

22. Ibid.

23. "Wide World of Sports (U.S. TV Series)," *Wikipedia*, last modified on April 26, 2016, https://en.wikipedia.org/wiki/Wide_World_of_Sports_(U.S._TV_series).

24. Associated Press, "MLB's Average Salary Eclipses $3M," ESPN.com, December 13, 2010, accessed September 14, 2014, http://espn.go.com/mlb/news/story?id=5915468.

25. Michael Haupert, "MLB's Annual Salary Leaders, 1874–2012," Society for American Baseball Research, SABR.org, updated March 30, 2013, accessed June 9, 2016, http://sabr.org/research/mlbs-annual-salary-leaders-1874-2012.

26. Associated Press, "MLB Average Salary Is $3.39M," ESPN.com, December 18, 2013, accessed September 14, 2014, http://espn.go.com/mlb/story/_/id/10158314/mlb -average-salary-54-percent-339-million.

27. Michael Haupert, "MLB's Annual Salary Leaders, 1874–2012."

28. "Los Angeles Clippers," *Wikipedia*, last modified on June 6, 2016, https:// en.wikipedia.org/wiki/Los_Angeles_Clippers#1978.E2.80.9384:_San_Diego_Clippers.

29. "Super Bowl XLVIII Draws 111.5 Million Viewers, 25.3 Million Tweets," Nielsen, nielsen.com, February 3, 2014, accessed June 9, 2016, http://www.nielsen.com/us/en /insights/news/2014/super-bowl-xlviii-draws-111-5-million-viewers-25-3-million- tweets.html.

30. "Study: Rise in Youth Football Participation Bucks Overall Sports Trend," *Sporting News*, n.d., accessed September 14, 2014, http://www.sportingnews.com /nfl/news/youth-football-participation-2013-usa-football-sfia-concussions/ gwm17kikor3b1e2b3lxnh3738.

31. Doug Wilson, in discussion with the author, June 2015.

32. Ibid.

33. Dave Seminara, "Vinko Bogataj and the Ecstasy of Defeat."

34. Ibid.

1 / Joan Benoit: The Advent of Arthroscopic Surgery

1. Kenny Moore, "A Joyous Journey for Joan," *Sports Illustrated*, May 21, 1984, accessed December 10, 2014, http://www.si.com/vault/1984/05/21/627368/a-joyous -journey-for-joan.

2. Ibid.

3. Ibid.

4. Ibid.

5. Amby Burfoot, "A Brief Chat with Joan Benoit Samuelson," *Runner's World*, April 9, 2013, accessed December 10, 2014, http://www.runnersworld.com/newswire/a-brief -chat-with-joan-benoit-samuelson/.

6. Bob Sevene, in discussion with the author, August 2015.

7. Kenny Moore, "A Joyous Journey for Joan."

8. Bob Sevene, in discussion with the author, August 2015.

9. Kenny Moore, "A Joyous Journey for Joan."

10. Joe Henderson, "Benoit's Knee," *Running Commentary*, JoeHenderson.com, December 22, 2011, accessed August 30, 2014, http://joehenderson.com/archive/home .php?article=2378.

11. Bob Sevene, in discussion with the author, August 2015.

12. Ibid.

13. Kenny Moore, "A Joyous Journey for Joan."

14. Bob Sevene, in discussion with the author, August 2015.

15. Kenny Moore, "A Joyous Journey for Joan."

16. Frank Litsky, "Ailing Joan Benoit May Miss Trials," *New York Times*, April 25, 1984, accessed August 30, 2014, http://www.nytimes.com/1984/04/25/sports/ailing -joan-benoit-may-miss-trials.html.

17. Ibid.

18. Bob Sevene, in discussion with the author, August 2015.

19. Kenny Moore, "A Joyous Journey for Joan."

20. Wesley M. Nottage, Norman F. Sprague III, Burt J. Auerbach, and Hesmet Shahriaree, "The Medial Patellar Plica Syndrome," *American Journal of Sports Medicine* 11, no. 4 (July–August 1983): 211–14.

21. John D. Dorchak, Robert L. Barrack, Jeffrey S. Kneisl, and A. Herbert Alexander, "Arthroscopic Treatment of Symptomatic Synovial Plica of the Knee: Long-Term Followup," *American Journal of Sports Medicine* 19, no. 5 (September–October 1991): 503–7.

22. Bob Sevene, in discussion with the author, August 2015.

23. Ibid.

24. Ibid.

25. Ibid.

26. Kenny Moore, "A Joyous Journey for Joan."

27. Joe Henderson, "Benoit's Knee."

28. Bob Sevene, in discussion with the author, August 2015.

29. "The Impact of the Arthroscopy Association of North America on the Development of Arthroscopic Surgery," Arthroscopy Association of North America, n.d., accessed March 8, 2016, http://www.aana.org/Portals/o/History/earlyhistory.pdf.

30. Ibid.

31. "Knee Arthroscopy," American Academy of Orthopaedic Surgeons, March 2010, accessed June 9, 2016, http://orthoinfo.aaos.org/topic.cfm?topic=a00299.

32. "Shoulder Surgery," American Academy of Orthopaedic Surgeons," August 2009, accessed June 9, 2016, http://orthoinfo.aaos.org/topic.cfm?topic=a00066.

33. Jeff Venables, "Joan Samuelson Tackles Final Olympic Marathon Trials in

Boston," American Running Association, April 20, 2009, accessed August 30, 2014, http://www.americanrunning.org/w/article/joan-samuelson-tackles-final-olympic -marathon-trials-in-boston.

34. Amby Burfoot, "A Brief Chat with Joan Benoit Samuelson."

35. "Joan Benoit Samuelson," Internet FAQ Archives, n.d., accessed online June 9, 2016, http://www.faqs.org/sports-science/Ba-Ca/Samuelson-Joan-Benoit.html#b.

36. Amby Burfoot, "A Brief Chat with Joan Benoit Samuelson."

37. Bob Sevene, in discussion with the author, August 2015.

38. Jeff Venables, "Joan Samuelson Tackles Final Olympic Marathon Trials in Boston."

39. Bob Sevene, in discussion with the author, August 2015.

40. "30 Years Later, Samuelson Finishes Marathon Within 30 Minutes of Her Winning Time," CBS Boston, April 15, 2013, accessed December 13, 2014, http://boston.cbslocal.com/2013/04/15/30-years-later-samuelson-finishes-marathon-within -30-minutes-of-her-winning-time/.

2 / Bernard King: Return to Elite Sports after ACL Injury

1. Tim Povtak, "The Comeback King: They Said He Was Washed Up, But Bernard King Has Silenced His Critics by Earning a Date with the All-Stars," *Orlando Sentinel*, February 10, 1991, accessed September 12, 2014, http://articles.orlandosentinel.com /1991-02-10/sports/9102100673_1_bernard-king-comeback-king-scott.

2. Ibid.

3. Ibid.

4. Andrew MacDougall, "Bernard King Says He's Most Proud of Grueling Comeback," *Newsday*, September 9, 2013, accessed August 21, 2014, http://www .newsday.com/sports/basketball/knicks/bernard-king-says-he-s-most-proud-of -grueling-comeback-1.6030658.

5. Sean Deveney, "Little by Little, Bernard King Defined Hall of Fame Legacy Through Will, Determination," *Sporting News*, September 9, 2013, accessed August 21, 2014, http://www.sportingnews.com/nba-news/4523446-bernard-king-hall-of-fame-knicks-nets-bullets-stats-gary-payton-jerry-tarkanian.

6. Dana Pennett, "Demise of Cunningham, Barkley Have Pain, Irony in Common," *Chicago Tribune*, December 12, 1999, accessed August 30, 2014, http://articles .chicagotribune.com/1999-12-12/sports/9912120114_1_charles-barkley-sixers-billy -cunningham.

7. Ibid.

8. Dania Sweitzer, in discussion with the author, July 2015.

9. Ibid.

10. Associated Press, "Bernard King to Undergo Surgery," *Ocala Star Banner*, March 25, 1985, accessed August 21, 2014, https://news.google.com/newspapers?id=re80 AAAAIBAJ&sjid=bQYEAAAAIBAJ&pg=4242%2C6163172.

11. "Surgery Is Urged for King," *New York Times*, March 26, 1985, accessed September 12, 2014, http://www.nytimes.com/1985/03/26/sports/surgery-is-urged-for-king.html.

12. Ibid.

13. Andrew MacDougall, "Bernard King Says He's Most Proud of Grueling Comeback."

14. "King to Undergo Surgery," *New York Times*, April 1, 1985, accessed September 12, 2016, http://www.nytimes.com/1985/04/01/sports/king-to-undergo-surgery.html.

15. P. Colombet, M. Allard, V. Bousquet, C. de Lavigne, and P. H. Flurin, "The History of ACL Surgery," n.d., accessed August 11, 2012, http://www.maitrise-orthop.com/corpusmaitri/orthopaedic/87_colombet/colombetus.shtml.

16. Ibid.

17. Ibid.

18. Ibid.

19. Ibid.

20. Dania Sweitzer, in discussion with the author, July 2015.

21. Chris Ekstrand, "How Today's ACL Surgery Saves NBA Careers," *Hoop Magazine*, April 1998, accessed August 21, 2014, http://www.apbr.org/forum/viewtopic.php?t=3533.

22. Donald Shelbourne, in discussion with the author, June 2015.

23. Dania Sweitzer, in discussion with the author, July 2015.

24. Norman Scott, in discussion with the author, June 2015.

25. Chris Ekstrand, "How Today's ACL Surgery Saves NBA Careers."

26. Sean Deveney, "Little by Little, Bernard King Defined Hall of Fame Legacy Through Will, Determination."

27. Dania Sweitzer, in discussion with the author, July 2015.

28. Ibid.

29. Donald Shelbourne, in discussion with the author, June 2015.

30. Stephen Lombardo, in discussion with the author, July 2015.

31. Julie Eibensteiner, in discussion with the author, October 2015.

32. Dania Sweitzer, in discussion with the author, July 2015.

33. Andrew MacDougall, "Bernard King Says He's Most Proud of Grueling Comeback."

34. Tim Povtak, "The Comeback King."

35. Dania Sweitzer, in discussion with the author, July 2015.

36. Joshua D. Harris, Brandon J. Erickson, Bernard R. Bach Jr., Geoffrey D.

Abrams, Gregory L. Cvetanovich, Brian Forsythe, Frank M. McCormick, Anil K. Gupta, and Brian J. Cole, "Return-to-Sport and Performance after Anterior Cruciate Ligament Reconstruction in National Basketball Association Players," *Sports Health: A Multidisciplinary Approach* 5, no. 6 (November 2013): 562–68, doi:10.1177/1941738113495788.

37. James P. Bradley, John J. Klimkiewicz, Michael J. Rytel, and John W. Powell, "Anterior Cruciate Ligament Injuries in the National Football League: Epidemiology and Current Treatment Trends among Team Physicians," *Arthroscopy* 18, no. 5 (May–June, 2002): 502–9.

38. Vishal M. Shah, James R. Andrews, Glenn S. Fleisig, Christopher S. McMichael, and Lawrence J. Lemak, "Return to Play after Anterior Cruciate Ligament Reconstruction in National Football League Athletes," *American Journal of Sports Medicine* 38, no. 11 (November 2010): 2233–39, doi:10.1177/0363546510372798.

39. James L. Carey, G. Russell Huffman, Selene G. Parekh, and Brian J. Sennett, "Outcomes of Anterior Cruciate Ligament Injuries to Running Backs and Wide Receivers in the National Football League," *American Journal of Sports Medicine* 34, no. 12 (December 2006): 1911–17.

40. Kirk A. McCullough, Kevin D. Phelps, Kurt P. Spindler, Matthew J. Matava, Warren R. Dunn, Richard D. Parker, MOON Group, and Emily K. Reinke, "Return to High School—and College-Level Football after Anterior Cruciate Ligament Reconstruction: A Multicenter Orthopaedic Outcomes Network (MOON) Cohort Study," *American Journal of Sports Medicine* 40, no. 11 (November 2012): 2523–29, doi:10.1177/0363546512456836.

41. Vehniah K. Tjong, M. Lucas Murnaghan, Joyce M. Nyhof-Young, and Darrell J. Ogilvie-Harris, "A Qualitative Investigation of the Decision to Return to Sport after Anterior Cruciate Ligament Reconstruction: To Play or Not to Play," *American Journal of Sports Medicine* 42, no. 2 (February 2014): 336–42, doi:10.1177/0363546513508762.

42. Erin Shannon, in discussion with the author, June 2015.

43. Harvey Araton, "Scars from Knee Surgery Fade, But There's Pain in Every Step," *New York Times*, May 8, 2012, accessed August 11, 2012, http://www.nytimes.com/2012/05/09/sports/basketball/for-bernard-king-scars-from-knee-surgery-fade-but-pain-remains.html.

44. Tim Povtak, "The Comeback King."

45. Michael Lee, "Bernard King Calls Comeback with Washington Bullets 'My Basketball Legacy,'" *Washington Post*, September 9, 2013, accessed August 21, 2014, https://www.washingtonpost.com/news/wizards-insider/wp/2013/09/09/bernard-king-calls-comeback-with-washington-bullets-my-basketball-legacy/.

3 / Hines Ward: Use of Platelet-Rich Plasma and Stem Cells for Active People

1. "Super Bowl XLVIII Draws 111.5 Million Viewers, 25.3 Million Tweets," Nielsen, nielsen.com, February 3, 2014, accessed June 9, 2016, http://www.nielsen.com/us /en/insights/news/2014/super-bowl-xlviii-draws-111-5-million-viewers-25-3-million -tweets.html.

2. Andrea Kremer, in discussion with the author, July 2015.

3. Ibid.

4. Mike Florio, "Hines Ward's Blood Treatment," *Pro Football Talk*, February 3, 2009, accessed November 7, 2014, http://profootballtalk.nbcsports.com/2009/02/03 /hines-wards-blood-treatment/.

5. Reid Kerr, "Super Bowl XLIII Timeline: Pittsburgh Steelers 27, Arizona Cardinals 23," AXS, n.d., accessed November 7, 2014, http://www.examiner.com/article/super -bowl-xliii-timeline-pittsburgh-steelers-27-arizona-cardinals-23.

6. Andrea Kremer, in discussion with the author, July 2015.

7. Colin Dunlap, "New Therapy Gave Ward's Knee Rapid Relief," *Pittsburgh Post-Gazette*, February 6, 2009, accessed November 7, 2014, http://www.post-gazette .com/sports/2009/02/06/New-therapy-gave-Ward-s-knee-rapid-relief/stories /200902060154.

8. James Bradley, in discussion with the author, July 2015.

9. Colin Dunlap, "New Therapy Gave Ward's Knee Rapid Relief."

10. Ibid.

11. James Bradley, in discussion with the author, July 2015.

12. Alan Schwarz, "A Promising Treatment for Athletes, in Blood," *New York Times*, February 16, 2009, accessed November 6, 2014, http://www.nytimes.com/2009/02/17 /sports/17blood.html.

13. James Bradley, in discussion with the author, July 2015.

14. Andrea Kremer, in discussion with the author, July 2015.

15. Alan Schwarz, "A Promising Treatment for Athletes, in Blood."

16. Ibid.

17. Monte Burke, "Average Player Salaries in the Four Major American Sports Leagues," *Forbes*, Forbes.com, December 7, 2012, accessed June 10, 2016, http://www .forbes.com/sites/monteburke/2012/12/07/average-player-salaries-in-the-four-major -american-sports-leagues/#465ebed13497.

18. Alan Schwarz, "A Promising Treatment for Athletes, in Blood."

19. Alan Schwarz, in discussion with the author, July 2015.

20. Andrea Kremer, in discussion with the author, July 2015.

21. Gina Kolata, "As Sports Medicine Surges, Hope and Hype Outpace Proven

Treatments," *New York Times*, September 4, 2011, accessed November 7, 2014, http://www.nytimes.com/2011/09/05/health/05treatment.html.

22. Bruce Reider, "Proceed with Caution," *American Journal of Sports Medicine* 37, no. 11 (November 2009): 2099–2101, doi:10.1177/0363546509352786.

23. Edward M. Wojtys, "Sports Science vs 'Boutique Medicine,'" *Sports Health: A Multidisciplinary Approach* 3, no. 6 (November 2011): 496–97.

24. Gina Kolata, "As Sports Medicine Surges, Hope and Hype Outpace Proven Treatments."

25. Ibid.

26. Timothy E. Foster, Brian L. Puskas, Bert R. Mandelbaum, Michael B. Gerhardt, and Scott A. Rodeo, "Platelet-Rich Plasma: From Basic Science to Clinical Applications," *American Journal of Sports Medicine* 37, no. 11 (November 2009): 2259–72, doi:10.1177/0363546509349921.

27. Luga Podesta, Scott A. Crow, Dustin Volkmer, Timothy Bert, and Lewis A. Yocum, "Treatment of Partial Ulnar Collateral Ligament Tears in the Elbow with Platelet-Rich Plasma," *American Journal of Sports Medicine* 41, no. 7 (July 2013): 1689–94, doi:10.1177/0363546513487979.

28. A. Hamid, Mohamad Shariff, Mohamed Razif Mohamed Ali, Ashril Yusof, John George, and Leena Poh Chen Lee, "Platelet-rich Plasma Injections for the Treatment of Hamstring Injuries: A Randomized Controlled Trial," *American Journal of Sports Medicine* 42, no. 10 (October 2014): 2410–18, doi:10.1177/0363546514541540.

29. Bruce Hamilton, Johannes L. Tol, Emad Almusa, Sirine Boukarroum, Cristiano Eirale, Abdulaziz Farooq, Rodney Whiteley, and Hakim Chalabi, "Platelet-rich Plasma Does Not Enhance Return to Play in Hamstring Injuries: A Randomised Controlled Trial," *British Journal of Sports Medicine* 49, no. 14 (July 2015): 943–50, doi:10.1136/bjsports-2015-094603.

30. G. Reurink, G. J. Goudswaard, M. H. Moen, A. Weir, J. A. Verhaar, S. M. Bierma-Zeinstra, M. Maas, J. L. Tol, and Dutch HIT-study Investigators, "Rationale, Secondary Outcome Scores and 1-Year Follow-up of a Randomised Trial of Platelet-rich Plasma Injections in Acute Hamstring Muscle Injury: The Dutch Hamstring Injection Therapy Study," *British Journal of Sports Medicine* 49, no. 18 (September 2015):1206–12, doi:10.1136/bjsports-2014-094250.

31. James Bradley, in discussion with the author, July 2015.

32. Allan K. Mishra, Nebojsa V. Skrepnik, Scott G. Edwards, Grant L. Jones, Steven Sampson, Doug A. Vermillion, Matthew L. Ramsey, et al., "Efficacy of Platelet-Rich Plasma for Chronic Tennis Elbow: A Double-Blind, Prospective, Multicenter, Randomized Controlled Trial of 230 Patients," *American Journal of Sports Medicine* 42, no. 2 (February 2014): 463–71, doi:10.1177/0363546513494359.

33. Thøger Persson Krogh, Ulrich Fredberg, Kristian Stengaard-Pedersen, Robin

Christensen, Pia Jensen, and Torkell Ellingsen, "Treatment of Lateral Epicondylitis with Platelet-Rich Plasma, Glucocorticoid, or Saline: A Randomized, Double-Blind, Placebo-Controlled Trial," *American Journal of Sports Medicine* 41, no. 3 (March 2013): 625–35, doi:10.1177/0363546512472975.

34. Suzan de Jonge, Robert J. de Vos, Adam Weir, Hans T. M. van Schie, Sita M. A. Bierma-Zeinstra, Jan A. N. Verhaar, Harrie Weinans, and Johannes L. Tol, "One-Year Follow-up of Platelet-rich Plasma Treatment in Chronic Achilles Tendinopathy: A Double-blind Randomized Placebo-controlled Trial," *American Journal of Sports Medicine* 39, no. 8 (August 2011): 1623–29, doi:10.1177/0363546511404877.

35. Jason L. Dragoo, Amy S. Wasterlain, Hillary J. Braun, and Kevin T. Nead, "Platelet-Rich Plasma as a Treatment for Patellar Tendinopathy: A Double-Blind, Randomized Controlled Trial," *American Journal of Sports Medicine* 42, no. 3 (March 2014): 610–18, doi:10.1177/0363546513518416.

36. Serdar Kesikburun, Arif Kenan Tan, Bilge Yilmaz, Evren Yasar, and Kamil Yazicioglu, "Platelet-Rich Plasma Injections in the Treatment of Chronic Rotator Cuff Tendinopathy: A Randomized Controlled Trial with 1-Year Follow-Up," *American Journal of Sports Medicine* 41, no. 11 (November 2013): 2609–16, doi:10.1177/0363546513496542.

37. James Bradley, in discussion with the author, July 2015.

38. Ibid.

39. Ibid.

40. "Arthritis: Data and Statistics," Centers for Disease Control and Prevention, last updated April 14, 2016, accessed June 10, 2016, http://www.cdc.gov/arthritis/data_statistics/index.htm.

41. "Arthritis: Cost Statistics," Centers for Disease Control and Prevention, last updated October 28, 2015, accessed June 10, 2016, http://www.cdc.gov/arthritis/data_statistics/cost.htm.

42. Elena Losina, Thomas S. Thornhill, Benjamin N. Rome, John Wright, and Jeffrey N. Katz, "The Dramatic Increase in Total Knee Replacement Utilization Rates in the United States Cannot Be Fully Explained by Growth in Population Size and the Obesity Epidemic," *Journal of Bone and Joint Surgery* 94, no. 3 (February 2012): 201–7, doi:10.2106/JBJS.J.01958.

43. Steven Kurtz, Kevin Ong, Edmund Lau, Fionna Mowat, and Michael Halpern, "Projections of Primary and Revision Hip and Knee Arthroplasty in the United States from 2005 to 2030," *Journal of Bone and Joint Surgery* 89, no. 4 (April 2007): 780–85, doi:10.2106/JBJS.J.01958.

44. "Knee Replacement Procedures," Bone and Joint Initiative USA, n.d., accessed June 10, 2016, http://www.boneandjointburden.org/2014-report/ive1/knee-replacement-procedures.

45. "Hip Replacement Procedures," Bone and Joint Initiative USA, n.d., accessed June 10, 2016, http://www.boneandjointburden.org/2014-report/ive2/hip-replacement -procedures.

46. Hilal Maradit Kremers, Dirk R. Larson, Cynthia S. Crowson, Walter K. Kremers, Raynard E. Washington, Claudia A. Steiner, William A. Jiranek, and Daniel J. Berry, "Prevalence of Total Hip and Knee Replacement in the United States," *Journal of Bone and Joint Surgery* 97, no. 17 (September 2015): 1386–97.

47. "Total Knee Replacement," American Academy of Orthopaedic Surgeons, last updated August 2015, accessed June 10, 2016, http://orthoinfo.aaos.org/topic.cfm ?topic=a00389.

48. Alberto Gobbi, Georgios Karnatzikos, Vivek Mahajan, and Somanna Malchira, "Platelet-Rich Plasma Treatment in Symptomatic Patients with Knee Osteoarthritis: Preliminary Results in a Group of Active Patients," *Sports Health: A Multidisciplinary Approach* 4, no. 2 (March 2012): 162–72.

49. James Bradley, in discussion with the author, July 2015.

50. J. Bruce Moseley, Kimberly O'Malley, Nancy J. Petersen, Terri J. Menke, Baruch A. Brody, David H. Kuykendall, John C. Hollingsworth, et al., "A Controlled Trial of Arthroscopic Surgery for Osteoarthritis of the Knee," *New England Journal of Medicine* 347, no. 2 (July 2002): 81–88.

51. Alexandra Kirkley, Trevor B. Birmingham, Robert B. Litchfield, J. Robert Giffin, Kevin R. Willits, Cindy J. Wong, Brian G. Feagan, et al., "A Randomized Trial of Arthroscopic Surgery for Osteoarthritis of the Knee," *New England Journal of Medicine* 359, no. 11 (September 11, 2008): 1097–1107, doi:10.1056/ NEJMoa0708333.

52. Surena Namdari, Keith Baldwin, Okechukwu Anakwenze, Min-Jung Park, G. Russell Huffman, and Brian J. Sennett, "Results and Performance after Microfracture in National Basketball Association Athletes," *American Journal of Sports Medicine* 37, no. 5 (May 2009): 943–48, doi:10.1177/0363546508330150.

53. Bert Mandelbaum, in discussion with the author, July 2015.

54. James Bradley, in discussion with the author, July 2015.

55. "Diffusion of Innovation Theory," Boston University, n.d., accessed November 1, 2015, http://sphweb.bumc.bu.edu/otlt/MPH-Modules/SB/SB721-Models/SB721 -Models4.html.

56. Bert Mandelbaum, in discussion with the author, July 2015.

57. James Bradley, in discussion with the author, July 2015.

58. Ibid.

4 / Phillip Hughes: Use of Protective Equipment in Sports

1. "Phillip Hughes: Australia Batsman the Victim of 'Incredibly Rare' Injury," BBC, November 27, 2014, accessed January 8, 2015, http://www.bbc.com/sport/cricket /30224091.

2. Scyld Berry, "Phillip Hughes' Death Has Shocked Cricket's Very Soul and Made It the Sport's Most Traumatic Week in Peacetime," *Telegraph*, November 30, 2014, accessed May 22, 2015, http://www.telegraph.co.uk/sport/cricket/11263332/Phillip -Hughes-death-has-shocked-crickets-very-soul-and-made-it-the-sports-most- traumatic-week-in-peacetime.html.

3. "Phillip Hughes: Cricket Australia Says Safety a Priority," BBC, November 28, 2014, accessed January 8, 2015, http://www.bbc.com/sport/cricket/30241930.

4. Peter Brukner, in discussion with the author, July 2015.

5. B. R., "The Bravery of the Batsman," *The Economist*, November 26, 2014, accessed June 10, 2016, http://www.economist.com/blogs/gametheory/2014/11/safety-cricket.

6. Rishi Iyengar, "Two Deaths Within a Week Makes Cricket Safety Conversation Get Louder," *Time*, December 1, 2014, accessed January 8, 2015, http://time.com /3611344/cricket-phillip-hughes-safety-debate-israeli-umpire/.

7. Ibid.

8. "Phillip Hughes: Cricket Australia Says Safety a Priority."

9. Peter Brukner, in discussion with the author, July 2015.

10. A. S. McIntosh and D. Janda, "Evaluation of Cricket Helmet Performance and Comparison with Baseball and Ice Hockey Helmets," *British Journal of Sports Medicine* 37, no. 4 (August 2003): 325–30.

11. B. R., "The Bravery of the Batsman."

12. Craig Ranson, Nicholas Peirce, and Mark Young, "Batting Head Injury in Professional Cricket: A Systematic Video Analysis of Helmet Safety Characteristics," *British Journal of Sports Medicine* 47, no. 10 (July 2013): 644–48, doi:10.1136/ bjsports-2012-091898.

13. Huw Richards, "How Protected Do Cricket Players Need to Be?" *New York Times*, November 27, 2014, accessed March 4, 2015, http://www.nytimes.com/2014 /11/28/sports/cricket/how-protected-do-cricket-players-need-to-be.html.

14. David Schoenfield, "Stanton's HBP Shows the Danger of Baseball," ESPN.com, September 12, 2014, accessed March 8, 2015, http://espn.go.com/blog/sweetspot/post /_/id/51391/stantons-hbp-shows-the-danger-of-baseball.

15. "Giancarlo Stanton HBP in Face," ESPN.com, September 12, 2014, accessed March 8, 2015, http://espn.go.com/mlb/story/_/id/11510777/giancarlo-stanton-miami -marlins-hit-face-pitch-exits-stretcher.

16. Ibid.

17. Gary Green, in discussion with the author, August 2015.

18. Buster Olney, "Stanton's Injury Could Cause MLB Change," ESPN.com, September 12, 2014, accessed May 22, 2015, http://insider.espn.go.com/blog/buster -olney/insider/post?id=8058.

19. "Brandon McCarthy Shows Good Signs," ESPN.com, September 6, 2012, accessed September 7, 2012, http://espn.go.com/mlb/story/_/id/8346548/oakland -athletics-brandon-mccarthy-alert-surgery-skull-fracture.

20. Jorge L. Ortiz, "A's Brandon McCarthy Has Skull Fracture, Surgery," *USA Today*, September 6, 2012, accessed March 8, 2015, http://content.usatoday.com/communities /dailypitch/post/2012/09/brandon-mccarthy-skull-fracture-brain-surgery/1# .VyfKxPkrIdW.

21. Aaron Gleeman, "Brandon McCarthy Cleared for 'Normal Baseball Activities,'" NBC Sports, November 14, 2012, accessed March 8, 2015, http://mlb.nbcsports.com /2012/11/14/brandon-mccarthy-cleared-for-normal-baseball-activities/.

22. "Coolbaugh, 35, Dies after Being Struck by Ball," ESPN.com, July 24, 2007, accessed March 8, 2015, http://espn.go.com/minorlbb/news/story?id=2945798.

23. "Coolbaugh's Death Prompts MLB to Adopt Helmets for Base Coaches," ESPN. com, November 8, 2007, accessed January 8, 2015, http://espn.go.com/mlb/news/story ?id=3100278.

24. Gary Green, in discussion with the author, August 2015.

25. Ibid.

26. Ibid.

27. Ira Boudway, "Why Doesn't Major League Baseball Use Pitchers' Helmets?," Bloomberg, March 20, 2014, accessed March 8, 2015, http://www.bloomberg.com /news/articles/2014-03-20/why-doesn-t-major-league-baseball-use-pitchers-helmets.

28. William Weinbaum, "MLB Won't Approve Padded Caps," ESPN.com, March 28, 2013, accessed March 4, 2015, http://espn.go.com/espn/otl/story/_/id/9106204/mlb -not-ready-approve-padded-cap-lining-opening-day.

29. Gary Green, in discussion with the author, August 2015.

30. Mike Oliver, in discussion with the author, July 2015.

31. Gary Green, in discussion with the author, August 2015.

32. Ibid.

33. Barry P. Boden, Robin Tacchetti, and Fred O. Mueller, "Catastrophic Injuries in High School and College Baseball Players," *American Journal of Sports Medicine* 32, no. 5 (July–Aug 2004): 1189–96.

34. Ibid.

35. Christy L. Collins and R. Dawn Comstock, "Epidemiological Features of High School Baseball Injuries in the United States, 2005–2007," *Pediatrics* 121, no. 6 (June 2008): 1181–87, doi:10.1542/peds.2007-2572.

36. Stephen G. Rice, Joseph A. Congeni, and Council on Sports Medicine

and Fitness, "Baseball and Softball." *Pediatrics* 129, no. 3 (March 2012): e842–56, doi:10.1542/peds.2011-3593.

37. Philip Caulfield, "High School Baseball Player, Thomas Adams, Dies after Being Hit in Chest by Pitch During Practice," *New York Daily News*, December 6, 2010, accessed March 4, 2015, http://www.nydailynews.com/news/national/high-school-baseball-player-thomas-adams-dies-hit-chest-pitch-practice-article-1.469819.

38. Jeff Roberts and Barbara Williams, "Equipment May Not Have Been Enough to Save Garfield Teen's Life," *The Record*, December 7, 2010, accessed June 10, 2016, http://www.northjersey.com/sports/equipment-won-t-save-teens-lives-experts-say-1.938490?page=all.

39. Luis E. Palacio and Mark S. Link, "Commotio Cordis," *Sports Health: A Multi-Disciplinary Approach* 1, no. 2 (March 2009): 174–79.

40. Jordan Metzl, in discussion with the author, August 2015.

41. Mark S. Link, "Mechanically Induced Sudden Death in Chest Wall Impact (Commotio Cordis)," *Progress in Biophysics and Molecular Biology* 82, nos. 1–3 (2003): 175–86; Barry J. Maron, Thomas E. Gohman, Susan B. Kyle, N. A. Mark Estes III, and Mark S. Link, "Clinical Profile and Spectrum of Commotio Cordis," *Journal of the American Medical Association* 287, no. 9 (2002): 1142–46.

42. Joseph J. Doerer, Tammy S. Haas, N. A. Mark Estes III, Mark S. Link, and Barry J. Maron, "Evaluation of Chest Barriers for Protection against Sudden Death Due to Commotio Cordis," *American Journal of Cardiology* 99, no. 6 (March 2007): 857–59.

43. Mike Oliver, in discussion with the author, July 2015.

44. Jordan Metzl, in discussion with the author, August 2015.

45. Peter Brukner, in discussion with the author, July 2015.

46. Jordan Metzl, in discussion with the author, August 2015.

47. Gary Green, in discussion with the author, August 2015.

48. Scyld Berry, "Phillip Hughes' Death Has Shocked Cricket's Very Soul and Made It the Sport's Most Traumatic Week in Peacetime."

49. "Sean Abbott Returns to Action Following Phillip Hughes's Death," BBC, December 9, 2014, accessed June 10, 2016, http://www.bbc.com/sport/cricket/30371699.

5 / Marc Buoniconti: Catastrophic Injuries in Football

1. "'An Injury Worse Than Stingley's,'" *Chicago Tribune*, October 31, 1985, accessed August 21, 2014, http://articles.chicagotribune.com/1985-10-31/sports/8503140675_1_herman-jacobs-marc-buoniconti-nick-buoniconti.

2. Susan Donaldson James, "Spinal-Cord Injury Therapy OK'd by FDA Could Lead to Cures," ABC News, July 31, 2012, accessed June 10, 2016.

3. Marc Buoniconti, "Paralyzed in a Football Game, a Star Tackles His New Life,"

People, September 15, 1986, accessed August 21, 2014, http://www.people.com/people /archive/article/0,,20094529,00.html.

4. Barry Boden, in discussion with the author, July 2015.

5. "'An Injury Worse Than Stingley's.'"

6. "Marc Buoniconti Undergoes Surgery," *Tuscaloosa News*, November 8, 1985, accessed August 30, 2014, https://news.google.com/newspapers?nid=1817&dat =19851108&id=LjsdAAAAIBAJ&sjid=NaYEAAAAIBAJ&pg=4064,2769296&hl=en.

7. Marc Buoniconti, "Paralyzed in a Football Game, a Star Tackles His New Life."

8. Jeff Hartsell, "Buoniconti, Jacobs Reunited 22 Years after Fateful Injury," *Post and Courier*, October 13, 2007, accessed August 21, 2014, http://www.postandcourier.com /article/20071013/ARCHIVES/310139989.

9. "'An Injury Worse Than Stingley's.'"

10. Barry P. Boden, Robin L. Tacchetti, Robert C. Cantu, Sarah B. Knowles, and Frederick O. Mueller, "Catastrophic Cervical Spine Injuries in High School and College Football Players," *American Journal of Sports Medicine* 34, no. 8 (August 2006): 1223–32.

11. Frederick Mueller, in discussion with the author, July 2015.

12. Jimmy Stamp, "Leatherhead to Radio-head: The Evolution of the Football Helmet," *Smithsonian*, October 1, 2012, accessed August 30, 2014, http://www.smithsonian mag.com/arts-culture/leatherhead-to-radio-head-the-evolution-of-the-football -helmet-56585562/?no-ist.

13. Robert C. Cantu and Frederick O. Mueller, "Catastrophic Spine Injuries in American Football, 1977–2001," *Neurosurgery* 53, no. 2 (August 2003): 358–62.

14. Frederick Mueller, in discussion with the author, July 2015.

15. Gary Green, in discussion with the author, August 2015.

16. Barry Boden, in discussion with the author, July 2015.

17. Barry P. Boden et al., "Catastrophic Cervical Spine Injuries in High School and College Football Players."

18. Erik Brady, "Finally, Buoniconti, Citadel Reconcile," *USA Today*, September 19, 2006, accessed August 21, 2014, http://usatoday30.usatoday.com/sports/college /football/southern/2006-09-18-marc-buoniconti_x.htm.

19. Ibid.

20. "What Is SCI? Statistics," The Miami Project, n.d., accessed August 21, 2014, http://www.themiamiproject.org/page.aspx?pid=374.

21. "Spinal Cord Injury Facts and Figures at a Glance," NSCISC National Spinal Cord Injury Statistical Center, February 2010, accessed August 21, 2014, https://www .nscisc.uab.edu/PublicDocuments/nscisc_home/pdf/Facts%20and%20Figures%20 at%20a%20Glance%202010.pdf.

22. Erik E. Swartz, Barry P. Boden, Ronald W. Courson, Laura C. Decoster, Mary Beth Horodyski, Susan A. Norkus, Robb S. Rehberg, and Kevin N. Waninger, "National Athletic Trainers' Association Position Statement: Acute Management of

the Cervical Spine–Injured Athlete," *Journal of Athletic Training* 44, no. 3 (May–June 2009): 306–31, doi:10.4085/1062-6050-44.3.306.

23. "Spinal Cord Injury Facts and Figures at a Glance."

24. Barry Boden, in discussion with the author, July 2015.

25. Erik Brady, "Marc Buoniconti Paralyzed on the Field, But Not in Life," *USA Today*, September 24, 2010, accessed August 11, 2014, http://usatoday30.usatoday.com /sports/football/2010-09-23-marc-buoniconti-citadel-paralyzed-miami-project_N.htm.

26. Ibid.

27. Jay Searcy, "Living with Broken Dreams Project May Mean Hope for Buoniconti," *Philly Inquirer*, January 12, 1986, accessed August 21, 2014, http://articles.philly .com/1986-01-12/sports/26054760_1_herman-jacobs-marc-buoniconti-miami-project.

28. Tom Canavan, "Marc Buoniconti Recalls Injury 25 Years Later," *Washington Times*, October 26, 2010, accessed August 21, 2014, http://www.washingtontimes.com /news/2010/oct/26/marc-buoniconti-recalls-injury-25-years-later/.

29. M. Dididze, B. A. Green, W. Dalton Dietrich, S. Vanni, M. Y. Wang, and A. D. Levi, "Systemic Hypothermia in Acute Cervical Spinal Cord Injury: A Case-Controlled Study," *Spinal Cord* 51, no. 5 (May 2013): 395–400, doi:10.1038/sc.2012.161.

30. "Doctors Perform First Schwann Cell Transplant for Spinal Cord Injury," The Miami Project to Cure Paralysis, January 23, 2013, accessed June 10, 2016, http://www .themiamiproject.org/first-schwann-cell-transplant/

31. Erik Brady, "Finally, Buoniconti, Citadel Reconcile."

6 / Sarah Burke: The Dangers of Extreme Sports

1. Gretchen Bleiler, "Burke's Accident Leaves Questions in Its Wake," ESPN.com, January 16, 2012, accessed January 16, 2012, http://espn.go.com/espnw/athletes-life /article/7461820/gretchen-bleiler-sarah-burke-accident-leaves-questions-wake.

2. "Burke in Critical Condition after Fall," ESPN.com, January 12, 2012, accessed January 23, 2015, http://espn.go.com/action/freeskiing/story/_/id/7447871/freeskier -sarah-burke-seriously-injured-utah-halfpipe-fall.

3. "Sarah Burke Dies from Injuries," ESPN.com, January 20, 2012, accessed June 10, 2016, http://xgames.espn.go.com/xgames/action/freeskiing/article/7466421/sarah -burke-dies-injuries-suffered-utah.

4. Eli Saslow, "One Light Will Not Go Out," ESPN.com, June 1, 2012, accessed January 22, 2015, http://espn.go.com/espnw/news-commentary/article/7984690 /freeskier-sarah-burke-leaves-lasting-legcacy-women-sports-espn-magazine.

5. "Sarah Burke Dies from Injuries."

6. "Sarah Burke and Rory Bushfield," The Ski Channel, March 11, 2013, accessed November 6, 2015, http://www.webmasterask.info/Sarah-Burke-and-Rory-Bushfield -Part-2-of-3(jXuGNcfIgXU).

7. "Burke in Critical Condition after Fall."

8. Colin Cathrea, "Technically Outdoors—Sarah Burke—A Superstar Hangs on to Life," *Edmonton Journal*, January 15, 2012, accessed June 10, 2016, http://edmonton journal.com/health/diet-fitness/technically-outdoors-sarah-burke-a-superstar-hangs -on-to-life.

9. "Sarah Burke Dies from Injuries."

10. Patrick A. Dowling, "Prospective Study of Injuries in United States Ski Association Freestyle Skiing 1976–77 to 1979–80," *American Journal of Sports Medicine* 10, no. 5 (September–October 1982): 268–75.

11. Tonje Wåle Flørenes, Stig Heir, Lars Nordsletten, and Roald Bahr, "Injuries among World Cup Freestyle Skiers," *British Journal of Sports Medicine* 44, no. 11 (September 2010): 803–8, doi:10.1136/bjsm.2009.071159.

12. Sophie E. Steenstrup, Tone Bere, and Roald Bahr, "Head Injuries Among FIS World Cup Alpine and Freestyle Skiers and Snowboarders: A 7-Year Cohort Study," *British Journal of Sports Medicine* 48, no. 1 (January 2014): 41–45, doi:10.1136 /bjsports-2013-093145.

13. Tom Hackett, in discussion with the author, August 2015.

14. Amy Parlapiano, "Before Injury, Kevin Pearce Was Set to Challenge Shaun White," *Post Game*, December 12, 2013, accessed January 22, 2015, http://www .thepostgame.com/blog/men-action/201312/crash-reel-kevin-pearce-lucy-walker -snowboarding-documentary.

15. Mike Miller, "Halfpipe Podium Points to Sky in Sarah Burke Tribute," NBC Sports, February 20, 2014, accessed June 10, 2016, http://olympics.nbcsports .com/2014/02/20/halfpipe-podium-points-to-sky-in-sarah-burke-tribute/.

16. Ibid.

17. "Why Are Fans Paying Medical Bills for World-Class Skier Sarah Burke?," NBC News, February 1, 2012, accessed January 22, 2015, http://usnews.nbcnews .com/_news/2012/02/01/10291483-why-are-fans-paying-medical-bills-for-world-class -skier-sarah-burke.

18. Rory Bushfield, in discussion with the author, July 2015.

19. Eli Saslow, "One Light Will Not Go Out."

20. "X Games 2012 Ratings Soar," Transworld Business, February 09, 2012, accessed June 10, 2016, http://business.transworld.net/news/x-games-2012-ratings -soar/#sR798S3EWK77IcDP.97.

21. Brent Rose, "It's Only a Matter of Time Before Someone Dies at the X Games [UPDATE]," *Deadspin*, January 31, 2013, accessed February 5, 2013, http://deadspin. com/5980175/its-only-a-matter-of-time-before-someone-dies-at-the-x-games.

22. Jason Blevins, "Caleb Moore in Desperate Condition after X Games Snowmobile Crash," *Denver Post*, January 28, 2013, accessed January 22, 2015, http://

www.denverpost.com/wintersports/ci_22467159/caleb-moore-crash-x-games
-snowmobile.

23. Ibid.

24. Colin Bane, "Autopsy Finds Caleb Moore Died of Chest Trauma," ESPN
.com, May 8, 2013, accessed January 8, 2015, http://xgames.espn.go.com/xgames
/article/9252843/autopsy-x-games-snowmobiler-caleb-moore-died-blunt-chest
-trauma.

25. Ibid.

26. Jason Blevins, "Caleb Moore in Desperate Condition after X Games
Snowmobile Crash."

27. Colin Bane, "Autopsy Finds Caleb Moore Died of Chest Trauma."

28. J. J. Pierz, "Snowmobile Injuries in North America," *Clinical Orthopaedics and
Related Research* 409 (April 2003): 29–36.

29. Plog, Benjamin A., Clifford A. Pierre, Vasisht Srinivasan, Kaushik Srinivasan,
Anthony L. Petraglia, and Jason H. Huang, "Neurologic Injury in Snowmobiling,"
Surgical Neurology International 5, no. 87 (2014), doi:10.4103/2152-7806.134074.

30. Brent Rose, "It's Only a Matter of Time Before Someone Dies at the X Games
[UPDATE]."

31. Jason Blevins, "ESPN to Review X Games' Snowmobile Contests after Caleb
Moore's Death," *Denver Post*, February 1, 2013, accessed January 22, 2015, http://www
.denverpost.com/ci_22495062/espn-review-x-games-snowmobile-contests-after-caleb.

32. Ibid.

33. Tom McCarthy, "X Games Safety in Spotlight after Snowmobiler Caleb Moore's
Death," *The Guardian*, February 1, 2013, accessed June 10, 2016, https://www
.theguardian.com/world/2013/jan/31/caleb-moore-death-x-games-injuries.

34. Dr. Tom Hackett, in discussion with the author, August 2015.

35. Billy Witz, "Little Call for Change after Skier's Death," FOX Sports, February 8,
2012, accessed June 10, 2016, http://www.foxsports.com/olympics/story/Sarah-Burke
-halfpipe-death-leaves-hard-questions-for-extreme-sports-020812.

36. M. Alison Brooks, Michael D. Evans, and Frederick P. Rivara, "Evaluation of
Skiing and Snowboarding Injuries Sustained in Terrain Parks Versus Traditional
Slopes," *Injury Prevention* 16, no. 2 (April 2010): 119–22, doi:10.1136/ip.2009.022608.

37. Jeff Blair, "Celebrating a Life on the Edge," *Globe and Mail*, January 19, 2012,
accessed January 22, 2015, http://www.theglobeandmail.com/sports/more-sports
/celebrating-a-life-on-the-edge/article4420289/.

38. Jason Blevins, "ESPN to Review X Games' Snowmobile Contests after Caleb
Moore's Death."

39. Billy Witz, "Little Call for Change after Skier's Death."

40. Rory Bushfield, in discussion with the author, July 2015.

41. Rachel George, "Autopsy Released for Snowmobiler Caleb Moore," *USA Today*, May 6, 2013, accessed January 22, 2015, http://www.usatoday.com/story/sports/olympics /2013/05/06/snowmobiler-x-games-caleb-moore-autopsy-cause-of-death/2138747/.

42. Ibid.

43. Rory Bushfield, in discussion with the author, July 2015.

44. Cindy Boren, "Caleb Moore X Games Crash: 'When Is Enough Enough?,'" *Washington Post*, January 30, 2013, accessed January 22, 2015, https://www .washingtonpost.com/news/early-lead/wp/2013/01/30/caleb-moore-x-games-crash -when-is-enough-enough/.

45. Gretchen Bleiler, "Burke's Accident Leaves Questions in Its Wake."

46. Rory Bushfield, in discussion with the author, July 2015.

47. Tom Hackett, in discussion with the author, August 2015.

48. Rory Bushfield, in discussion with the author, July 2015.

7 / Dave Duerson: Long-Term Brain Damage in Football

1. Dan Pompei, "The Final Days of Dave Duerson," *Chicago Tribune*, February 26, 2011, accessed January 26, 2015, http://articles.chicagotribune.com/2011-02-26/sports/ct -spt-0227-dave-duerson-final-days--20110226_1_dave-duerson-alicia-duerson-tregg.

2. Paul Solotaroff, "Dave Duerson: The Ferocious Life and Tragic Death of a Super Bowl Star," *Men's Journal* (May 2011), accessed January 27, 2015, http://www .mensjournal.com/magazine/dave-duerson-the-ferocious-life-and-tragic-death-of-a -super-bowl-star-20121002.

3. Ibid.

4. Dan Pompei, "The Final Days of Dave Duerson."

5. Ibid.

6. Robert Cantu, in discussion with the author, July 2015.

7. Ann McKee, in discussion with the author, July 2015.

8. Paul Solotaroff, "Dave Duerson."

9. Robert Cantu, in discussion with the author, July 2015.

10. Ann C. McKee, Thor D. Stein, Christopher J. Nowinski, Robert A. Stern, Daniel H. Daneshvar, Victor E. Alvarez, Hyo-Soon Lee, et al., "The Spectrum of Disease in Chronic Traumatic Encephalopathy," *Brain* 136 (January 2013): 43–64, doi:10.1093/ brain/aws307.

11. Paul Solotaroff, "Dave Duerson."

12. Ibid.

13. Ibid.

14. Jane Leavy, "The Woman Who Would Save Football," Grantland, August 17, 2012, accessed January 26, 2015, http://grantland.com/features/neuropathologist-dr -ann-mckee-accused-killing-football-be-sport-only-hope/.

15. Alan Schwarz, "Duerson's Brain Trauma Diagnosed," *New York Times*, May 2, 2011, accessed January 26, 2015, http://www.nytimes.com/2011/05/03/sports /football/03duerson.html.

16. Jane Leavy, "The Woman Who Would Save Football."

17. Alan Schwarz, "Duerson's Brain Trauma Diagnosed."

18. Ira R. Casson, Elliot J. Pellman, and David C. Viano, "Correspondence: Chronic Traumatic Encephalopathy in a National Football League Player," *Neurosurgery* 58, no. 5 (May 2006): E1003.

19. Kenneth C. Kutner, "Correspondence: Chronic Traumatic Encephalopathy in a National Football League Player," *Neurosurgery* 58, no. 5 (May 2006): E1152.

20. David C. Viano, Ira R. Casson, Elliot J. Pellman, Cynthia A. Bir, Liying Zhang, Donald C. Sherman, and Marilyn A. Boitano, "Concussion in Professional Football: Comparison with Boxing Head Impacts—Part 10," *Neurosurgery* 57, no. 6 (December 2005): 1154–72.

21. Steve Fainaru and Mark Fainaru-Wada, "Mixed Messages on Brain Injuries," ESPN.com, November 16, 2012, accessed December 29, 2014, http://espn.go.com /espn/otl/story/_/page/OTL-Mixed-Messages/nfl-disability-board-concluded -playing-football-caused-brain-injuries-even-officials-issued-denials-years.

22. Ibid.

23. Ann McKee, in discussion with the author, July 2015.

24. Ibid.

25. Robert Stern, in discussion with the author, September 2015.

26. Robert Cantu, in discussion with the author, July 2015.

27. Mike Oliver, in discussion with the author, July 2015.

28. Ann McKee, in discussion with the author, July 2015.

29. Ibid.

30. Robert Cantu, in discussion with the author, July 2015.

31. Gary W. Small, Vladimir Kepe, Prabha Siddarth, Linda M. Ercoli, David A. Merrill, Natacha Donoghue, Susan Y. Bookheimer, et al., "PET Scanning of Brain Tau in Retired National Football League Players: Preliminary Findings," *American Journal of Geriatric Psychiatry* 21, no. 2 (February 2013): 138–44, doi:10.1016/j.jagp.2012.11.019.

32. Ira R. Casson, David C. Viano, E. Mark Haacke, Zhifeng Kou, and Danielle G. LeStrange, "Is There Chronic Brain Damage in Retired NFL Players? Neurora-diology, Neuropsychology, and Neurology Examinations of 45 Retired Players," *Sports Health: A Multidisciplinary Approach* 6, no. 5 (September 2014): 384–95, doi:10.1177/1941738114540270.

33. Edward M. Wojtys, "Better News!," *Sports Health: A Multidisciplinary Approach* 6, no. 5 (September 2014): 382–83, doi:10.1177/1941738114546835.

34. "SN Concussion Report: Losing Grip on Reality a Fear That Never Stops," *Sporting News*, August 16, 2012, accessed January 27, 2015, http://www.sportingnews

.com/nfl-news/4035342-nfl-concussion-effects-former-players-dementia-brain
-trauma-report.

35. Jason M. Breslow, "The NFL's Concussion Problem Still Has Not Gone Away," PBS, September 19, 2014, accessed December 29,2014, http://www.pbs.org/wgbh /frontline/article/the-nfls-concussion-problem-still-has-not-gone-away/.

36. Kevin M. Guskiewicz, Stephen W. Marshall, Julian Bailes, Michael McCrea, Herndon P. Harding, Amy Matthews, Johna Register Mihalik, and Robert C. Cantu, "Recurrent Concussion and Risk of Depression in Retired Professional Football Players," *Medicine & Science in Sports & Exercise* 39, no. 6 (June 2007):903–9.

37. Kevin M. Guskiewicz, Stephen W. Marshall, Julian Bailes, Michael McCrea, Robert C. Cantu, Christopher Randolph, and Barry D. Jordan, "Association between Recurrent Concussion and Late-Life Cognitive Impairment in Retired Professional Football Players," *Neurosurgery* 57, no. 4 (October 2005): 719–726.

38. Everett J. Lehman, Misty J. Hein, Sherry L. Baron, and Christine M. Gersic, "Neurodegenerative Causes of Death among Retired National Football League Players," *Neurology* 79, no. 19 (November 6, 2012): 1970–74.

39. Robert Stern, in discussion with the author, September 2015.

40. Paul Solotaroff, "Dave Duerson."

41. Ibid.

42. Ibid.

43. Associated Press, "Dave Duerson's Family Sues NFL over His Suicide," *USA Today*, February 23, 2012, accessed January 27, 2015, http://usatoday30.usatoday.com /sports/football/nfl/story/2012-02-23/dave-duerson-death-lawsuit/53228680/1.

44. Associated Press, "Judge Gives Her Preliminary OK," ESPN.com, July 7, 2014, accessed January 27, 2015, http://espn.go.com/nfl/story/_/id/11188140/us-district -judge-anita-brody-gives-preliminary-ok-nfl-concussion-settlement.

45. Ken Belson, "Appeals Court Affirms Landmark N.F.L. Concussion Settlement," *New York Times*, April 18, 2016, accessed June 11, 2016, http://www.nytimes .com/2016/04/19/sports/football/nfl-concussion-lawsuit.html.

46. Mark Fainaru-Wada and Steve Fainaru, "Duerson Family Objects to Settlement," ESPN.com, October 14, 2014, accessed January 27, 2015, http://espn .go.com/espn/otl/story/_/id/11702872/dave-duerson-family-files-objection-nfl- concussion-settlement.

47. Mark Fainaru-Wada and Steve Fainaru, "NFL Reports Remain Inconsistent," ESPN.com, December 13, 2012, accessed December 29, 2014, http://espn.go.com/espn /otl/story/_/id/8706409/nfl-concussion-program-marked-inconsistencies-making -difficult-assess-whether-league-making-progress-issue.

48. Ira R. Casson, David C. Viano, John W. Powell, and Elliot J. Pellman, "Twelve Years of National Football League Concussion Data," *Sports Health: A Multidisciplinary Approach* 6, no. 2 (November/December 2010): 471–83.

49. Ann McKee, in discussion with the author, July 2015.

50. David Remnick, "Going the Distance," *New Yorker*, January 27, 2014, accessed June 11, 2016, http://www.newyorker.com/magazine/2014/01/27/going-the-distance -david-remnick.

51. "NFL Concussion Poll: 56 Percent of Players Would Hide Symptoms to Stay on Field," *Sporting News*, November 12, 2012, accessed December 29, 2014, http://www .sportingnews.com/nfl/story/2012-11-11/nfl-concussions-hide-symptoms-sporting- news-midseason-players-poll.

52. "Concussion Confidential," *ESPN the Magazine*, December 19, 2010, accessed June 11, 2016, http://espn.go.com/espn/news/story?id=5925876.

53. Jason M. Breslow, "High School Football Players Face Bigger Concussion Risk," *PBS Frontline*, October 31, 2013, accessed December 29, 2014, http://www.pbs.org /wgbh/frontline/article/high-school-football-players-face-bigger-concussion-risk/.

54. Robert Cantu, in discussion with the author, July 2015.

55. Robert Stern, in discussion with the author, September 2015.

56. Robert Cantu, in discussion with the author, July 2015.

57. Brandi Chastain, in discussion with the author, July 2015.

58. Robert Cantu, in discussion with the author, July 2015.

59. Kevin Grier and Tyler Cowen, "What Would the End of Football Look Like?," Grantland, February 13, 2012, accessed October 5, 2012, http://grantland.com/features /cte-concussion-crisis-economic-look-end-football/.

60. "Poll: Parents Uncomfortable with Kids Playing Football," FOX News, August 28, 2014, accessed December 29, 2014, http://www.foxnews.com/health/2014/08/28 /poll-parents-uncomfortable-with-kids-playing-football.html.

61. Paula Lavigne, "Concussion News Worries Parents," ESPN.com, August 26, 2012, accessed December 4, 2012, http://espn.go.com/espn/otl/story/_/id/8297366 /espn-survey-finds-news-coverage-concussions-leads-majority-parents-less-likely -allow-sons-play-youth-football-leagues.

62. "Barack Obama Is Not Pleased," *New Republic*, February 11, 2013, http://www .newrepublic.com/article/112190/obama-interview-2013-sit-down-president#.

63. Steve Fainaru and Mark Fainaru-Wada, "Youth Football Participation Drops," ESPN.com, November 14, 2013, accessed December 29, 2014, http://espn.go.com/espn /otl/story/_/page/popwarner/pop-warner-youth-football-participation-drops-nfl -concussion-crisis-seen-causal-factor.

64. Derrick Z. Jackson, "Mass. Leading a Retreat from Youth Football," *Boston Globe*, November 23, 2013, accessed August 20, 2016, http://www.bostonglobe.com /opinion/2013/11/23/football-slide-unpopularity-boxing/Dq99wTL1rxjrnPwOvhmSTL /story.html.

65. Paula Lavigne, "Concussion News Worries Parents."

66. Paul Solotaroff, "Dave Duerson."

67. Mike Oliver, in discussion with the author, July 2015.

68. Ibid.

69. Ibid.

70. Steven P. Broglio, Douglas Martini, Luke Kasper, James T. Eckner, and Jeffery S. Kutcher, "Estimation of Head Impact Exposure in High School Football: Implications for Regulating Contact Practices," *American Journal of Sports Medicine* 41, no. 12 (December 2013): 2877–84, doi:10.1177/0363546513502458.

71. Ann McKee, in discussion with the author, July 2015.

72. Michael Duerson, in discussion with the author, August 2015.

73. Ann McKee, in discussion with the author, July 2015.

8 / Sam Bowie: Medical Evaluation and Clearance of Athletes to Play

1. *1984 NBA Draft: Sam Bowie*, YouTube, uploaded July 25, 2008, accessed February 19, 2015, https://www.youtube.com/watch?v=2nERNj0afyY.

2. *Going Big*, ESPN Films, aired December 20, 2012.

3. Ibid.

4. Tom Friend, "Sam Bowie Doesn't Ask 'What If?,'" ESPN.com, December 20, 2012, February 18, 2015, http://espn.go.com/espn/espnfilms/story/_/id/8748334/espn-films-documentary-examines-sam-bowie-legacy.

5. Ibid.

6. Joe Freeman, "Sam Bowie Denies Lying to Blazers About His Health before the 1984 NBA Draft," *Oregonian*, December 12, 2012, accessed February 18, 2015, http://www.oregonlive.com/blazers/index.ssf/2012/12/sam_bowie_denies_lying_to_blazers_about_his_health.html.

7. *Going Big*.

8. Ibid.

9. Ibid.

10. Sam Bowie, in discussion with the author, July 2015.

11. Ibid.

12. *Going Big*.

13. Ibid.

14. Ibid.

15. Ibid.

16. Ibid.

17. Ibid.

18. "Oden Undergoes Microfracture Surgery," NBA.com, n.d., accessed February 18, 2015, http://www.nba.com/blazers/news/Oden_Undergoes_Microfracture_S-236705-1218.html.

19. "Oden's Recovery from Surgery Likely in Range of 6–12 Months," ESPN. com, September 14, 2007, accessed February 18, 2015, http://espn.go.com/nba/news/ story?id=3017538.

20. Ibid.

21. "What Exactly Happened to Greg Oden's Knee?" ESPN.com, September 13, 2007, accessed February 18, 2015, http://espn.go.com/blog/truehoop/post/_/id/3892/ what-exactly-happened-to-greg-oden-s-knee.

22. "Greg Oden Has Microfracture Surgery," ESPN.com, February 21, 2012, accessed February 15, 2015, http://espn.go.com/nba/story/_/id/7595246/surgery-greg-oden-portland-trail-blazers-turned-third-microfracture.

23. Ibid.

24. Tyler Conway, "Greg Oden's Doctor Recommended He Retire after Last Knee Surgery," *Bleacher Report*, August 13, 2013, accessed February 18,2015, http:// bleacherreport.com/articles/1736984-greg-odens-doctor-recommended-he-retire-after-last-knee-surgery.

25. "Blazers' Brandon Roy to Retire," ESPN.com, December 10, 2011, accessed February 20, 2015, http://espn.go.com/nba/story/_/id/7335092/brandon-roy-portland-trail-blazers-retire-due-knees.

26. Jason Quick, "Brandon Roy Opens Up about Why He Came Back, What It Means If He Never Plays Again," *Oregonian*, November 22, 2012, accessed February 20, 2015, http://www.oregonlive.com/blazers/index.ssf/2012/11/brandon_roy_opens_up_about_why_he_came_back_what_i.html.

27. Bill Walton, in discussion with the author, August 2015.

28. Ibid.

29. Lisette Hilton, "Walton Weathered Injuries to Win Titles," ESPN Classic, n.d., accessed February 18, 2015, http://espn.go.com/classic/biography/s/Walton_Bill.html.

30. Howard Beck, "Pain Gone, Walton Talks With Zeal Once Again," *New York Times*, May 6, 2010, accessed February 18, 2015, http://www.nytimes.com/2010/05/07/ sports/basketball/07walton.html.

31. Bill Walton, in discussion with the author, August 2015.

32. Ibid.

33. Stephen Lombardo, in discussion with the author, July 2015.

34. Matt Matava, in discussion with the author, July 2015.

35. Ibid.

36. James L. Carey, G. Russell Huffman, Selene G. Parekh, and Brian J. Sennett, "Outcomes of Anterior Cruciate Ligament Injuries to Running Backs and Wide Receivers in the National Football League," *American Journal of Sports Medicine* 34, no. 12 (December 2006): 1911–17.

37. Robert H. Brophy, Corey S. Gill, Stephen Lyman, Ronnie P. Barnes, Scott A.

Rodeo, and Russell F. Warren, "Effect of Anterior Cruciate Ligament Reconstruction and Meniscectomy on Length of Career in National Football League Athletes: A Case Control Study," *American Journal of Sports Medicine* 37, no. 11 (November 2009): 2102–7.

38. Robert H. Brophy, Eric L. Chehab, Ronnie P. Barnes, Stephen Lyman, Scott A. Rodeo, and Russell F. Warren, "Predictive Value of Orthopedic Evaluation and Injury History at the NFL Combine," *Medicine & Science in Sports & Exercise* 40, no. 8 (August 2008): 1368–72, doi:10.1249/MSS.0b013e31816f1c28.

39. Matt Matava, in discussion with the author, July 2015.

40. Sam Bowie, in discussion with the author, July 2015.

41. *Going Big*.

42. Sam Bowie, in discussion with the author, July 2015.

43. Howard Beck, "Curry Faces Tests to Evaluate Risk Factor," *New York Times*, October 5, 2005, accessed February 18, 2015, http://www.nytimes.com/2005/10/05/sports/basketball/curry-faces-tests-to-evaluate-risk-factor.html.

44. Ibid.

45. Timothy Epstein, in discussion with the author, July 2015.

46. Jay Z, "Hola' Hovito," *The Blueprint*, CD released on September 11, 2001.

47. *Going Big*.

9 / Michael Jordan: Return-to-Play Decisions in Sports

1. Bob Sakamoto, "Jordan Will Miss 6 Weeks," *Chicago Tribune*, November 5, 1985, accessed August 30, 2014, http://articles.chicagotribune.com/1985-11-05/sports/8503160399_1_bulls-success-cat-scan-bone.

2. Walter LaFeber, *Michael Jordan and the New Global Capitalism* (New York: W. W. Norton, 1999).

3. David Halberstam, *Playing for Keeps: Michael Jordan and the World He Made* (New York: Open Road Integrated Media, 2000).

4. Bob Sakamoto, "Jordan Will Miss 6 Weeks."

5. Ibid.

6. Ibid.

7. Louis C. Towne, Martin E. Blazina, and Lewis N. Cozen, "Fatigue Fracture of the Tarsal Navicular," *Journal of Bone and Joint Surgery* 52, no. 2 (March 1970): 376–78.

8. Alissa J. Burge, Stephanie L. Gold, and Hollis G. Potter, "Imaging of Sports-Related Midfoot and Forefoot Injuries," *Sports Health: A Multidisciplinary Approach* 4, no. 6 (November 2012): 518–34, doi:10.1177/1941738112459489.

9. David Halberstam, *Playing for Keeps*.

10. Jeff Stotts, in discussion with the author, July 2015.

11. "Incessant Pounding on Legs and Feet Has Caused an Epidemic of Stress Fractures in the NBA," *Sports Illustrated*, April 27, 1987, accessed August 11, 2012, http://sportsillustrated.cnn.com/vault/article/magazine/MAG1065890/index.htm.

12. Ibid.

13. Mike Sielski, "What Can Yao, Jordan Foot Injuries Tell Sixers about Embiid?," *Philly Inquirer*, July 5, 2014, accessed November 13, 2014, http://articles.philly.com/2014-07-05/sports/51078434_1_joel-embiid-jeff-van-gundy-brett-brown.

14. Letha Y. Hunter, "Stress Fracture of the Tarsal Navicular: More Frequent Than We Realize?," *American Journal of Sports Medicine* 9, no. 4 (July–August 1981): 217–19.

15. Joseph S. Torg, Helene Pavlov, Leroy H. Cooley, Michael H. Bryant, Steven P. Arnoczky, John Bergfeld, and Letha Y. Hunter, "Stress Fractures of the Tarsal Navicular: A Retrospective Review of Twenty-one Cases," *Journal of Bone and Joint Surgery* 64, no. 5 (June 1982): 700–712.

16. Karim M. Khan, Peter J. Fuller, Peter D. Brukner, Chris Kearney, and Hugh C. Burry, "Outcome of Conservative and Surgical Management of Navicular Stress Fracture in Athletes: Eighty-Six Cases Proven with Computerized Tomography," *American Journal of Sports Medicine* 20, no. 6 (November–December 1992): 657–66.

17. United Press International, "Doctor Says Jordan Shouldn't Play James: The Foot Could Potentially Require Surgery If He Reinjures It," *Orlando Sentinel*, April 23, 1986, accessed August 30, 2014, http://articles.orlandosentinel.com/1986-04-23/sports/0210450022_1_healing-process-jordan-broken-foot.

18. Ibid.

19. David Halberstam, *Playing for Keeps*.

20. United Press International, "Doctor Says Jordan Shouldn't Play James."

21. David Halberstam, *Playing for Keeps*.

22. James Litke, "Jordan Sidelined for Rest of Season," *Kentucky New Era*, February 11, 1986, accessed August 30, 2014, https://news.google.com/newspapers?nid=266&dat=19860211&id=CgMsAAAAIBAJ&sjid=aGoFAAAAIBAJ&pg=3576,5109236&hl=en.

23. David Halberstam, *Playing for Keeps*.

24. Ibid.

25. Bill Walton, in discussion with the author, August 2015.

26. Matt Matava, in discussion with the author, July 2015.

27. Rick Maese, "NFLPA Survey: Nearly Four in Five Football Players Don't Trust Team Medical Staffs," *Washington Post*, January 31, 2013, accessed July 3, 2013, https://www.washingtonpost.com/sports/redskins/nflpa-survey-nearly-four-in-five-football-player-dont-trust-team-medical-staffs/2013/01/31/d0cead20-6bb6-11e2-8f4f-2abd96162ba8_print.html.

28. Matt Matava, in discussion with the author, July 2015.

29. Ibid.

30. Ibid.

31. Ibid.

32. Sam Bowie, in discussion with the author, July 2015.

33. Bill Walton, in discussion with the author, August 2015.

34. Ibid.

35. D. J. Short, "Pedroia Seeks Second Opinion on Foot; Talks to Michael Jordan for Advice," NBC Sports, August 25, 2010, accessed November 13, 2014, http://mlb.nbcsports.com/2010/08/25/pedroia-seeks-second-opinion-on-foot-talks-to-michael-jordan-for-advice/.

10 / Hank Gathers: Sudden Cardiac Deaths and Universal Screening

1. "Twenty Years After: Hank Gathers Stirs Memories for His Family," AOL News, March 2, 2010, accessed August 25, 2012, http://www.aolnews.com/2010/03/02/twenty-years-after-hank-gathers-stirs-memories-for-his-family/.

2. Ibid.

3. Elliott Almond, "The Death of Hank Gathers: Doctor Says Gathers Was Well Enough to Be Playing Ball," Los Angeles Times, March 6, 1990, accessed August 25, 2012, http://articles.latimes.com/1990-03-06/sports/sp-1848_1_hank-gathers.

4. Lorenzo Benet, "College Star Hank Gathers Dies at the Height of His Powers," People, March 19, 1990, accessed August 25, 2012, http://www.people.com/people/archive/article/0,,20117101,00.html.

5. Lawrence K. Altman, "No Trace of Heart Medicine in Gathers, Autopsy Indicates," New York Times, March 16, 1990, accessed August 25, 2012, http://www.nytimes.com/1990/03/16/sports/no-trace-of-heart-medication-in-gathers-autopsy-indicates.html.

6. Rick Weinberg, "62: Hank Gathers Collapses, Dies of a Heart Condition," ESPN.com, July 8, 2004, accessed August 12, 2012, http://espn.go.com/espn/espn25/story?page=moments/62; Connor Letourneau, "25 Years Ago, OSU Trainer Tom Fregoso Tried to Save Hank Gathers' Life," The Oregonian, March 8, 2015, accessed August 20, 2016, http://www.oregonlive.com/beavers/index.ssf/2015/03/tom_fregoso_oregon_state_beave.html.

7. Ibid.

8. Paul Buker, "Gathers' Death Ends Tourney," The Oregonian, March 5, 1990, accessed August 25, 2012, http://blog.oregonlive.com/behindbeaversbeat/2010/03/remembering_hank_gathers_our_c.html.

9. Lawrence K. Altman, "No Trace of Heart Medicine in Gathers, Autopsy Indicates."

10. Robert Campbell, Stuart Berger, and Michael J. Ackerman, "Pediatric Sudden Cardiac Arrest," Pediatrics 129, no. 4 (April 2012): e1094–1102.

11. Domenico Corrado, Cristina Basso, Giulio Rizzoli, Maurizio Schiavon, and Gaetano Thiene, "Does Sports Activity Enhance the Risk of Sudden Death in Adolescents and Young Adults?," *Journal of the American College of Cardiology* 42, no. 11 (December 3, 2003): 1959–63.

12. Kimberly G. Harmon, Irfan M. Asif, Joseph J. Maleszewski, David S. Owens, Jordan M. Prutkin, Jack C. Salerno, Monica L. Zigman, et al., "Incidence, Cause, and Comparative Frequency of Sudden Cardiac Death in National Collegiate Athletic Association Athletes: A Decade in Review," *Circulation* 132, no. 1 (July 7, 2015): 10–19, doi:10.1161/CIRCULATIONAHA.115.015431.

13. Kimberly G. Harmon, Irfan M. Asif, David Klossner, and Jonathan A. Drezner, "Incidence of Sudden Cardiac Death in National Collegiate Athletic Association Athletes," *Circulation* 123, no. 15 (April 19, 2011): 1594–1600, doi:10.1161/CIRCULATIONAHA.110.004622.

14. Robert Campbell, Stuart Berger, and Michael J. Ackerman, "Pediatric Sudden Cardiac Arrest."

15. Robert J. Myerburg and Victoria L. Vetter, "Electrocardiograms Should Be Included in Preparticipation Screening of Athletes," *Circulation* 116, no. 22 (November 2007): 2616–26.

16. "Wes Leonard Collapsed on Court," ESPN.com, March 5, 2011, accessed June 11, 2016, http://espn.go.com/college-sports/highschool/news/story?id=6180469.

17. Eryn Brown, "Wes Leonard: High School Star's Cardiac Arrest Caused by Underlying Heart Condition," *Los Angeles Times*, March 4, 2011, accessed August 26, 2012, http://articles.latimes.com/2011/mar/04/news/la-heb-wes-leonard-cardiac-arrest-20110304.

18. "Miscellaneous (Rare) Cardiomyopathies," American Heart Association, n.d., accessed June 11, 2016, https://www.heart.org/idc/groups/heart-public/@wcm/@hcm/documents/downloadable/ucm_312226.pdf.

19. "HS Star Wes Leonard Dies after Winning Shot," CBS News, March 4, 2011, accessed September 8, 2012, http://www.cbsnews.com/news/hs-star-wes-leonard-dies-after-winning-shot/.

20. "Fennville Honors Late Basketball Star Wes Leonard at Graduation," *Detroit Free Press*, May 24, 2012, accessed August 26, 2012, http://www.freep.com/article/20120524/HSS/120525001/Fennville-honors-late-basketball-star-Wes-Leonard-at-graduation.

21. Christopher Matthew Smith and Michael C. Colquhoun, "Out-of-Hospital Cardiac Arrest in Schools: A Systematic Review," *Resuscitation* 96 (November 2015): 296–302.

22. Sherry L. Caffrey, Paula J. Willoughby, Paul E. Pepe, and Lance B. Becker, "Public Use of Automated External Defibrillators," *New England Journal of Medicine* 347 (October 17, 2002): 1242–47.

23. Ricardo A. Samson, Robert A. Berg, and Robert Bingham, "Use of Automated External Defibrillators for Children: An Update—An Advisory Statement From the Pediatric Advanced Life Support Task Force, International Liaison Committee on Resuscitation," *Pediatrics* 112, no. 1 (July 2003): 163–68.

24. Jonathan A. Drezner, Jordan S. D. Y. Chun, Kimberly G. Harmon, and Derminer, "Survival Trends in the United States Following Exercise-Related Sudden Cardiac Arrest in the Youth: 2000–2006," *Heart Rhythm* 5, no. 6 (June 2008): 794–99, doi:10.1016/j.hrthm.2008.03.001.

25. Douglas J. Casa, Kevin M. Guskiewicz, Scott A. Anderson, Ronald W. Courson, Jonathan F. Heck, Carolyn C. Jimenez, Brendon P. McDermott, et al., "National Athletic Trainers' Association Position Statement: Preventing Sudden Death in Sports," *Journal of Athletic Training* 47, no. 1 (January–February 2012): 96–118.

26. Domenico Corrado, Cristina Basso, Andrea Pavei, Pierantonio Michieli, Maurizio Schiavon, and Gaetano Thiene, "Trends in Sudden Cardiovascular Death in Young Competitive Athletes after Implementation of a Preparticipation Screening Program," *Journal of the American Medical Association* 296, no. 13 (October 4, 2006): 1593–1601.

27. Domenico Corrado, Antonio Pelliccia, Hans Halvor Bjørnstad, Luc Vanhees, Alessandro Biffi, Mats Borjesson, Nicole Panhuyzen-Goedkoop, et al., "Cardiovascular Pre-Participation Screening of Young Competitive athletes for Prevention of Sudden Death: Proposal for a Common European Protocol Consensus Statement of the Study Group of Sport Cardiology of the Working Group of Cardiac Rehabilitation and Exercise Physiology and the Working Group of Myocardial and Pericardial Diseases of the European Society of Cardiology," *European Heart Journal* 26, no. 5 (March 2005): 516–24.

28. Arne Ljungqvist, Peter Jenoure, Lars Engebretsen, Juan Manuel Alonso, Roald Bahr, Anthony Clough, and Guido De Bondt, "The International Olympic Committee (IOC) Consensus Statement on Periodic Health Evaluation of Elite Athletes March 2009," *British Journal of Sports Medicine* 43, no. 9 (September 2009): 631–43, doi:10.1136/bjsm.2009.064394.

29. Kevin M. Harris, Austin Sponsel, Adolph M. Hutter Jr., and Barry J. Maron, "Brief Communication: Cardiovascular Screening Practices of Major North American Professional Sports Teams," *Annals of Internal Medicine* 145, no. 7 (October 3, 2006): 507–11.

30. Barry J. Maron, Tammy S. Haas, Aneesha Ahluwalia, and Stephanie C. Rutten-Ramos, "Incidence of Cardiovascular Sudden Deaths in Minnesota High School athletes," *Heart Rhythm* 10, no. 3 (March 2013): 374–77, doi:10.1016/j.hrthm.2012.11.024.

31. Barry J. Maron, Paul D. Thompson, Michael J. Ackerman, Gary Balady, Stuart Berger, David Cohen, Robert Dimeff, et al., "Recommendations and Considerations

Related to Preparticipation Screening for Cardiovascular Abnormalities in Competitive Athletes, 2007 Update: A Scientific Statement from the American Heart Association Council on Nutrition, Physical Activity, and Metabolism, Endorsed by the American College of Cardiology Foundation," *Circulation* 115, no. 12 (2007): 1643–55.

32. Barry J. Maron, and Antonio Pelliccia, "The Heart of Trained Athletes : Cardiac Remodeling and the Risks of Sports, Including Sudden Death," *Circulation* 114, no. 15 (2006): 1633–44.

33. Domenico Corrado, Cristina Basso, and Gaetano Thiene, "Sudden Cardiac Death in Athletes: What Is the Role of Screening?," *Current Opinion in Cardiology* 27, no. 1 (January 2012): 41–48, doi:10.1097/HCO.0b013e32834dc4cb.

34. Barry J. Maron et al., "Recommendations and Considerations Related to Preparticipation Screening for Cardiovascular Abnormalities in Competitive Athletes."

35. Barry J. Maron, Richard A. Friedman, Paul Kligfield, Benjamin D. Levine, Sami Viskin, Bernard R. Chaitman, Peter M. Okin, et al., "Assessment of the 12-Lead ECG as a Screening Test for Detection of Cardiovascular Disease in Healthy General Populations of Young People (12–25 Years of Age): A Scientific Statement From the American Heart Association and the American College of Cardiology," *Circulation* 130, no. 15 (October 7, 2014): 1303–34, doi:10.1161/CIR.0000000000000025.

36. George P. Rodgers, Jamie B. Conti, Jeffrey A. Feinstein, Brian P. Griffin, Jerry D. Kennett, Svati Shah, Mary Norine Walsh, Eric S. Williams, and Jeffrey L. Williams, "ACC 2009 Survey Results and Recommendations: Addressing the Cardiology Workforce Crisis, a Report of the ACC Board of Trustees Workforce Task Force," *Journal of the American College of Cardiology* 54, no. 13 (September 22, 2009): 1195–1208.

37. Barry J. Maron, et al., "Recommendations and Considerations Related to Preparticipation Screening for Cardiovascular Abnormalities in Competitive Athletes."

38. Ibid.

39. Robert J. Myerburg and Victoria L. Vetter, "Electrocardiograms Should Be Included in Preparticipation Screening of Athletes," *Circulation* 116, no. 22 (November 27, 2007): 2616–26.

40. Colin M. Fuller, "Cost Effectiveness Analysis of Screening of High School Athletes for Risk of Sudden Cardiac Death," *Medicine & Science in Sports & Exercise* 32, no. 5 (2000): 887–90.

41. Jordan Metzl, in discussion with the author, August 2015.

42. Kimberly G. Harmon, Irfan M. Asif, David Klossner, and Jonathan A. Drezner, "Incidence of Sudden Cardiac Death in National Collegiate Athletic Association Athletes," *Circulation* 123, no. 15 (April 19, 2011): 1594–1600, doi:10.1161/CIRCULATION-AHA.110.004622.

43. Sharon Terlep, "In the NCAA, a Push to Reform Health Standards," *Wall Street*

Journal, March 4, 2015, accessed March 10, 2015, http://www.wsj.com/articles/in-the-ncaa-a-push-to-reform-health-standards-1425414886.

44. Kimberly G. Harmon, Irfan M. Asif, Joseph J. Maleszewski, David S. Owens, Jordan M. Prutkin, Jack C. Salerno, Monica L. Zigman, et al., "Incidence, Cause, and Comparative Frequency of Sudden Cardiac Death in National Collegiate Athletic Association Athletes: A Decade in Review," *Circulation* 132, no. 1 (July 7, 2015): 10–19, doi:10.1161/CIRCULATIONAHA.115.015431.

45. Sharon Terlep, "In the NCAA, a Push to Reform Health Standards."

11 / Korey Stringer: Exertional Heat Stroke

1. Thomas George, "PRO FOOTBALL; Heat Kills a Pro Football Player; N.F.L. Orders a Training Review," *New York Times*, August 2, 2001, accessed August 30, 2014, http://www.nytimes.com/2001/08/02/sports/pro-football-heat-kills-a-pro-football-player-nfl-orders-a-training-review.html.

2. Stringer v. Minnesota Vikings Football Club LLC MD, Court of Appeals of Minnesota, September 21, 2004, accessed June 12, 2016, http://caselaw.findlaw.com/mn-court-of-appeals/1267357.html; Stringer v. Minnesota Vikings Football Club LLC 30, Supreme Court of Minnesota, November 17, 2005, accessed June 12, 2016, http://caselaw.findlaw.com/mn-supreme-court/1075117.html.

3. Ibid.

4. Thomas George, "PRO FOOTBALL; Heat Kills a Pro Football Player; N.F.L. Orders a Training Review."

5. Ibid.

6. Douglas Casa, in discussion with the author, July 2015.

7. Ibid.

8. Thomas George, "PRO FOOTBALL; Heat Kills a Pro Football Player; N.F.L. Orders a Training Review."

9. Ibid.

10. Stringer v. Minnesota Vikings Football Club LLC 30, Supreme Court of Minnesota.

11. Appellants' brief, Minnesota.gov, n.d., accessed June 12, 2016, http://mn.gov/law-library-stat/briefs/pdfs/a031635scA.pdf.

12. Allyson S. Howe and Barry P. Boden, "Heat-Related Illness in Athletes," *American Journal of Sports Medicine* 35, no. 8 (August 2007): 1384–95.

13. Douglas Casa, in discussion with the author, July 2015.

14. Barry Boden, in discussion with the author, July 2015.

15. Yoram Epstein, Daniel S. Moran, Yair Shapiro, Ezra Sohar, and Joshua Shemer, "Exertional Heat Stroke: A Case Series," *Medicine & Science in Sports & Exercise* 31, no. 2 (February 1999): 224–28.

16. Clifton Brown, "Korey Stringer, 10 Years Later: 'Nobody Was Prepared for His Death,'" *Sporting News*, August 1, 2011, accessed August 30, 2014, http://www.sportingnews.com/nfl-news/193712-nobody-was-prepared-for-his-death.

17. Robert J. Murphy, "Heat Illness in the Athlete," *American Journal of Sports Medicine* 12, no. 4 (July–August 1984): 258–61.

18. Douglas J. Casa, Lawrence E. Armstrong, Susan K. Hillman, Scott J. Montain, Ralph V. Reiff, Brent S. E. Rich, William O. Roberts, and Jennifer A. Stone, "National Athletic Trainers' Association Position Statement: Fluid Replacement for Athletes," *Journal of Athletic Training* 35, no. 2 (2000): 212–24.

19. Douglas Casa, in discussion with the author, July 2015.

20. Barry P. Boden, Ilan Breit, Jason A. Beachler, Aaron Williams, and Frederick O. Mueller, "Fatalities in High School and College Football Players," *American Journal of Sports Medicine* 41, no. 5 (May 2013): 1108–16, doi:10.1177/0363546513478572.

21. Douglas J. Casa, David Csillan, and Inter-Association Task Force for Preseason Secondary School Athletics Participants, "Preseason Heat-Acclimatization Guidelines for Secondary School Athletics," *Journal of Athletic Training* 44, no. 3 (May–June 2009): 332–33, doi:10.4085/1062-6050-44.3.332.

22. Douglas Casa, in discussion with the author, July 2015.

23. Ibid.

24. Zachary Y. Kerr, Stephen W. Marshall, R. Dawn Comstock, and Douglas J. Casa, "Exertional Heat Stroke Management Strategies in United States High School Football," *American Journal of Sports Medicine* 42, no. 1 (January 2014): 70–77, doi:10.1177/0363546513502940.

12 / Brandi Chastain: Prevention of ACL Injuries

1. "Soccer Star Brandi Chastain Tells SCU Graduates to Be Impact Players," *San Francisco Chronicle*, June 17, 2014, accessed October 18, 2014, http://www.sfgate.com/opinion/openforum/article/Soccer-star-Brandi-Chastain-tells-SCU-graduates-5555971.php.

2. Joann Weiner, "America's Newest Soccer Hero Takes a Page from Brandi Chastain's Playbook," *Washington Post*, June 17, 2014, accessed October 18, 2014, https://www.washingtonpost.com/blogs/she-the-people/wp/2014/06/17/americas-newest-soccer-hero-takes-a-page-from-brandi-chastains-playbook/.

3. Brandi Chastain, in discussion with the author, July 2015.

4. Ibid.

5. Mark C. Anderson, "A Look at What Pushes Soccer Legend Brandi Chastain to Keep Playing," *Monterey County Weekly*, February 10, 2011, accessed May 22, 2015, http://www.montereycountyweekly.com/news/cover/article_708712c0-f6ee-56ca-908c-50ee1b253661.html.

6. "Soccer Star Brandi Chastain Tells SCU Graduates to Be Impact Players."

7. "Title IX," *Wikipedia*, last modified on June 9, 2016, accessed June 12, 2016, https://en.wikipedia.org/wiki/Title_IX.

8. Ibid.

9. "Title IX and Athletics: Proven Benefits, Unfounded Objections," The National Coalition for Women & Girls in Education, n.d., accessed June 12, 2016, http://www.ncwge.org/TitleIX40/Athletics.pdf.

10. "High School Participation Increases for 25th Consecutive Year," National Federation of State High School Associations, October 30, 2014, accessed June 12, 2016, http://www.nfhs.org/articles/high-school-participation-increases-for-25th-consecutive-year/.

11. "NCAA Participation Rates Going Up," NCAA, November 2, 2011, accessed May 5, 2015, http://www.ncaa.com/news/ncaa/article/2011-11-02/ncaa-participation-rates-going.

12. Timothy Hewett, in discussion with the author, June 2015.

13. Elizabeth Arendt and Randall Dick, "Knee Injury Patterns Among Men and Women in Collegiate Basketball and Soccer: NCAA Data and Review of Literature," *American Journal of Sports Medicine* 23, no. 6 (November–December 1995): 694–701.

14. Julie Agel, Elizabeth A. Arendt, and Boris Bershadsky, "Anterior Cruciate Ligament Injury in National Collegiate Athletic Association Basketball and Soccer: A 13-Year Review," *American Journal of Sports Medicine* 33, no. 4 (April 2005): 524–30.

15. David E. Gwinn, John H. Wilckens, Edward R. McDevitt, Glen Ross, and Tzu-Cheg Kao, "The Relative Incidence of Anterior Cruciate Ligament Injury in Men and Women at the United States Naval Academy," *American Journal of Sports Medicine* 28, no. 1 (January–February 2000): 98–102.

16. Eduardo Gomez, Jesse C. DeLee, and William C. Farney, "Incidence of Injury in Texas Girls' High School Basketball," *American Journal of Sports Medicine* 24, no. 5 (September–October 1996): 684–87.

17. Leanne C. S. Mihata, Anthony I. Beutler, and Barry P. Boden, "Comparing the Incidence of Anterior Cruciate Ligament Injury in Collegiate Lacrosse, Soccer, and Basketball Players: Implications for Anterior Cruciate Ligament Mechanism and Prevention," *American Journal of Sports Medicine* 34, no. 6 (June 2006): 899–904.

18. Mark Zeigler, "Women Athletes Suffering Torn Anterior Cruciate Ligaments at Alarming Rate," *San Diego Union Tribune*, May 26, 2003, accessed October 18, 2014, http://www.sandiegouniontribune.com/sports/soccer/20030526-9999_mz1s26acl.html.

19. R. Kevin Flynn, Cheryl L. Pedersen, Trevor B. Birmingham, Alexandra Kirkley, Dianne Jackowski, and Peter J. Fowler, "The Familial Predisposition Toward Tearing the Anterior Cruciate Ligament: A Case Control Study," *American Journal of Sports Medicine* 33, no. 1 (January 2005): 23–28.

20. Timothy Hewett, in discussion with the author, June 2015.

21. Ibid.

22. Alex Umeki, "Women's Soccer: The 'Pop' That Plagues Female Soccer Players," *Bleacher Report*, April 10, 2012, accessed June 12, 2016, http://bleacherreport.com/articles/1096690-womens-soccer-that-pop-sound-that-plagues-female-soccer-players.

23. Bert Mandelbaum, in discussion with the author, July 2015.

24. Jo Hannafin, in discussion with the author, July 2015.

25. Ibid.

26. Bert Mandelbaum, in discussion with the author, July 2015.

27. Charles Henning and ND Griffis, *Injury Prevention of the Anterior Cruciate Ligament* [videotape] (Wichita, KS: Mid-America Center for Sports Medicine, 1990).

28. Carl F. Ettlinger, Robert J. Johnson, and Jasper E. Shealy, "A Method to Help Reduce the Risk of Serious Knee Sprains Incurred in Alpine Skiing," *American Journal of Sports Medicine* 23, no. 5 (September–October 1995): 531–37.

29. G. Myklebust, S. Maehlum, I. Holm, and R. Bahr, "A Prospective Cohort Study of Anterior Cruciate Ligament Injuries in Elite Norwegian Team Handball," *Scandinavian Journal of Medicine & Science in Sports* 8, no. 3 (June 1998): 149–53.

30. Timothy E. Hewett, Thomas N. Lindenfeld, Jennifer V. Riccobene, and Frank R. Noyes, "The Effect of Neuromuscular Training on the Incidence of Knee Injury in Female Athletes," *American Journal of Sports Medicine* 27, no. 6 (November 1999): 699–706.

31. Bert Mandelbaum, in discussion with the author, July 2015.

32. Holly Silvers, in discussion with the author, June 2015.

33. Bert R. Mandelbaum, Diane S. Watanabe, John F. Knarr, Stephen D. Thomas, Letha Y. Griffin, Donald T. Kirkendall, and William Garrett Jr., "Effectiveness of a Neuromuscular and Proprioceptive Training Program in Preventing Anterior Cruciate Ligament Injuries in Female Athletes: 2-Year Follow-up," *American Journal of Sports Medicine* 33, no. 7 (July 2005): 1003–10.

34. Julie Gilchrist, Mandelbaum, Bert R., Heidi Melancon, George W. Ryan, Holly J. Silvers, Letha Y. Griffin, Diane S. Watanabe, et al., "A Randomized Controlled Trial to Prevent Noncontact Anterior Cruciate Ligament Injury in Female Collegiate Soccer Players," *American Journal of Sports Medicine* 36, no. 8 (August 2008): 1476–83, doi:10.1177/0363546508318188.

35. "Press Release: Alternative Warm-Up Program Reduces Risk of ACL Injuries for Female College Soccer Players," CDC Newsroom, July 25, 2008, accessed October 18, 2014, http://www.cdc.gov/media/pressrel/2008/r080725.htm.

36. Bert Mandelbaum, in discussion with the author, July 2015.

37. Lindsay DiStefano, in discussion with the author, July 2015.

38. Bert Mandelbaum, in discussion with the author, July 2015.

39. Robert H. Brophy, Leah Schmitz, Rick W. Wright, Warren R. Dunn, Richard D. Parker, Jack T. Andrish, Eric C. McCarty, et al., "Return to Play and Future ACL Injury Risk after ACL Reconstruction in Soccer Athletes, from the Multicenter Orthopaedic Outcomes Network (MOON) Group," *American Journal of Sports Medicine* 40, no. 11 (November 2012): 2517–22, doi:10.1177/0363546512459476.

40. John Orchard, Hugh Seward, Jeanne McGivern, and Simon Hood, "Intrinsic and Extrinsic Risk Factors for Anterior Cruciate Ligament Injury in Australian Footballers," *American Journal of Sports Medicine* 29, no. 2 (March 2001): 196–200.

41. Timothy Hewett, in discussion with the author, June 2015.

42. Dennis J. Caine and Yvonne M Golightly, "Osteoarthritis as an Outcome of Paediatric Sport: An Epidemiological Perspective," *British Journal of Sports Medicine* 45, no. 4 (April 2011): 298–303, doi:10.1136/bjsm.2010.081984.

43. Richard C. Mather III, Lane Koenig, Mininder S. Kocher, Timothy M. Dall, Paul Gallo, Daniel J. Scott, Bernard R. Bach Jr., and Kurt P. Spindler, "Societal and Economic Impact of Anterior Cruciate Ligament Tears," *Journal of Bone and Joint Surgery* 95, no. 19 (October 2, 2013): 1751–59.

44. Donald Shelbourne, in discussion with the author, June 2015.

45. J. Herbert Stevenson, Chad S. Beattie, Jennifer B. Schwartz, and Brian D. Busconi, "Assessing the Effectiveness of Neuromuscular Training Programs in Reducing the Incidence of Anterior Cruciate Ligament Injuries in Female Athletes: A Systematic Review," *American Journal of Sports Medicine* 43, no. 2 (February 2015): 482–90, doi:10.1177/0363546514523388.

46. Herbert Stevenson, in discussion with the author, July 2015.

47. Lindsay DiStefano, in discussion with the author, July 2015.

48. Timothy Hewett, in discussion with the author, June 2015.

49. Holly Silvers, in discussion with the author, June 2015.

50. Lindsay DiStefano, in discussion with the author, July 2015.

51. Holly Silvers, in discussion with the author, June 2015.

52. Gregory D. Myer, Dai Sugimoto, Staci Thomas, and Timothy E. Hewett, "The Influence of Age on the Effectiveness of Neuromuscular Training to Reduce Anterior Cruciate Ligament Injury in Female Athletes: A Meta-Analysis," *American Journal of Sports Medicine* 41, no. 1 (January 2013): 203–15, doi:10.1177/0363546512460637.

53. Holly Silvers, in discussion with the author, June 2015.

54. Darin A. Padua, Lindsay J. DiStefano, Stephen W. Marshall, Anthony I. Beutler, Sarah J. de la Motte, and Michael J. DiStefano, "Retention of Movement Pattern Changes After a Lower Extremity Injury Prevention Program Is Affected by Program Duration," *American Journal of Sports Medicine* 40, no. 2 (February 2012): 300–306, doi:10.1177/0363546511425474.

55. Lindsay DiStefano, in discussion with the author, July 2015.

56. Holly Silvers, in discussion with the author, June 2015.

57. Brandi Chastain, in discussion with the author, July 2015.

13 / Tommy John: Tommy John Surgery and Youth Sports Injuries

1. Tommy John, *T.J.: My 26 Years in Baseball* (New York: Bantam, 1991).

2. Ibid.

3. Todd Sperry, "Tommy John Accepts Role in Baseball and Medical History," CNN, April 24, 2012, February 3, 2013, http://www.cnn.com/2012/04/24/health/tommy-john -surgery/index.html.

4. John, *T.J.: My 26 Years in Baseball.*

5. Ibid.

6. Ibid.

7. Ibid.

8. Todd Sperry, "Tommy John Accepts Role in Basball and Medical History."

9. Reid Forgrave, "Pitcher, Doctor Change Baseball," FOX Sports, February 20, 2012, accessed January 5, 2013, http://www.foxsports.com/mlb/story/Tommy-John -surgery-Dr-Frank-Jobe-changed-baseball-gave-new-life-to-pitchers-022012.

10. Mark A. Vitale and Christopher S. Ahmad, "The Outcome of Elbow Ulnar Collateral Ligament Reconstruction in Overhead Athletes: A Systematic Review," *American Journal of Sports Medicine* 36, no. 6 (June 2008): 1193–1205, doi:10.1177/0363546508319053.

11. E. Lyle Cain Jr., James R. Andrews, Jeffrey R. Dugas, Kevin E. Wilk, Christopher S. McMichael, James C. Walter II, Reneé S. Riley, et al., "Outcome of Ulnar Collateral Ligament Reconstruction of the Elbow in 1281 Athletes: Results in 743 Athletes with Minimum 2-Year Follow-up," *American Journal of Sports Medicine* 38, no. 12 (December 2010): 2426–34, doi:10.1177/0363546510378100.

12. Lyle Cain, in discussion with the author, July 2015.

13. Brett W. Gibson, David Webner, G. Russell Huffman, and Brian J. Sennett, "Ulnar Collateral Ligament Reconstruction in Major League Baseball Pitchers," *American Journal of Sports Medicine* 35, no. 4 (April 2007): 575–81.

14. George A. Paletta Jr. and Rick W. Wright, "The Modified Docking Procedure for Elbow Ulnar Collateral Ligament Reconstruction: 2-Year Follow-up in Elite Throwers," *American Journal of Sports Medicine* 34, no. 10 (October 2006): 1594–98.

15. Stan A. Conte, Glenn S. Fleisig, Joshua S. Dines, Kevin E. Wilk, Kyle T. Aune, Nancy Patterson-Flynn, and Neal ElAttrache, "Prevalence of Ulnar Collateral Ligament Surgery in Professional Baseball Players," *American Journal of Sports Medicine* 43, no. 7 (July 2015): 1764–69, doi:10.1177/0363546515580792.

16. Reid Forgrave, "Pitcher, Doctor Change Baseball."

17. Associated Press, "Stephen Strasburg Has Torn Ligament," August 28, 2010, accessed February 3, 2013, http://espn.go.com/mlb/news/story?id=5502866.

18. Tommy John, in discussion with the author, December 2012.

19. Tommy John, *T.J.: My 26 Years in Baseball*.

20. Pedro Gomez, "Stephen Strasburg Limit Decided," ESPN, July 20, 2012, accessed January 29, 2013, http://espn.go.com/mlb/story/_/id/8180037/washington -nationals-plan-shut-all-star-stephen-strasburg.

21. Steven Cuce, "Leo Mazzone on Nationals Shutting Down Stephen Strasburg: 'It's Absolutely Pathetic; To Shut Him Down Would Be Totally Ridiculous,'" 95.7 The Game in San Francisco [sports radio interview], August 16, 2012, accessed August 21, 2012, http://sportsradiointerviews.com/2012/08/16/leo-mazzone-national-shutting -down-stephen-strasburg/.

22. Thomas Boswell, "Stephen Strasburg Shutdown Debate Masks the Washington Nationals' True Story," *Washington Post*, August 14, 2012, accessed August 21, 2012, https://www.washingtonpost.com/sports/nationals/stephen-strasburg-shutdown- debate-masks-the-washington-nationals-true-story/2012/08/14/d09ea3ee-e63e-11e1 -8741-940e3f6dbf48_story.html?wprss=rss_homepage.

23. Stan A. Conte et al., "Prevalence of Ulnar Collateral Ligament Surgery in Professional Baseball Players."

24. Nathan E. Marshall, Robert A. Keller, Jonathan R. Lynch, Michael J. Bey, and Vasilios Moutzouros, "Pitching Performance and Longevity after Revision Ulnar Col- lateral Ligament Reconstruction in Major League Baseball Pitchers," *American Journal of Sports Medicine* 43, no. 5 (May 2015): 1051–56, doi:10.1177/0363546515579636.

25. Joshua S. Dines, Lewis A. Yocum, Joshua B. Frank, Neal S. ElAttrache, Ralph A. Gambardella, and Frank W. Jobe, "Revision Surgery for Failed Elbow Medial Collateral Ligament Reconstruction," *American Journal of Sports Medicine* 36, no. 6 (June 2008): 1061–65, doi:10.1177/0363546508314796.

26. Thomas Boswell, "Stephen Strasburg Shutdown Debate Masks the Washington Nationals' True Story."

27. "Nats Shut Down Stephen Strasburg," ESPN.com, September 8, 2012, accessed September 8, 2012, http://espn.go.com/mlb/story/_/id/8351235/washington-nationals- shutting-stephen-strasburg-immediately-davey-johnson-says.

28. Lindsay Berra, "Force of Habit," ESPN.com, March 23, 2012, accessed August 21, 2012, http://espn.go.com/mlb/story/_/id/7712916/tommy-john-surgery-keeps- pitchers-game-address-underlying-biomechanical-flaw-espn-magazine.

29. Glenn Fleisig, in discussion with the author, July 2015.

30. Lyle Cain, in discussion with the author, July 2015.

31. Christopher Smith, "More Young Pitchers Face Big League Arm Trouble," *Eagle Tribune*, November 26, 2011, accessed January 5, 2013, http://www.eagletribune.com/

sports/more-young-pitchers-face-big-league-arm-trouble/article_a62a159c-95e3-5434-804c-4a54003f5c11.html.

32. "Prevention and Misconception Are Chief Concerns in Battling Youth Sports Injuries," *Orthopedics Today* (May 2010), accessed January 5, 2013, http://www.healio.com/orthopedics/pediatrics/news/print/orthopedics-today/%7B1df10dfe-9589-42bc-ab5c-f699264f8106%7D/prevention-and-misconception-are-chief-concerns-in-battling-youthsports-injuries.

33. Lyle Cain, in discussion with the author, July 2015.

34. Damon H. Petty, James R. Andrews, Glenn S. Fleisig, and E. Lyle Cain, "Ulnar Collateral Ligament Reconstruction in High School Baseball Players: Clinical Results and Injury Risk Factors," *American Journal of Sports Medicine* 32, no. 5 (July–August 2004): 1158–64.

35. Glenn Fleisig, in discussion with the author, July 2015.

36. Glenn S. Fleisig and James R. Andrews, "Prevention of Elbow Injuries in Youth Baseball Pitchers," *Sports Health: A Multidisciplinary Approach* 4, no. 5 (September/October 2012): 419–24.

37. Matthew Muench, "Dr. James Andrews Talks Tommy John," ESPN.com, February 8, 2012, accessed January 5, 2013, http://espn.go.com/blog/high-school/baseball/post/_/id/1091/dr-james-andrews-talks-tommy-john.

38. Jere Longman, "Fit Young Pitchers See Elbow Repair as Cure-All," *New York Times*, July 20, 2007, accessed January 5, 2013, http://www.nytimes.com/2007/07/20/sports/baseball/20surgery.html.

39. Christopher S. Ahmad, William Jeffrey Grantham, and R. Michael Greiwe, "Public Perceptions of Tommy John Surgery," *Physician and Sportsmedicine* 40, no. 2 (May 2012): 64–72, doi:10.3810/psm.2012.05.1966.

40. Gary Green, in discussion with the author, August 2015.

41. Lyle Cain, in discussion with the author, July 2015.

42. Glenn Fleisig, in discussion with the author, July 2015.

43. Lindsay Berra, "Force of Habit."

44. Glenn Fleisig, in discussion with the author, July 2015.

45. Gary Green, in discussion with the author, August 2015.

46. Ibid.

47. Brandon J. Erickson, Joshua D. Harris, Matthew Tetreault, Charles Bush-Joseph, Mark Cohen, and Anthony A. Romeo, "Is Tommy John Surgery Performed More Frequently in Major League Baseball Pitchers from Warm Weather Areas?," *Orthopaedic Journal of Sports Medicine* 27, no. 2 (October 2014): 2325967114553916, doi:10.1177/2325967114553916.

48. Jason L. Zaremski, Mary Beth Horodyski, Robert M. Donlan, Sonya Tang Brisbane, and Kevin W. Farmer, "Does Geographic Location Matter on the Prevalence of Ulnar Collateral Ligament Reconstruction in Collegiate Baseball Pitchers?,"

Orthopaedic Journal of Sports Medicine 3, no. 11 (November 2015): 2325967115616582, doi:10.1177/2325967115616582.

49. American Medical Society for Sports Medicine, "Effectiveness of Early Sport Specialization Limited in Most Sports, Sport Diversification May Be Better Approach at Young Ages," *ScienceDaily*, April 23, 2013, accessed June 12, 2016, https://www.sciencedaily.com/releases/2013/04/130423172601.htm.

50. Brandi Chastain, in discussion with the author, July 2015.

51. Ibid.

52. Gary Green, in discussion with the author, August 2015.

53. Christopher Smith, "More Young Pitchers Face Big League Arm Trouble."

54. Glenn Fleisig, in discussion with the author, July 2015.

55. Todd Sperry, "Tommy John Accepts Role in Basball and Medical History."

Conclusion

1. Bill Walton, in discussion with the author, August 2015.

2. Matthew Pouliot, "Dr. Frank Jobe: 'It Could Have Been Sandy Koufax Surgery,'" NBCSports.com, July 14, 2012, accessed August 23, 2016, http://mlb.nbcsports.com/2012/07/14/dr-frank-jobe-it-could-have-been-sandy-koufax-surgery/.

3. Stan A. Conte, Glenn S. Fleisig, Joshua S. Dines, Kevin E. Wilk, Kyle T. Aune, Nancy Patterson-Flynn, and Neal ElAttrache, "Prevalence of Ulnar Collateral Ligament Surgery in Professional Baseball Players," *American Journal of Sports Medicine* 43, no. 7 (July 2015): 1764–69, doi:10.1177/0363546515580792.

4. Norman Scott, in discussion with the author, June 2015.

5. Robert E. Leach, "Job Auction," *American Journal of Sports Medicine* 23, no. 4 (July–August 1995): 379.

6. American Orthopaedic Society for Sports Medicine, "Principles for Selecting Team Medical Coverage" (unpublished manuscript, 2005).

7. Erin Shannon, in discussion with the author, June 2015.

8. Ibid.

9. Gregg Williams, in discussion with the author, June 2015.

10. Erin Shannon, in discussion with the author, June 2015.

11. Riana R. Pryor, Douglas J. Casa, Lesley W. Vandermark, Rebecca L. Stearns, Sarah M. Attanasio, Garrett J. Fontaine, and Alex M. Wafer, "Athletic Training Services in Public Secondary Schools: A Benchmark Study," *Journal of Athletic Training* 50, no. 2 (February 2015): 156–62, doi: 10.4085/1062-6050-50.2.03.

12. Julian Sonny, "The Statistical Breakdown of Becoming a Professional Athlete Will Make You Keep Your Day Job," *Elite Daily*, February 26, 2014, accessed

September 4, 2015, http://elitedaily.com/sports/odds-going-pro-sports-will-make-rethink-day-job/.

13. "Youth Sports Injuries Statistics," STOP Sports Injuries, 2016, accessed June 12, 2016, http://www.stopsportsinjuries.org/STOP/Resources/Statistics/STOP/Resources/Statistics.aspx?hkey=24daffdf-5313-4970-a47d-ed621dfc7b9b.

14. Brandi Chastain, in discussion with the author, July 2015.

15. National Federation of State High School Associations, "The Case for High School Activities," accessed August 20, 2016, https://www.nfhs.org/articles/the-case-for-high-school-activities/.

16. Alana Glass, "Ernst & Young Studies the Connection Between Female Executives and Sports," *Forbes*, June 24, 2013, accessed June 12, 2016, http://www.forbes.com/sites/alanaglass/2013/06/24/ernst-young-studies-the-connection-between-female-executives-and-sports/#28ad94883f98.

17. Bert Mandelbaum, in discussion with the author, July 2015.

18. Glenn Fleisig, in discussion with the author, July 2015.

INDEX

athletic trainers, 242–43

autografts, 31, 35

autologous conditioned plasma (ACP), 43–45

automated external defibrillators (AEDs),
171–72

Aybar, Erick, 68

Bailes, Julian, 125

Ballmer, Steve, 6

ball-striking injuries, 7

Barkley, Charles, 133, 150, 163

Barta, Chuck, 181

baseball: ball-striking injuries in, 7; and
commotio cordis, 74–76; freak accidents
in, 72–76; head injuries and helmets in,
67–77, 243; and home plate collisions, 84;
and long-toss programs, 221; and navicular
fractures, 165; and overuse of pitchers,
226–27; and pitching mechanics, 224–26;
and youth injuries, 216–32. See also John,
Tommy; UCL (ulnar collateral ligament)
injuries

baseballs, safety of, 76

baseline concussion tests, 125–26, 128

basketball: and marketing relationships,
161–62; and medical evaluations, 132,
143–44, 148–50, 240; participation statistics
of, 243–44; and players' agents, 160; and
return-to-play decisions, 151–65; short-
term vs. long-term health balance in, 163–
65; and team doctors, 159–63. See also ACL
injuries; Bowie, Sam; elite sports; Gathers,
Hank; Jordan, Michael; King, Bernard;
sudden cardiac death

Basle, Tina, 49

Battersby, Ashley, 97

Battersby, Rose, 97

Bay Area Women's Sports Initiative (BAWSI),
214–15

Bayh, Birch, 197

Beard, Butch, 26

Beck, Howard, 143, 149

Ben-David, Ron, 104

Benoit, Joan, 7, 9–24; and 1984 Olympics

marathon, 22; and 2008 US Women's
Olympics marathon trials, 24; and Achilles
tendonitis, 23–24; arthroscopic knee
surgery, 233; arthroscopic knee surgery of,
15–17; background of, 9–10; and Boston
Marathons, 23–24; Nike sponsorship of, 22;
original knee injury of, 10–12; post-surgery
training of, 17–18

Bergfeld, John, 49, 156

beta blockers, 167

Bias, Len, 158

"The Bill of Rights for the College Athlete," 5

Bircher, Eugen, 20

Bird, Larry, 25, 144, 157, 163

Birk, Matt, 181

Bissinger, Buzz, 124

Bleiler, Gretchen, 88, 100–101

Blevins, Jason, 99

blood doping, 43. See also platelet-rich plasma
(PRP) treatment

bobblehead doll effect, 122

Boden, Barry, 72, 80–81, 84–85, 187, 190

Bogataj, Vinko, 1–3, 6, 8

Boren, Cindy, 100

Boston Marathon, 11, 23–24

Boswell, Thomas, 223

bouncers, cricket, 63–66, 77

Bowie, Sam, 7, 131–50; background of, 133–34;
drafted by Portland Trailblazers, 131–33,
150; and Going Big, 132, 136, 148, 150; and
medical evaluations, 131, 147–48; on
physical demands of professional sports,
163; stress fracture injuries of, 131–36

Bowman, Maddie, 93, 100

boxing and boxers, 107, 110, 113, 123, 241

Boyd, Brent, 117–18

Bozzini, Phillipp, 20

Bradley, James, 43–46, 51, 53–54, 57, 60–62

Bradshaw, Terry, 124

Brady, Eric, 86–87

Brady, Tom, 202

Breuer, Randy, 157

Brody, Anita, 119

Broglio, Steven P., 127–28

Sanchez, Tino, 69

Santa Clara Institute of Sports Law and Ethics, 123

Santangelo, F. P., 225

SCD (sudden cardiac death), 7, 166–80

Schaefer, Robert, 167–68

Schaeffer, Benjamin, 168

Schmorl, George, 20

Schwann cell transplantation, 87

Schwarz, Alan, 46–48, 109

Scott, Norman, 28–32, 37, 154, 234

screening, cardiovascular, 7, 172–80

screening of athletes, 239–40. *See also* medical evaluations; preparticipation physical exams (PPEs)

Scurry, Brianna, 196–97

Seigert, Shaun, 64

self-reporting of injuries, 120–21, 125, 129, 148–49

Selig, Bud, 229

Seminara, Dave, 1

Sevene, Bob, 9–12, 15, 17–19, 23–24

Shannon, Erin, 39, 240–41

Shelbourne, Donald, 33–34, 210

short-term vs. long-term health balance, 163–65, 238–39

Silvers, Holly, 204–5, 212–13

single-sport specialization, 229–30

skateboarding, 99

skiing, 1–8, 204

slopestyle skiing, 88–89, 97, 100

Small, Gary W., 114

Smith, Christopher, 231

Smith, Dean, 132

Smith, DeMaurice, 160–61

Snook, George A., 4

snowboarding, 3, 88, 91–93, 99–100, 243

snowmobiling, 7, 95–100, 241, 243

soccer: and ACL injuries, 195–215; participation statistics of, 244; and physical demands on youth players, 164; and risk of concussions/CTE in, 122–23. *See also* Chastain, Brandi

Solotaroff, Paul, 103–4, 108–9, 117–18

spearing and spear tackling, 82–84, 87

Spencer, Michael, 94

spinal cord injuries, 78–87

sports franchises, marketing relationships with, 161–62

sports injuries: financial burdens of, 85–86; legal ramifications of, 84–85. *See also specific injuries and sports*

Sports Legacy Institute, 105, 123, 129

sports medicine: American origins of, 4–5; and appropriateness of treatment, 238–39; doctor-team-patient relationship in, 237–38; future of, 7; mental and emotional aspects of, 240–41; origins of, 4; overview, 233–34; and preparticipation physical exams (PPEs), 239–40; and role of coaches and athletic trainers, 242–43; role of surgeons and doctors in, 235–37; and rule changes to decrease injuries, 241–42; and screening of athletes, 239–40; short-term vs. long-term health balance in, 238–39; surgeons' and physicians' responsibility to educate, 245–46. *See also specific sports, injuries, and treatments*

sports psychology, 240–41

sports statistics, 6

spotters, concussion, 121

Stanton, Giancarlo, 67–69

statistics, sports, 6

Steadman, Richard, 59, 138

stem cell treatments, 50, 54–55, 60–61, 245

Sterling, Donald, 6

Stern, David, 131, 137

Stern, Robert, 105, 112, 116, 122

steroids, 45, 57, 62. *See also* cortisone

Stevens, Mal, 5

Stevenson, J. Herbert, 210

STOP Sports Injuries campaign, 244

Stotts, Jeff, 154

Strasburg, Stephen, 220–25

stress fractures, 7, 131–36, 152–58

Dr. David Geier is an orthopaedic surgeon and sports medicine specialist who provides education and commentary on sports and exercise injuries to athletes and active people to help them stay healthy and perform their best.

After spending eight years serving as director of sports medicine at an academic medical center, he left to start his own practice. He currently serves as medical director of sports medicine at a private hospital outside of Charleston, South Carolina. He holds a board certification from the American Board of Orthopaedic Surgery in orthopaedic surgery as well as a subspecialty certification in orthopaedic sports medicine.

Currently he serves as the Communications Council chair for the American Orthopaedic Society for Sports Medicine (AOSSM) Board of Directors. He also serves as chairman of the publications committee for AOSSM. He serves on the outreach committee for the STOP Sports Injuries campaign and the medical aspects of sports committee for the South Carolina Medical Association. He has previously served as the chairman of the public relations committee for AOSSM and as a member of the sports medicine evaluation committee for the American Academy of Orthopaedic Surgeons.

He started writing articles on his website—DrDavidGeier.com—in August 2010 as a hobby. His goal at the time was simple: to share sports medicine and wellness information in easy-to-understand language for athletes, parents, coaches, and other health-care providers.

What he never expected to find back in 2010 was a passion for communicating this information. Despite long hours in clinic and surgery, he is still excited to open his laptop and write. He now writes a regular column for the daily Charleston newspaper, *The Post and Courier*. He records videos every week answering questions from his audience, and he produces a weekly sports medicine podcast. He also created a networking and educational site for health-care professionals who work with athletes and active people, Sports Medicine University. As of this writing, over 200,000 unique visitors come to his website every month.

For more information about Dr. Geier, or for more information on sports and exercise injuries and injury treatments and prevention, check out DrDavidGeier. com and his Sports Medicine Simplified online courses.

DATE

PRINTED IN U.S.